ADVANCES IN PSYCHOSOMATIC MEDICINE

ADVANCES IN
PSYCHOSOMATIC
MEDICINE

Symposium of the Fourth European Conference
on Psychosomatic Research.
4ᵈ, Hamburg, 1959.

edited by

ARTHUR JORES

HELLMUTH FREYBERGER

Robert Brunner, Inc.
PUBLISHERS   NEW YORK

Published in the United States of America by
Robert Brunner, Inc., 1961
Library of Congress Catalog Card No. 61-11029
MANUFACTURED IN THE UNITED STATES OF AMERICA

Preface

In 1955 the European Conferences for Psychosomatic Medicine were created by Dr. Denis Leigh, London, and Dr. J. Groen, Amsterdam. The first meeting was held in the Maudsley Hospital in London. A number of research workers and physicians who had done scientific studies in the field of psychosomatic medicine were invited by the founders. The meeting was received so well by the participants that it was decided to repeat it. Thus, in 1956 one gathered for a second time in Amsterdam, and again in 1957 in Copenhagen. The fourth conference was held from April 21st to April 25th, 1959, in Hamburg.

Although participation in these conferences has grown steadily, it never exceeded a number that would have interfered with personal communication and discussion. All Western European countries are represented at our meetings. We consequently agreed on English as the sole official language and this has proved successful. It is for this reason that this report, with one exception, is given in English.

We feel that the publication of this series of monographs dealing with the problems of psychosomatic medicine fulfills a genuinely needed task. The essence of the matter in question leads to types of scientific investigations which, because of their range, are not suitable for journal publication. Detailed case histories are the material on which psychosomatic research is based. We hope that this publication will further contribute to the advance of psychosomatic research—of research in scientific problems that are of considerable importance from the point of view of practical medicine.

ARTHUR JORES
HELLMUTH FREYBERGER

Contents

ADVANCES IN PSYCHOSOMATIC MEDICINE

Some Basic Remarks on the Occasion of the Opening of the 4th European Conference of Psychosomatic Medicine

A. JORES, Hamburg

The psychosomatic approach to disease is still fighting for genuine recognition and a firm place in the teachings of modern medicine. Two obstacles, in my opinion, are essential *hindrances:* firstly, that medicine based on the natural sciences cannot understand why it should leave its time-tried and reliable aspects and methods of research, which undeniably have been so successful; the second is, that the same demands are made on psychological research as on that of natural science, i.e. the verification of results by experiment and exact observation. The first per se is erroneous, the second is based on false premises. A brief elucidation of this statement follows:

1. It is an error to assume that todays medicine, with its predominantly somatic approach is able to convey a well rounded and complete picture (of the nature and dynamics) of disease. Such an assumption is justified only in disease with a clearcut exogenous etiology, i.e. essentially infectious and parasitic disease, which today, however, are only of minor importance. With respect to all other diseases, representing the great majority of diseases occupying the physician today, somatic medicine is unable to present an answer to the question concerning the cause of disease.

In view of the intensive research carried on during the last decades in the entire world this is an astonishing fact. Could the reason for this be, that the cause of the disease is not located in the domain accessible to the research methods of natural science, the domain of external reality? Due to a lack of truly etiological knowledge most of the patients populating the waiting rooms of practitioners today are receiving only symptomatic and not causal treatment. A great portion of these patients never regains real health. Consequently the number of the chronically ill and prematurely disabled increases continously. It must also be realized that our clinical methods are fairly crude. Before they indicate a pathological process a long period of development not accessible to these methods has often already taken place. The French surgeon LÉRICHE once gave a good comparison in stating that todays medicine is in the position of a visitor of a theatre in which the first two acts took place in darkness, with the stage lights not switched on before the third act. This gap in the knowledge of modern medicine is overbridged in a most fortuitous manner by the psychological point of view. The latter is infinitely more differentiated than the somatic approach, above all capable of something impossible for the somatic approach: an access to the past. Thus in taking case histories we often learn that the first act has already taken place in childhood, with a long pause following during which nothing happened. Then a certain life situation turned up and when this approached the culmination point, complaints set in. Only now is the moment in which the stage lights go on for somatic methods. Now the roentgenologist is able to find the ulcer on his photographic films. It would be erroneous to assume, however, that up to this moment nothing had happened in the somatic domain. The alterations which have already ensued are merely inaccessible to present methods. In view of this, is it not merely a matter of sound and practical common sense to employ psychological methods which lead further and enable more subtle analysis? The same pertains to therapy. Here also, entirely new possibilities, of which modern medicine as yet has scarcely made any use, appear, not only of symptomatic value, but capable of restoring complete health.

2. Many doctors experience difficulties in accepting the results of psychological research because they have been schooled on the principles of natural science and endowed with a sceptical attitude towards all socalled subjective methods. Psychological research unquestionably is subjective. The object of its research is a subject, and the researcher himself is a subject. In natural science the subjective is considered unreliable, even more, as a playground of illusions. Consequently research based on the natural sciences is striving for an objective basis, a fixation of results in pictures, measurements and numbers, and experimental verification. All of these possibilities,

prerequisite as proof for a statement in the realm of natural science, are non-existent in psychology. Here the question must be raised, however, whether the suspicion, that the subjective is unreliable, is justified. Does the world really acknowledge only those things as true which can be fixed in terms of measurement and numbers? Certainly not. Every individual possesses a fund of truth accumulated by experience. These truths are far more convincing than mathematical proofs. It is therefore urgently necessary to again recognize and employ experience as the most important and reliable source of information of man. The reason for its being discredited is probably the fact that certain rationally inaccessible factors play a role in the formation of experience. If experience is recognized as a source of human knowledge, then the results of psychological research must also be recognized, and it must be added that many of these results cannot be proved by the methods of natural science. This is due to the non-substantive and unmeasurable elements involved. To begin with, the conception of the soul: hardly anyone is able to give a real definition of the soul. It is not accessible to photography, measurement or expression in terms of numbers. For this reason the natural scientist does not speak of the soul. It does not occur in his reference system of external reality. This is justified. Life, and especially the existence of man presents a wealth of phenomena from which the existence of a soul can be deducted. Nevertheless, the soul remains an *auxiliary hypothesis* in the realm of natural science. The soul can be perceived, however, in my own experience and that of my fellow humans, and this perception is absolutely unequivocal and convincing. With this I leave the realm of the natural sciences and approach the realm of the psychology. The majority of doctors trained according to the principles of natural sciences shy lack from this step because they feel that they are submitting to pure speculation. The sceptic who is unwilling to accept the statements of psychological medicine as true must make his own way with the methods worked out by this discipline, he will then experience the validity of these statements. For this personal experience there is no substitute. Nevertheless, even in the psychological domain the attempt will be made to "objectivate" as much as possible. The possibilities for this are limited, however.

One of them is the experiment in the animal and the experiment in hypnosis. To both types of experiment we owe important information, yet the deductions possible remain limited. This also applies to all attempts to objectivate psychological facts by the use of statistics

or by psychological tests. Unquestionably, important deductions have
been made with both methods, but we must realize, however, that the
possibilities of these methods in their turn are limited, limited because
psychological factors at the basis of disease are almost always psychologically too differentiated to be grasped in a statistical *scheme*. The same
applies to psychological tests. It is not the purpose of my statements
to deal beforehand with the conclusions of various speakers of this
meeting who will present reports especially on the questions concerning
limits and possibilities. When one reads the results obtained in various
parts of the world in the sector of psychology, the picture that presents
itself is remarkably uniform. Naturally there are differences. These
are due to the complicated nature and variability of factors involved.
They are also due to the fact that psychotherapists already beginning
with FREUD have made the mistake of not restricting themselves to
the registration of psychological findings, but of proceeding directly
to the interpretation of these findings and the construction of a
system of learning with regard to the structure of the soul. There
remained not only one system, new and different systems followed.
It is clear, of course, that psychological findings of necessity had to
vary depending on the point of view from which they were obtained.
The basic principle in disease according to my opinion is relatively
simple, the variability of phenomena almost unlimited, however.
Thus there always is the great danger that researchers in the somatic
as well as in the psychological domain become lost in this vast
variability of phenomena and are no longer able to recognize the
underlying principle. Often researchers in medicine appear to me like
individuals who have climbed too high up into the branches of a
great tree and, sitting at its peak somewhere, are ardently inspecting
every little twig and leaf, but are no longer able to see the stem of
the tree. My wish for this meeting is that we may not make a mistake
of this kind, but that we may gain full sight of the stem and roots of
human disease and that our discussion may be fruitful. I herewith open
the Fourth European Conference on Psychosomatic Medicine.

Author's address: PROF. DR. A. JORES, II. Medizinische Universitätsklinik und Poliklinik, *Hamburg* (Germany).

I
Methods and Principles of Research on Psychosomatic Fundamentals

Psychopharmacology in the Psychosomatic Fundamentals

M. PFLANZ, Giessen

"The contribution of neuropharmacology to psychosomatic basic research" was the subject of a paper by LOPEZ IBOR at the 1956 Amsterdam-conference. Tab. 1 shows the various topics he dealt

Table 1. Topics dealt with by LÓPEZ IBOR 1956, in his lecture "Contribution of neuro-pharmacology to psychosomatic research"

Model psychoses
Placebo problem
Specific therapeutic value of drugs in the treatment of neuroses and psychosomatic disturbances
Neurogenic roots of mood (anxiety, depression)
Reserpine and Chlorpromazine
Reticular system

with. Although all these topics are still, today, at the focal point of research, psychopharmacology has materially widened its scope during the last few years. Tab. 2 contains some of the topics which

Table 2. Some experimental fields of contemporary psychopharmacology

Model psychoses (Mescaline, *d*-Lysergic Acid Diethylamide, Adrenochrome, Bufotenine, Psilocybine, Taraxein, Ceruloplasmin)
Metabolism of the central nervous system
Metabolism of psychoses

Biochemistry of the model psychoses
Search for the "schizophrenogenic agent"
Development of methods for selection of drugs for the therapy of psychoses
(with animals, healthy people, sick people)
Development of new drugs for the therapy of psychoses with greater effectiveness
and lesser toxicity
Development of new drugs against depression
Development of drugs for the therapy of neuroses
Psychological experiments on the effects of drugs (hypnotics, stimulants, hormones)
Psychodynamic experiments on the effect of drugs
Interaction between pharmacotherapy and psychotherapy

are being investigated by the psychopharmacology today. It demonstrates that its area extends from purely biochemical over pharmacological and animal-psychological questions, as far as the field of human
behaviour and, lastly, to the interaction between pharmacotherapy
and psychotherapy. The increase in quantity of psychopharmacological experiments has only little influence on psychosomatic basic
research, as long as, at least in part, the question is not gone into more
deeply, both methodologically, experimentally, and terminologically.
In such investigation, however, a closer co-operation between the
psychopharmacologist and the psychosomatic researcher, which up
till now is just beginning, is necessary. Therefore one can, in this
report, speak not so much of the already available results of such co-
operation than of the areas to which the future will bring more intensive treatment. Tab. 3 shows us those topics to be dealt with in
this report.

Table 3. Topics in which psychopharmacology can contribute to psychosomatic
fundamentals

Significance of brain functions for the psychosomatic research
Integration of neural and humoral mechanisms in the chain of psychosomatic
pathogenesis
Physiology of emotions
Rôle of personality, motivation, mood and sociopsychological environment
in pharmacological and biochemical effects
Examination of psychosomatic patterns, pharmacologically released
Influence on perception
            memory
            motivation
            symbolic significance of percepts
            readyness to act
            symbolic processes
            body image
by pharmacological and biochemical agents

"Toxicology of the personality" vs. psychodynamic concepts in some psychosomatic illnesses
Pharmacotherapy of psychosomatic affections
Search for methods to objectivate therapeutically produced personality changes
and improvement of symptoms

I want to remind you of a well-known scheme which shows
neural connections between the cortex reacting on the viscera via
diencephalon. We all know that this scheme is only a cursory supple-
mentary introduction, posing for us more questions than it answers.
But we know how to appreciate such a scheme which actually opens
the way for psychosomatic questions to many of our colleagues, who
are purely somatically orientated. One branch of psychosomatic
medicine is concerned with the question of the significance of single
brain structures in psychosomatic occurence. I would only remind
you of those papers which interpret the diencephalon as psychosomatic
connection-area par excellence. They also examine the lines of connections from the cerebral cortex and its functions to the limbic
system and its influence on somatic functions. I would also remind
you of those theories, which see in the ascending reticular system the
link between organic sensations and consciousness, or which attribute
a decisive rôle in psychosomatic reactions to the temporal lobe. It
seemed as though psychopharmacology could contribute materially
to such questions. This hope was justified as long as one had the
conception that every drug has a specific area of its effects, that particularly the psychologically effective substances have an influence on
quite definite anatomically and functionally separated substrates in the
central nervous system. This hope has been disappointed. If one
wishes to summarise these papers in the supposed area of the effects
of central acting substances, than one can only say that there is no
substance which affects only one single anatomical substrate. If we
take chlorpromazine as an example, then we find that it influences in
the periphery the gamma system of the reflex control; further more
centrally the reticular system and also-certainly in toxic doses—the
extrapyramidal system. Therefore the effect of chlorpromazine is
similar in many ways to the deconnection between the frontal lobe
and the remaining parts of the cerebral cortex. Its vegetative effects
infer an influence on the hypothalamic centres, and probably the
cerebral cortex itself is also involved. It would serve little purposes to
name the various areas affected by it. One can better express its
effects, as with all the other psychotropic substances, in terms of the

functional interplay. This is an important hint that even the neuro-physiologically inclined psychiatrists must get used to the idea that single parts of the brain do not have a specific relationship to human behaviour and somatic functions but that we can only comprehend functional integration and its disturbances scientifically. However, the terminology necessary for this, is still missing in part.

Recollecting once more the scheme of neural connections between the brain and the viscera we will find that this scheme is liable to correction in another respect. The neurophysiological scheme cannot be understood in the sense of more or less modified lines of impulses along premarked paths of conduction, to which idea we could be led by electrophysiological investigations. Physical and chemical processes are inseparably allied in the whole proceedings. Previous neuro-chemical investigation gives only a slight impression of the complexity of this problem. We only know fragments of the interplay of electro-lytes, neurohumoral transmitters and hormones, as well as the enzyme system which releases, activates or destroys these important sub-stances. The psychosomatic pathogenetic chain is therefore to be seen as neither purely neural nor purely humoral, also neither accord-ing to PAWLOW's nor to CANNON's concept; but both ways, as the neural and the humoral are closely integrated. But, they can also separate and influence themselves simultaneously in one direction. For this there is a schematic example: Sympathin, identical with noradrenaline, originates at the endings of sympathetic nerves. But noradrenaline influences the sympathetic ganglia. Finally, the sym-pathetic nerve system can produce under strongly affective stimuli, first of all, the preponderantly neural rise of blood pressure, tachycardia and other symptoms, until, after some seconds or minutes, the nor-adrenaline, in the meantime mobilised, together with adrenaline, maintains the symptoms further. If, after few minutes, the amine oxidase has destroyed the catechol amines, the thyroid gland can be activated through the pituitary or the ergotropic centres of the hypo-thalamus, and now maintains the accompanying symptoms of the psychic affect for a period of days or months together with the sympa-thetic system. Although this example is very crude, it shows, however, that examinations of the psychosomatic pathways must take simul-taneously existant neural and humoral mechanisms into consideration. Whereas the complicated interaction between psychological and physiological functions is left out—if I may express it in such bold mechanistic terms.

Table 4. "Physiology of Emotions"

under examination	–	connection between emotions and biochemical constellation (Particularly: pituitary hormones adrenal hormones gonadal hormones neurochemical transmitters)
has to be examined	–	connection between emotions and hormon-like substances (e.g. serotonin, histamin) hormonal catabolites (e.g. adrenochrome) enzymes which release or destroy the hormones substances of the liver metabolism electrolytes acid – base – balance
met with difficulties	–	qualitative and quantitative differenciation and registration of emotions is still not satisfactory possible impossibility to examine all concerned biochemical substances the reciprocal regulation of the biochemical mechanisms makes it difficult to find out the essential substances only exceptionally "pure" emotions can be produced pharmacologically

The biochemical part of this pathogenetic chain has been given particular attention during recent years. Thus the hormonal constellations, among these again the pituitary and adrenal hormones, have been specially investigated. Whereas the part played by hormone-like substances, various catabolits, the releasing, activating and destroying enzymes, just as thoses of the elctrolytes and the acid-base-balance has been neglected. The chemic feed-back mechanisms makes it difficult to analyse exactly the processes, which are of importance in the release and maintenance of psychosomatic happenings. Therefore the differentiation between essential and unessential substances is hard to find. Particularly the research, concerned with the physiology of emotions must suffer in this way. It is a tempting idea to study the correlation between clearly defined emotions and physiological and biochemical mechanisms. There are certain proofs of the connections between fear and noradrenaline, rage and adrenaline, tension and acetylcholin, resentment and an acetylcholin-like substance. But, for the moment, we are still dealing with rather crude results. In spite of many attempts, there has still been no satisfactory success in comprehending differentiated emotions qualitatively, not to mention quantitatively, which is, however, a prerequisite for a physiology of the emotions. Also the biochemist can only examine one substance or another on a hit and miss basis. Just the same, one should not give up hope to finding that, one day, we shall know and understand these correlations better than we do today. This trend of research will, perhaps, actually enable us, on the basis of a biochemical analysis, to find differences within the apparently similar emotions. This could be of great use, for example, in the case of depressions and fear. It cannot yet be decided whether experimental "pure" emotions, which permit simultaneous psychological and physiological analysis, can be successfully produced by pharmacopsychological means. Of course, the drug can produce considerably alterations, yet there is hardly a substance which regularly elicits a definite mood.

The question, of whether there is a specific relationship between the emotions and the humoral changes accompanying them, is a very crucial one. The conceptions of most of us, and the views given in many books, do not question such a strong specifity. Just the same, it must be said that the conception has not yet been empirically proved. On the basis of its experiments, psychopharmacology was able to provide new facts in the tendency of medicine today, to abandon more and more the strict conception of specifity—a tendency which is also to be increasingly observed in psychosomatic medicine.

Table 5. Psychopharmacological effects of some substances

Amphetamine, Methamphetamine: Loss of appetite, alertness
Caffeine: alertness, mental stimulation
Alcohol: gladness, diminished mental capacity, diminished selfcriticism
Barbiturates: restriction of thought sequence, sleepiness
LSD 25: nausea, hallucinations, illusions, delusions
Chlorpromazine, Reserpine: ataraxia, tranquilization

We all possess fixed conceptions of the psychopharmacological effect of certain drugs. Amphetamine makes people alert and spoils the appetite, caffeine stimulates, alcohol produces merriment, barbiturate paralyses the thoughts and makes one sleepy, LSD 25 produces hallucinations, illusions and delusions, chlorpromazine erects a wall between the person and his conflicts and makes him indifferent—all these statements have a positive foundation. But there are many exceptions for these rules, which are very important to psychosomatic research.

Table 6. Psychopharmacological effect does not only depend on the substance, administered or endogenous produced, but also on –

somatic factors   dose
                           route of administration

rate of absorption
condition of the vegetative nervous system
substances previously administered
unexplained factors in tachyphylaxy and addiction

Psychological factors   basic personality
a) primary
b) secondary: subjective interpretation of the drug effects
(psychological superstructure)
motivation
previous experiences
mood
sociopsychological environment

First of all, the psychopharmacological effect of an administered or endogenously produced substance depends on purely somatic factors, on the given dose, the route of administration, the rate of absorption, also on the condition of the vegetative nervous system, previously given substances and on some little-explained processes as in the case of tachyphylaxia or addiction, in the pharmacological sense. Then there are, however, the factors which are of much more importance to psychosomatic research. The personality of the subject, difficult though it is to define, is particularly decisive for the psychological effect which we can observe after the administration of the drug. First of all, a primary effect appears, which is, in its qualitative and quantitative form, materially determined by the basic personality. Thus, methamphetamine can make an inert person more active; it can fill a mentally alert person with a stream of thoughts which renders him inactive; a neurotic person experiences the strongest feelings of apathy, a brave person will be still braver, an anxious person more anxious; it can make an addict sleep or fight against imaginary bugs, calm a person with strong libido and stimulate a weak one, to mention only a few possibilities. As it is so difficult to make reliable statements on basic personality and to collect together a sufficient number of subjects with similar personality structures, our knowledge in spite of promising beginnings, is more casuistical than systematical.

After this primary effect of the drug a secondary quickly follows, which depends on the first in the subjective interpretation of the drug effect and which can be described as forming a psychological superstructure. If, after the giving of a hypnotic a phase of stimulation with an increased need of speaking occurs, one need not necessarily explain this with a central release from inhibition, as pharmacologists do, but it can be a question of an attempt on the part of the person to overcompensate the oncoming sleepiness. Here we are certainly leaving empirical ground as neither self-observation, nor indirect or direct objective observation can register this secondary effect regularly or reliably.

The incidental mood of a person also materially determines the psychopharmacological effect. Someone who is hungry looses his feelings of hunger after amphetamine, whereas in the case of a satiated person the oral region is not affected. All emotions and affects cannot only themselves be changed by drugs, but can also modify the effect of drugs.

The sociopsychological environment, which also shapes the psychopharmacological effect, is very good to investigate experimentally. It is possible to determine fundamental differences according to whether an experiment is carried out in social isolation, or in the presence of the doctor carrying out the experiment, or in a group, and also according to interpersonal contacts. The most common example is the effect of alcohol, which usually manifests itself quite differently in company, from what it does in isolation. Here an opportunity presents itself of examining exactly the meaning of sociopsychological factors in the psychosomatic happening which are better to define exactly than are personality and mood. On the other hand one may also establish that sociopsychological occurences may be influenced pharmacologically.

Even if the methodological difficulties are not to be underestimated, the possibility exists of analysing in model experiments, the interactions between personality, mood, sociopsychological environment, external stimuli and humoral reactions which are very significant in clinical psychosomatic medicine. This interaction can only be inferred retrospectively in clinical cases, if at all possible.

This does not limit the value of the psychopharmacological experiment, as we are dealing here with an unequivocally somatogenic factor, whereas clinical psychosomatics is generally engaged with psychogenic factors. In the above-mentioned performances the drug merely plays the part of a releasing factor in psychopharmacological experiments whereas the essential complete happening is, at the same time, of a psychological and physiological nature. This complete happening does not differ fundamentally from that which takes place in emotions, in an acute conflict-situation and probably also does not differ from the happening in case of a chronic condition with acute exacerbation, as with asthma, ulcer, paroxysmal tachycardia, colitis or migraine. This indicates how meaningless it is, in the case of psychosomatic disturbances, to differentiate according to the factor of release in somatogenic or psychogenic forms. The factor of release is of little importance in comparison with the very powerful preformed patterns which are modified simultaneously by somatic and psychic factors. The jump from psychic to somatic or vice-versa from somatic to psychic cannot be explained in a mechanistical way, however many brain-physiology or neurochemical theories we may desire to quote.

Very material points of view in psychosomatic basic research may be gained from psychopharmacological results which have proved the radical influences of drugs on perception, memory, motivation, symbolic significance of percepts, readiness to act, the symbolic processes and the body image. Here you will be thinking primarily of the experiments with psychomimetic, hallucinogenic substances. It is not necessary to quote these toxic and very effective drugs, which have been, up till now, of no great importance to psychosomatic medicine. Daily consumed drugs contained in tea and coffee or in the cigarette, tablets against pain, antihistamines, harmless ataractics, bromide and barbiturate preparations can influence the quoted psychic functions. It is, moreover just these insignificant effects, which are, as a rule, so integrated in the personality, that they cannot be easily registered either through introspection, or by an interviewing or experimenting doctor which are so interesting. As hunger cuts an "oral sector" out of the realm of perception, so drugs can guide perception, itself, in a particular direction, or can strengthen the defense of perception which prevents, delays, or weakens the perception of particular elements. Further, the symbolic meaning of percepted objects and also of remembered experiences can be changed by drugs. It is possible, for example, that a previously uninteresting scientific book can be of lively interest after the ingestion of amphetamine, phenmetrazine, or methylphenidate, or that a disegreable, sad experience presents only its positive aspects after the ingestion of the same drugs. Such occurences can play a part in the psychoanalytical examination of psychosomatic patients. This is not only noticeable when a patient has taken stimulants or other drugs, without the doctor's knowledge, but also particularly in endocrinological illnesses. It is possible, for example, that a patient with a thyreotoxicosis volunteers quite different childhood memories before or after thyreostatic treatment or a strumectomy.

Psychosomatic medicine, especially in the case of endocrinological illnesses, also of tuberculosis, has to clarify whether the observed changes in personality are to be explained toxicologically. Though the toxicological interpretation was preferred in former times, today there is a decided preference for a psychodynamic explanation or, at least, for a combination of both. Psychopharmacology can contribute much to this problem. The question of whether permanent personality changes can be attained by pharmacological methods cannot be answered with a definite "yes" or "no". Temporary changes in personality can, without doubt, be elicited with drugs. It is also possible to promote a development of personality or to limit an unfavourable development pharmacologically. But it is not yet satisfactorally explored whether it is possible to produce a complete change of the personality by giving particular substances. Theoretically this possibility cannot be completely discarded. It is possible that substances will be developed which can display therapeutically or experimentally such effects. However, it is an other question whether we can take the responsibility to manipulate human beings to such an extent.

In conclusion, the contribution of psychopharmacology to the therapy of psychosomatic disturbances has to be reviewed. It is concerned with a general treatment which should primarily influence the psychic functions in order to, secondarily, thereby improve the functional disturbances or organic injuries. Many psychosomatic doctors are sceptical about every somatic therapy, and rely exclusively on psychotherapy. Due to many personal, economic, sociological and psychological reasons, it will not be possible in the next few decades to treat all the patients, needing this kind of therapy, psychotherapeutically. For this reason, it is necessary to acquire an alleviation, for the remaining patients, which is not purely palliative but rather one which has a lasting effect. The experiments made, up till now, with bromides, barbiturates, phenothiazines, reserpine, meprobamate, methylpentinol carbamate, benactyzyl and other substances show that this method is practicable in single cases, but that the rate of failures is still very high and we still do not know any differentiated indications. It is desirable that more and more psychotherapeutically employed psychosomatic doctors gain unbiased experience of these drugs and examine the results with their criteria. It is not yet definite that unwanted influences on the psychodynamic constellation, like displacement of symptoms, repressions, and substitution symptoms can occur through drug therapy, but it has not yet been satisfactorily proved scientifically. It is to be wished that the pharmaceutical industry will, in the future, go new ways in the production of drugs which can help the patient, who, for some reasons, cannot be treated psycho-therapeutically. Such drugs will probably deviate in their effect from those known up till now. They will more likely display an effect which may be compared with that of alcohol, amphetamine or morphine without sharing their strong tendency towards habit or addiction forming and toxic effects. It is not impossible that such drugs further advance the ability for self-knowledge and activate the mental powers of self-healing. Thus they could, in a psychodynamic respect, enter into a certain competition with psychotherapy. At the moment, one can only speculate on this, as such drugs do not yet exist.

In order to evaluate such pharmacotherapy in the case of psycho-somatic disturbances, the existing methods must be refined. The crude classification in "improved" and "not improved", is un-satisfactory. It is a future task in which psychopharmacology, psycho-logy, psychosomatic medicine and psychiatry must take part to develop new methods in order to be able to objectivate the success of a therapy in its various stages. These methods will also be material in estimating the success of psychotherapy. It would be necessary for them to register slight changes in mood and behaviour and they should be highly independent of every kind of transference and affective contact.

Author's address: DR. M. PFLANZ, Medizinische Universitäts-Poliklinik, *Giessen* (Germany).

Test Methods in Psychosomatic Research

J. T. BARENDREGT, Amsterdam

Nowadays psychological tests are generally applied in research of psychiatry and psychosomatics. Their usefulness is evidently recognized so widely that it would hardly seem worthwhile to spend a lot of words on this fact. I do think it worthwhile to discuss the most important purpose of the application of tests. This purpose is the obtaining of norms or standards.

The behaviour of a human being is always related to a situation. Consequently it is impossible to study this behaviour without taking the situation into account. Less systematic observation gives rise to the problem that situations tied to certain behaviour may vary to such a degree that we no longer have means to compare the behaviour of different persons. It has been attempted to eliminate this difficulty by means of psychological tests in which the situations used are as similar as possible. In this way we can, to a certain degree, render comparable either the behaviour of different patients, or the behaviour of one patient at different times. This enables the investigator to obtain the required norms.

It is apparent in our literature how much we want norms for our research. I dont want to deal with an enumeration of a great amount of publications on this subject. There can be no doubt about the poor reliability and the poor validity of psychiatric diagnosis. Unreliable, because one patient may be considered neurotic by one psychiatrist and normal by another. Hardly valid, because few of the predictions based on those diagnoses are confirmed by facts.

It seems hardly possible to apply successfully intuition in estimating the part played by the diverging circumstances of the patients. Without explicit norms no investigator has yet been proved capable of evaluating his psychological data correctly.

Small wonder that the application of tests has been generally acclaimed, the more so since several of them have proved to produce explicit and reliable norms, enabling us to make useful predictions.

However, tests also have drawbacks. For the time being they do not provide us with norms for many aspects of human behaviour, which we should like to include in our investigations. It may be true that the results of tests are more reliable than the diagnoses of psychiatrists, yet only too often we have to depend on their diagnoses, simply because no tests are available for many of the fields of human behaviour. No tests, i.e. tests that produce explicit and reliable norms.

This has led to sharp contrasts in psychology. We know tests, and I am particularly thinking of the projective techniques, in which few restrictions are made as to the fields of behaviour they are supposed to cover. But unfortunately these tests provide us with few norms. And no matter in how subtle a way they are handled, literature shows that neither the reliability, nor the validity of these tests is any better than psychiatric diagnoses. In these tests, too, it is the investigator who, through his intuition, must evaluate the data and this is something which no one is able to achieve.

The contrast in the test psychology has led to rivalry between the clinical and the statistical methods. This rivalry resulted, with few exceptions, in the defeat of the clinical method. Psychologists have to choose now whether they want to know much badly, or little comparatively well. It may often be difficult in applied psychology to make this choice, but it stands to reason that research people will prefer to know little comparatively well.

Now, what do we learn from psychosomatic literature? It is true, tests are generally being applied, but then the tests applied are mostly projective tests. In other words, although the psychologist handles tests, in fact he is only an extension of the psychiatrist and he handles subjective methods exactly as the psychiatrist does. If you insist on a strict conception of the aim of testing, I have to take back what I said in the beginning. I ought to have said: In psychosomatic research psychological tests are seldom applied. As a psychological test I should like to consider a test of which the result is reliable and does not depend on the investigator's interpretation. I shall give you an example:

We read in psychosomatic literature that for instance one investigator classified 60% of his peptic ulcer patients as psychoneurotics. The value of such a number becomes rather dubious if we look at the diagnoses in American Recruting Centers during the last war. For what we see there, is that in one center 2.7% of those refused for the army on psychiatric grounds were declared psychoneurotic. Whereas 90.2% were labelled with this diagnosis in another center. The diagnosis "psychopathic" varied from zero to 81%. Now one may argue that all the investigators wanted to do was to screen out those who were unfit from a psychiatric point of view. But the percentage of refusals on psychiatric grounds turned out to be varying from 0.5% in one center to 51% in another. Needless to say, that the validity of these judgments was practically nil. Now one may object again, arguing that medical examination for military purposes is a poor example. But other examples described in the literature on this subject also fail to support the reliability of psychiatric diagnosis. I should like to extend my last argument to all those investigations in which projective tests were applied. It is true, objections may be made against many of the studies, of which the results are negative, but we are still waiting for positive proof that a reliable and valid diagnosis of psychoneurosis can be made by means of projective tests.

So, investigating the question of whether psychosomatic patients are neurotics, we did not rely on results of interviews, nor on results of projective techniques. We used the Two Factor Personality Inventory of HERON. This inventory turned out to have a high correlation with the inventory used by EYSENCK in his factorial analysis studies, from which it was demonstrated that the inventory showed a high loading in the factor neuroticism. The items, offered in writing, had to be marked true or not true. Fourty-two of the 110 items are concerned with neuroticism. They have been selected from a great number of questions. Everyone of them has been statistically investigated on its usefulness in distinguishing between normals and neurotics. For this purpose the psychiatric diagnoses of normal and neurotic were accepted. So, it is true, a number of misclassifications was taken into the bargain, but all the same we may assume that the group of subjects classified by the psychiatrists as neurotics did contain a few more neurotics than the group classified by the psychiatrists as normal. Now the neuroticism-score is defined as the number of so-called neurotic answers to these 42 items. These scores are obviously not influenced by the investigator. A test-retest investigation at an interval of one month gave a correlation of .86, which, of course, is most reliable. We validated the inventory on the following groups of subjects:

1. 25 normal men between 20 and 50 years. They answered to the following criteria:

a) They all had a job.

b) None of them had ever been in prison.

c) None of them had ever been treated for a chronic disease.

d) None of them had ever been treated by a psychiatrist.

2. 100 male patients, who had reported at the Psychoanalytical Institute of Amsterdam, applying for treatment of psychological difficulties.

The normal group has a mean neuroticism-score of 6.1 with s of 4. The neurotic group has a mean score of 16.5 with s of 7. Statistically this difference is highly significant. So this test is not only reliable and not influenced by the investigator, but it is also a valid instrument to distinguish normals from neurotics.

Applying this instrument, we found the scores of 25 peptic ulcer patients to be 17.2 with s of 8. We cross-validated these results on female groups.

We found the scores of 30 normal females to be:

$$M = \ 7.3 \qquad s = 5$$

100 neurotic females	$M = 19.1$	$s = 7$
79 female asthmatics	$M = 18.5$	$s = 7$

The similarity with the results found in the male groups is apparent. I will not go further into the matter of the significance of the results. All I want to do is to convey, that reliable and valid tests, not influenced by the investigator, are available to distinguish between neurotics and normals.

With the next figures the same subjects are concerned, but the results reflect a different personality dimension. HERON's inventory contains two scales. The second one is called introversion-extraversion by EYSENCK and sociability by HERON. The score is determined by 36 of the 110 items of HERON's inventory. This score has a high loading in the factor introversion-extraversion, as was demonstrated by EYSENCK's factorial analysis studies. The groups of subjects mentioned before produced the following scores:

Male groups:

Peptic ulcer	$M = 18.2$	$s = 7$
Neurotic	$M = 15.2$	$s = 6$
Normal	$M = 21.5$	$s = 6$

Female groups:

Asthmatic	$M = 19.6$	$s = 5$
Neurotic	$M = 14.8$	$s = 6$
Normal	$M = 19.7$	$s = 5$

On this variable the psychosomatic patients do not go along with the neurotics, but more with the normals.

Whether or not we may draw the conclusion that psychosomatic patients are neurotics even if socially adjusted neurotics, showing their neurosis not so much in their social behaviour as in a somatic way—, whether or not we may draw this desirable conclusion, we do not know.

Besides, this does not concern us here. The idea was to demonstrate once again a few findings, resulting from—I repeat—reliable tests.

At the beginning of this paper I said that the application of psychological tests in psychosomatic research was generally accepted. Afterwards I took this back and said that, on the contrary, little use is made of tests in psychosomatic research. This is especially true in so far as investigation of the hypothesis of psychosomatic specificity is concerned. A very great number of publications on this subject can be found admittedly. But the tests applied in these cases are mostly projective tests. In addition the practice of cross-validation is comparatively rare as far as projective techniques are concerned.

Last year we did a cross-validation research of some 60 Rorschach results described in literature. Not more than three of those results were reasonably confirmed. Yet this hypothesis of specificity can be excellently verified by means of psychological tests. This appears from an investigation made by POSER. He inserted a pin in the cuff of a bloodpressure apparatus. Increasing the pressure, he asked his subjects to tell him when they felt pain. Peptic ulcer and ulcerative colitis patients showed no differences in this respect. The difference appeared when POSER continued increasing the pressure and asked his patients to tell him when they could hardly bear the pain. The point of warning turned out to be much lower for the colitis patients than for the ulcer patients. The possibility of verifying the hypothesis by tests has also become apparent from studies made by HECHT AND RAIFMANN. They asked their patients what score they expected to make in performing a certain task. After they had been informed of the score they actually made, they were asked to predict their score, if they had to perform the same task again. In this case the expectation of the ulcer patient in relation to his preceding achievement was higher than the expectation of the colitis patient.

It is not difficult to determine the reliability of these tests, nor is it difficult to determine how much the investigator may influence the issue. The scores can easily be approached with statistical techniques.

Curiously enough such investigations can hardly be found in psychosomatic literature. Yet it seems that the validity of the hypothesis of psychosomatic specificity would appear to depend on them very much.

Judging from the literature one must admit that discussions on the validity of this hypothesis seem to be of less current interest than a few years ago. There would appear to be an armistice between supporters and opponents, each side maintaining his point of view just the same. For the problem is not solved. Nor could it be expected after so many more discussions than investigations on the subject. Despite the amount of publications on the hypothesis of psychosomatic specificity, its investigation has hardly begun, because until now so little use has been made of psychological tests.

Author's address: DR. J.T. BARENDREGT, Psychologisch Laboratorium der Universiteit van *Amsterdam* (Netherlands).

Hypnosis as a Method and Principle of Research on Psychosomatic Fundamentals

B. Stokvis, Leyden

In this address I propose to discuss the possibilities which hypnosis offers—more especially from an experimental point of view—in our endeavours at scientific objectification of the psychosomatic course of events. In other words, what essential significance should we attach to our experiences with hypnosis—either experimentally or therapeutically applied, that might give us a better understanding of the psychosomatic interrelation. Where are the possibilities, and where do the limits lie?

I here use the expression "psychosomatic course of events" in order to avoid, in principle, terms such as psycho-physical interaction, accompanying physiopsychological phenomena, influence of the mind on the body or vice-versa, physiological processes as expressions of emotional impulses within the organism. Within the scope of the modern totality conception both the psychic and the physical factor can be simultaneously cause and effect. There exists, in fact, no essential separation between the mind and the organism, since the psychic condition may be determined by the state of the organism, and conversely. What happens is a process which is simultaneously psychic *and* somatic.

In investigating the "psychosomatic fundamentals", therefore, one has to take this total psychosomatic course of events as one's starting point. In essence, this amounts to an investigation into the action of affects. This affective happening is manifested in the experience of a feeling, and in a physical utterance or expression. And for the purpose of such an investigation, hypnosis provides us with the means *par excellence*. For, in the first place, hypnosis is itself a psychosomatic sequence; secondly, it acts psychosomatically, and thirdly, the experimental situation in hypnosis can be repeated ad infinitum—although never completely unchanged in one and the same subject.

Let me first clarify the significance of hypnosis as an experimental method of psychosomatic investigation in general.

As I said just now, hypnosis is itself a psychosomatic sequence; it is coupled with an affective influencing or auto-influencing of the consciousness, in which the psycho-physical totality of the person undergoes certain changes. Formerly, these affective changes of consciousness used to be called the "lowering" and "narrowing" of consciousness: the person who is being hypnotized directs his attention to the hypnotist,—so it was thought—and this created the term "lowering of the narrowed consciousness". Within our own conception, that of the totality of the mind-body duality, we prefer to speak of a condition of active relaxation, which is expressed psychosomatically by simultaneously occurring electro-encephalographic changes and altered muscular contraction, on the one hand, and the subject's experience of being relaxed on the other hand.—The psychophysical phenomena that occur in the hypnotic state are expressed in affectively determined changes in thinking, feeling and willing, and, further, in all vegetative functions. At the same time, there is a marked regression: our experiments taught us that it is possible for regressive changes to occur in which even the Oedipus situation and castration anxiety are re-actualized; the regression to the primitive and archaic, moreover, is reflected in the vegetative system. We found in our experiments that there may occur profound changes, *inter alia* in the functioning of the cardio-vascular system, the respiratory apparatus, and the gastrointestinal canal.

As I said before, hypnosis acts psychosomatically. Under the spell of the now antiquated conceptions of the psychosomatic relationship—in the sense of the dualistic view, with a reciprocal causal interaction, we have for many years described hypnosis, quite unsatisfactorily, as a condition brought about through the psychic influence on the sleep centres; the associative link between the oculomotor nucleus and the sleep centres was supposed to explain the action of the fixation methods used to induce hypnosis. And the fact that the sleep centres happen to be in the vicinity of the vegetative centres and the diencephalon was thought sufficient to explain the fact that the subject's animal processes could be influenced by hypnosis. To-day, however, we endeavour to apply the totality conception of man as a psychosomatic unity also to the theory of hypnosis, we see the point of attack of hypnosis in its inherent affective action. Its influence creates an increased neuro-secretory activity of the ganglion cells of the hypothalamic areas, and in this way the impulses of the central nervous system are transferred to the endocrine system by chemical action (1). The old view, that hypnosis causes vegetative changes via the diencephalic "commutator stations" becomes less vague with the aid of the modern micro-biochemical investigation.

The third advantage of hypnosis as a means to investigate the psychosomatic interconnexion is that the experimental conditions can be varied as often as necessary; with the aid of suggestions, different affective situations can be created over and over again, enabling one to study affective actions on the organism. The drawback of this, however, is that a change of testee completely alters the affective situation; and that, therefore, entirely new experimental conditions have arisen. The same applies to the repetition of the experiment with the same testee, in view of possible changes in the transfer relationship. Comparison with previous experiments in other testees thereby becomes difficult. Neither is it scientifically justifiable to make comparisons with the experimental results obtained by other authors. This explains the great differences in the findings that are published in the literature. (Reviews of the literature by FL. DUNBAR (5), I. H. SCHULTZ (15), O. SCHWARZ (16), B. STOKVIS (18, 19, 21).) Fruitless discussions result when the significance of changing the affective relationship in the hypnotic experiment is lost sight of; the transference-counter-transference conditions may well be of very great importance.

After these introductory remarks, let us proceed to discuss the possibilities which hypnosis offers, in an experimental respect, when we seek to objectify the psychosomatic course of events. Here, experimental medical psychology presents three possibilities: 1. the so-called physio-psychological examination; 2. the clinical-psychological—or psychodiagnostic—examination; and 3. the experimental-psychological clinical examination.

ad a. *As regards the "physio-psychological" examination.* As early as the eighteen-nineties, numerous European investigators endeavoured, with the aid of simple instruments, to study the psycho-somatic interconnexions experimentally by means of hypnosis. If one turns over the leaves of some old books on hypnosis, such as BERNHEIM's

(2), O. STOLL's (25), and A. MOLL's (11) classic works, one is struck with the large number of experiments that were made in this field.

But these were—if I may use this term—"atomistic" investigations: isolated from the subject's life history. They bore a strictly experimental character, and these authors confined themselves to reporting physical findings only; minute descriptions of—chiefly—"changes in the circulatory and respiratory tracts", under the influence of hypnosis as they were wont to put it. The pejorative qualification of "soulless psychology" is, indeed, quite apposite here. The study of the width of the range of action of hypnosis—and notably that of therapeutically intended hypnosis—was regarded as the true objective of these investigations. One can hardly say, however, that these investigations have contributed anything to the deepening of our knowledge of the psychosomatic sequence, however great our respect may be for the pioneering work of these former research workers.

The investigations entered upon a new phase in the nineteen-twenties, when it was endeavoured to discover a connexion between the nature of the suggested affect and changes in the digestive tract. A good many names might be mentioned here, but I will confine myself to recalling the investigations of HEYER (7), and, later, those of WITTKOWER (26). The purpose of these experiments was more than a mere demonstration of motorial changes in the stomach, or changes in the gastric juice and in the bile in the hypnotic state; it was seriously endeavoured to view these physical phenomena within the totality of the mind-body situation as it is changed in the hypnotic state. As such these experiments may be regarded as forerunners of the later, more purposive experimental psychosomatic research work.

At this point I may also mention our own physio-psychological investigations made at Leyden during the nineteen-thirties. The purpose of this work was to find a connexion between physical changes under hypnosis and the personality structure. To this end we used the uninterruptedly registered changes in the blood pressure in the hypnotic state in both healthy subjects and sufferers from essential hypertonia, endeavouring to view these changes in their totality-relationship to certain qualities of the subjects' personality, that is, their temperamental condition. It was found that there exist certain psychosomatic correlatives—which, however, have nothing whatever to do with the so-called specificity problem in psychosomatics. We found that the degree in which the affect expresses itself in the subject's organic condition goes hand in hand with a certain temperamental constitution. Thus, in sufferers from essential hypertension we found, through experimental hypnosis, a psychic determination which could be traced by the peculiar shape of the blood-pressure curves. The subject's receptivity to emotions, on the one hand, and his emotional state, on the other hand, could be followed, during the hypnotic experiment, as separately recognizable configurations in the physio-psychological picture of the blood-pressure curves.

From our hypnotic investigations—but also from those of WITTKOWER, all of which, therefore, were made before the beginning of the actual development of psychosomatic medicine—it is evident that emotions may be coupled with different physical changes. These changes, however, differ only quantitatively, not qualitatively. If one knows the vegetative changes, it is quite possible to determine the "intensity" of the emotional experience in question, but not its specific nature. This finding has recently been confirmed by V. BLOCH (3). A further discovery was that, in addition to hypertonia, which I mentioned before, various syndromes that are nowadays called psychosomatic affections—such as bronchial asthma, and "manager's disease"—may be provoked through excitement. By means of methodically applied rest-treatment-hypnosis, active tonus regulation, autogenic training—we found it possible, already in those early days, to exercise a favourable influence on the body-mind condition of this type of patients (Literature: E. D. WITTKOWER (26), B. STOKVIS (18, 19, 20).

In quite a special category are the numerous investigations of I. H. SCHULTZ, with which he started as early as fifty years ago. His meaningful, finely elaborated method of autogenic training, which I mentioned just now, comprises a series of (auto)hypnotic experiments, which has considerably enriched our knowledge of the psychosomatic interconnexion in a state of concentrated autorelaxation, which SCHULTZ calls "Versenkung" (immersion).

All these investigations, which I have enumerated, constituted a transition to the present-day physio-psychological examination in the hypnotic state. Before discussing this, however, I should like to say that it is precisely through the work of the older hypnotists, and the so-called "rational" psychotherapists, that the general significance of psychic determinants in medical science has been brought to the fore. To the psychoanalysts must be granted the great merit of having elaborated these classical findings in an understandingly psychological manner, and of having advocated the deep-psychological treatment, in medicine, of organic phenomena.—To-day, the psychosomatic idea is the guiding principle in hypnotic experimental technique; one endeavours to study the mental and bodily action of affective conversations or situations, and thereby to obtain a better knowledge of the person's life-history and, in this case, the history of his experiences, in their psychosomatic significance.

For this purpose, certain suitable fragments from the person's life-history may be experienced affectively once again by him in the hypnotic state. This may enable us to discover whether, and to what extent, these events acted psycho-traumatically at the time, both as regards the person's mental reaction and as regards the physical utterance, or manner of expression, of the affects in question. And this may be of psychotherapeutic, but also of psychohygienic importance. Here, we might again make honourable mention of a number of names; for example: F. DEUTSCH (4), W. EBBECKE (6), E. H. HSÜ (8), H. KLEINSORGE (9), B. PASQUARELLI BLAISE and N. BULL (12), H. SCHLOSBERG (14), I. STEVENSON (17), and E. D. WITTKOWER (27).

At Leyden we have recently acquired an electronic polygraph, which enables us to register, with eight channels, different vegetative changes simultaneously. By this means it is possible to study the patient's typological nature; 1. his receptivity to emotional experiences, i.e. his emotionality (a quality!) or, respectively, his sensitivity, 2. the degree of his emotionalism (i.e. his being emotionalized [condition!]), and 3. the degree in which possible pent-up affects are being repressed.

ad 2. *As regards the clinical psychological examination.* Let us now proceed to discuss our experiences with hypnosis during the psychodiagnostic examination in psychosomatics. In our Leyden Psychosomatic Centre we attach great importance to the structure-analytical examination, as such, of psychosomatic patients. In some cases we repeat such an examination with the patient in the hypnotic state, in order to find out experimentally, how the sufferer psycho-dynamically "digests" some very particular affective state which he once passed through and which he now once again experiences with the aid of hypnotic suggestions. I here refer to something different from the concept of "hypnodiagnosis" which was recently introduced by MARCUSE AND HAGGERTY (10), and which amounts to the application of hypnosis for the psychodiagnostic examination of the personality. On this subject, many investigators have done meritorious work; but a summary of their findings (STOKVIS (23, 24)) can nevertheless teach us but little concerning the psychosomatic interconnexion.

As I said just now, we here refer to something different. With this range of investigations we also class the technique of "hypnotic age regression", which we merely regard as an autosuggestive, hypnotic representation of a previously experienced period of life. I will refer to this anon. With the aid of this technique it is possible to study the psychodynamic conditions governing conflict situations in the early childhood of psychosomatic patients. In our own experience, however, this method has experimental rather than psychotherapeutic importance.

ad 3. *As regard the third point: The experimental-psychological clinical examination.* By this we understand experimental investigations with the aid of hypnosis in the clinic, in order to get to know more about the patient's behaviour when under certain states of experience. At this point I would again refer to the technique of "age-regression" which, in our opinion, is wrongly regarded—by, among others, PLATONOW (13)—as a "genuine" regression. In this state both psychological and physiological changes may occur that are important for our knowledge of the psychosomatic interrelation.

This class of investigations comprises the whole area of the experimental study of affective action with the aid of hypnosis. On this subject we reported extensively and in detail some time ago (20, 23). These experiments enable us to generate physical phenomena by suggestive action, and, moreover, to cause certain psychological changes, for example, in order to obtain a clearer insight into psychological happenings. Theoretically, the possibilities open to hypnosis to influence the organism, are as great as those open to the affects; they are potentially unlimited, but nevertheless, practically more or less limited; that is, by resistances such as anxiety, suspicion, doubt, or negative suggestibility, on the part of the testee; and further, because of the insufficiency of possibilities which, after all, is inherent in the technique itself. Studying the psychological happenings in these states of profound regression of the personality offered us further possibilities for increasing our knowledge of the psychosomatic interrelation (21, 22, 23).

On reviewing the essential significance of all these investigations, one cannot doubt that hypnosis is an important means towards the objectification of psychosomatic factors and processes. Indeed, by the application of the hypnotic technique we directly touch upon the foundations of the psychosomatic course of events. None the less, one should not—and this happens only too often—indulge in uncritical over-estimation. Nor should we overrate the significance of hypnosis as a form of psychosomatic therapy. However, a discussion of this aspect would be outside the scope of my address.

To sum up, considerable value may be attached to hypnosis in helping us better to understand the psychosomatic interrelation. But it must not be expected that by hypnosis alone, as if it were some magical process, the enigma of this interrelation can be solved.

Summary

In the psychosomatic course of events there exists, in fact, no essential seperation between the mind and the organism. What happens is a process which is simultaneously psychic and somatic. An investigation into this psychosomatic course of events amounts, in essence, to an investigation into the action of affects. This affective happening is manifested in the experience of a feeling and in a physical utterance or expression. And for the purpose of such an investigation, hypnosis provides us with the means par excellence. For the first place, hypnosis is itself a psychosomatic sequence; secondly, hypnosis acts psychosomatically, and thirdly, the experimental stituation in hypnosis can be repeated ad infinitum, although never completely unchanged in one and the same subject in view of possible changes in the transference relationship.

After ample discussion of the significance of hypnosis in general, the speaker proceeds to discuss the possibilities which hypnosis offers in an experimental respect, when we seek to objectify the psychosomatic course of events. Here, experimental medical psychology presents three possibilities:

1. the so-called physio-psychological examination,
2. the clinical-psychological,—or psychodiagnostic—examination, and
3. the experimental-psychological clinical examination.

The speaker discusses these three possibilities in view of data from literature as well as from his own investigations during the nineteen-thirties and later. Presently the psychosomatic view is indicated in the hypnotic experimental technique. Certain suitable fragments from the person's life-history may be experienced affectively once again by him in the hypnotic state. This may enable us to discover whether, and to what extent, these events acted psycho-traumatically at the time. By means of the polygraph, built in Leyden, the speaker is able to study:

1. the patients typological nature;
2. his receptivity to emotional experiences;
3. the degree of his emotionalism, i.e. his being emotionalized before, during and after hypnotism;
4. the degree in which possible pent-up affects are being repressed.

Summarizing the speaker comes to the conclusion that it is evident that hypnosis is an important means towards the objectification of psychosomatic factors and processes. One should not, however,—which is done too often—overrate the significance of hypnosis.

Bibliography

1. BARGMANN, W. ET AL.: 2. Int. Symposium über Neurosekretion 1957 (Springer, Berlin 1958).
2. BERNHEIM, H.: Die Suggestion und ihre Heilwirkung (translated by Sigmund Freud) (F. Deuticke, Leipsic/Vienna 1888).
3. BLOCH, V.: Sur les conceptions actuelles de l'émotion. J. Psychol. norm. path., 47–51; 79–90 (1954).
4. DEUTSCH, F.: Thus speaks the body. Acta med. orient. *10*: 67–86 (1951).
5. DUNBAR, F.: Emotions and bodily changes (Columbia Univ. Press, 3rd ed. New York 1949, p. 419).
6. EBBECKE, W.: Psychische Beeinflussung körperlicher Vorgänge. Naturwissenschaften *39*: 49 (1952). Abstr. Zbl. ges. Neurol. Psychiat. *121*: 267 (1953).
7. HEYER, G.R.: Psychogene Funktionsstörungen des Verdauungstraktes. In: O. SCHWARZ *16*: 228–258.
8. HSÜ, E.H.: Comparative study of factor patterns, physiologically and psychologically determined. J. gen. Psychol. *47*: 105–128 (1952).
9. KLEINSORGE, H.: Neue Forschungsergebnisse über psychophysische Zusammenhänge. In E. SPEER: Vortr. 3. Lindauer Psychotherapiewoche 1952, p. 62–74 (Thieme, Stuttgart 1953).
10. MARCUSE, F.L., and HAGGERTY, A.: Hypnodiagnosis. In M.V. KLINE: The annual review of hypnosis literature. Vol. I and II, 1950/51 (Woodrow Press, New York 1953).
11. MOLL, A.: Der Hypnotismus, mit Einschluss der Psychotherapie und der Hauptpunkte des Okkultismus. 5th ed. (Kornfeld, Berlin 1924).
12. PASQUARELLI, B., and BULL, N.: Experimental investigation of the body-mind continuum in affective states. J. nerv. ment. Dis. *113*: 512–521 (1951).
13. PLATONOW, K.I.: J. gen. Psychol. Worchester *9*: 190 (1933).
14. SCHLOSSBERG, H.: Three dimensions of emotion. Psychol. Rev. *61*: 81–88 (1954). Abstr. Psychol. Abstr. *28*: 8509 (1954).

15. SCHULTZ, I. H.: Das autogene Training (Konzentrative Selbstentspannung). 9th ed. (Thieme, Stuttgart 1956).

16. SCHWARZ, O.: Psychogenese und Psychotherapie körperlicher Symptome (Springer, Vienna 1925).

17. STEVENSON, I.: Physical symptoms during pleasurable emotional states. Psychosom. Med. *12*: 2 (1950).

18. STOKVIS, B.: Hypnose, psyche en bloeddruk (Tijdstroom, Lochem 1937) (with 1430 references).

19. STOKVIS, B.: Psychologie und Psychotherapie der Herz- und Gefässkranken. (Tijdstroom, Lochem 1941)(with 898 references).

20. STOKVIS, B.: Die Bedeutung der experimentellen Psychologie für die psychische Hygiene. In: MENG, H. ET AL.: Praxis der seelischen Hygiene (Benno Schwabe, Basel 1943).

21. STOKVIS, B.: Hypnose in der ärztlichen Praxis (S. Karger, Basel/New York 1955) (with 679 references).

22. STOKVIS, B.: Brit. J. med. Hypnot. *7*: 1, p. 13–20 (1955).

23. STOKVIS, B.: Allgemeine Überlegungen zur Hypnose. Handbuch der Neurosenlehre und Psychotherapie, p. 71–122 (Urban & Schwarzenberg, Munich/ Berlin 1957) (with 274 references).

24. STOKVIS, B.: Hypnose, Suggestion, Entspannungstherapie. In: STERN, E.: Die Psychotherapie in der Gegenwart, p. 143–185 (Rascher, Zürich 1958).

25. STOLL, O.: Suggestion und Hypnotismus in der Völkerpsychologie (2nd ed., Veit & Comp., Leipsic 1904).

26. WITTKOWER, E.: Einfluss der Gemütsbewegungen auf den Körper (Sensen Verlag, Vienna/Leipsic 1936), p. 92–107; 2nd ed. 1937.

27. WITTKOWER, E.: Predictive psychophysiological studies. Acta psychother. *6*: 11–22 (1958).

Author's address: DR. B. STOKVIS, Psychosomatic Center of the Leyden State University, *Leyden-Oegstgeest* (Netherands).

Methods and Principles of Research
on Psychosomatic Fundamentals

(The Contribution of Psycho-Analysis to Psychosomatic Medicine)

A. Mitscherlich, Heidelberg

As experiment is impossible in psycho-analysis, its theories must always be based on clinical observation. Of the many possible definitions of psychosomatic medicine I shall therefore—as a psychoanalyst—choose a simple, clinical pragmatical one. Psychosomatic patients go to the doctor complaining of physical or psychical symptoms, and these are susceptible of purely physical interpretation. Their illness faces us with a decision. Is it to be regarded as primarily somatic, or is the somatic symptomatology connected with mental experiences, and is it the latter which are the primary cause? By "experience" is meant a series of mental events which have led to an inner conflict or a "basic fault" (Balint) incapable of resolution by the ego. The general pathogenetic conception of psychosomatic illness is that instinctual wishes (id-wishes) have been mobilised into a state of conflict which has not been satisfactorily resolved. The normal or direct route to satisfaction of these wishes being barred by the ego, the id secures partial relief by enforcing a compromise. This is staged in the patient's own organism, with its multiplicity of organ functions. Thus we may say with Winnicott that where the "exploitation of the intellect" fails, there is a "counterpart psychosomatic disorder".

An over-all definition of this kind, however, tells us nothing about the specific nature of the conflicts or the "basic fault" and compromises associated with specific organic symptoms. Before I say anything about the highly controversial theme of specificity or symptom choice, I should like to linger for a moment over the decision with which we are faced when, as I have mentioned, an organic finding has been made in a patient. What is the next step? Are we to assume that the causes are organic and adopt a therapy based on removing it, or, if necessary, only its symptoms? Or are we to understand the symptom as a signal, a message, an effort at communication made by an individual in a state of conflict which makes it intellectually and emotionally impossible for him to communicate with us in speech?

This raises the question of the observer's purpose. But, more is involved in the question than a mere intellectual decision, for the questioner's emotions are deeply implicated. We never ask questions in a void; our questioning is limited by the bounds of what we believe to be possible. What we believe to be possible depends on a system of contemporary prejudices. Prejudices always indicate taboos, and taboos are collective rituals for warding off danger. That enables us to see why the new questions which have arisen with psychosomatic medicine have met with so much emotional and prejudiced opposition, open or concealed. It also enables us to see why psychosomatic medicine, under the guidance of American investigators, has grown more and more innocuous in the course of years, more and more experimental, more and more statistical, more and more similar to physical medicine. The danger of new questions, the fear of offending against collective scientific taboos, was evidently too great.

In trying to fight this fear, you come up against the well known fact that every science is determined by its system of observation. It is said that each of the three kinds of medicine—the magic, the scientific, the psychosomatic—deals with only a section of the vital phenomena available to observation. Scientific medicine claims, however, that it sees more, and with greater accuracy, than magic medicine does, while psychosomatic medicine claims that it sees more and farther than organic medicine.

Permit me to linger over familiar matters for a moment longer while I steer towards a highly controversial goal. Conventional medicine depends on experimental proof, and has accumulated innumerable data about the human organism. In addition to this, it has developed a philosophy, of which the principal tenet is that underlying all the human phenomena that we observe are physical processes, and that life itself is a result of these physical processes. Hence the sole aim of medical investigation is elucidation of the material processes underlying the physiological and pathological phenomena.

The psycho-analyst, whether his patient is psychoneurotic or somatic, uses a different system of observation, and fits his work into an entirely different frame of reference. In the first place the object of his observations is not the human body, but *human behaviour*. He regards a physical symptom as a diseased way of behaviour. His frame of reference is not the patient's somatic organisation, but his life history. Thus in one respect he is akin to the historian, for he is a student of sources. But his critical method is not weighing up and comparing different sources, but strengthening the critical capacity of the ego towards its own behaviour. Moreover, in comparison with the historian's the analyst's investigations are on a microscopic scale and, above all, his objective is different; he wishes, not to reconstruct the past for its own sake, but to alter events and influence future behaviour. He is a pragmatist; the past is material he uses to enable him to understand the present.

The underlying biochemical and biophysical processes are of relatively minor interest to him. They come within his field of vision only to the extent that they show him where lie the boundaries beyond which there can be no influencing the future. Constitutional limitations, irreversible decay of the higher functions, such a thing as a cancerous growth spreading at the expense of the whole organism, decreasing capacity due to age—all these are things to which the analyst, like any other physician, must bow. But, easy though it is to point to limiting conditions such as these, I should like to point out that it would be wrong to conclude that we can lay down hard and fast boundaries in our ordinary, everyday practice. War experiences for example have demonstrated over and over again the apparently extraordinary feats, both active and passive, of which the ordinary human being is capable, and the extent of the reserves at his disposal. To me it seems to be not the sheer threat to life that brings out these things, but a highly complex collective mental influence *. We find the same thing in the processes of adaptation of the whole period of childhood. in the greatly varying and often extremely burdensome family environments.

Thus it is clear that the psycho-analyst and the conventional physician are interested in very different aspects of one and the same

---

* A. JORES has shown us recently the same phenomenon on an example from the opposite, when he mentioned the rapid decay of strength and the precocity of death of individuals having lost the final aims of their lives.

individual, though the object of both is the same, namely freeing him from his illness. That brings me to expressing the controversial opinion that I do not expect much of team-work between psycho-analysts and conventional medical investigators, at any rate for the time being. In view of the tremendous expansion of the boundaries of knowledge in our time, the general trend is inevitably towards team-work. GRINKER (1) says that in the psychosomatic field, as in others, the "multidisciplinary attack", the "inter-disciplinary group", should be able to "give us clues as to the primary psychosomatic unity and subsequent specific somatic and psychological variations of function known as health or disease". After my brief initial remarks about the dependence of an observation on the method and view-point of the observer, it will be understood that as a psycho-analyst I find it rather hard to conceive of such team-work's being really integrated into psychosomatics and developing into something more than mere play with a "modern" idea. On the other hand I hold team-work by psycho-analysts among themselves to be essential, and one of the most regrettable weaknesses of our science seems to me to be that it is practised so little. Apart from that, I fail to see what results could be produced by a multidisciplinary team. Such results as I have seen have boiled down in practice to the adoption into the philosophy, the speculative superstructure, of natural science of some of the results of psycho-analytic observation; or, put more crudely, the enrichment of the experimental approach by some new problems or settings. The results, to the best of my knowledge, have never led to any greater precision or differentiation in the area of the subject covered, admittedly still primitively, by psychoanalytic enquiry. Another fact that can hardly be disputed is that those psycho-analysts who have joined such teams have increasingly abandoned their own viewpoint and become more and more undifferentiated in their own special field of observation.

What I am now saying boils down to an argument for *purism of method*. That is something which we should learn to accept more readily than hitherto on both sides. When I observe an individual's behaviour, that is to say, the formation, the displacements, and the disappearance of his symptoms and try to influence them therapeutic-ally, the organic processes by which they appear and disappear are immaterial, whether I am dealing with a compulsion, an eczema, or a stomach ulcer; in fact burdening the mind with physiological ideas about what is possible and what is not can be a hindrance rather than an aid. When GEORG GRODDECK (2), that brilliant pioneer of the psycho-analytic investigation of somatic symptoms, described premature ageing, for instance, and in particular premature growing grey, as the somatic assumption of a "father mask" (to look like the father), and incidentally pointed out that he had several times observed greyness coming on and passing away again, he was certainly describing an unusual physiological process. How such a thing was possible, indeed, whether it was possible at all according to established physiological ideas, was an altogether secondary question which did not interest him at all. I believe he was entirely right to ignore it. The humorist GEORGE MIKES once remarked that "life is full of problems if you know where to find them". Sometimes it is a good thing to turn a blind eye to a problem, and merely to note that grey hair is capable of returning to its original shade when the "father mask" is dropped.

I know that we are on the way to a scientific Esperanto, using the grammar of experimental research and statistics. As against this I should like to point to the value of independent families of scientific languages. In other words, premature methodological eclecticism seems to me to be harmful to psycho-analysis, and hence to be an impoverishment of psychosomatics as a whole. The latter must first reconcile itself to the fact that it contains within itself something entirely heterogeneous, something as heterogeneous as the word "psychosomatic" itself.

The displeasure that my rejection of team-work between physical medicine and psycho-analysis will certainly have roused among many of you, may cause the question to be asked whether turning one's back on team-work in this way does not involve putting oneself in a position of irresponsible isolation, whether the psychoanalyst, in his refusal to be impressed by clinical findings and his indifference to standard clinical therapy, is not overlooking the propitious moment and favourable opportunities for a successful cure. Is he not turning himself into an outsider, a quack? Such arguments rather tend to make one smile. For it is a rare experience for a patient suffering, say, from vague stomach pains to come to a psycho-analyst straight from the street. Such patients have normally made the rounds of many physicians' consulting rooms and have been subjected to innumerable examinations and treatments before the decision was made to direct them to us; and by that time, alas! only too often the propitious moment for our therapy has passed.

Thus, the fears nurtured in regard to us, are, to use our own terminology, at the very least projections of the guilt feelings of those who
handled the case before us.

However, I do not wish to underrate the problem. In the great
army of physicians, psycho-analysts are an advanceguard, with the
advantages and disadvantages of that position. Many of our present-
day ideas will in the course of time be revised or overtaken by new
discoveries. There is nothing remarkable in that, for it is impossible
to be a pioneer (or if you like a revolutionary) without being a product of the past which the pioneer (or revolutionary) desires to alter.
It was the same in the history of painting. CÉZANNE, VAN GOGH,
KANDINSKY, the Fauvists, the Cubists, the Abstract school, were all
told by their contemporaries that they could not paint. But is painting
repetition of the established style? Is any revolution that makes
history prepared by illiterates, or by people trained in the predominant
outlook of their time who are unable to reconcile with the latter what
they see before their eyes? Are we analysts, in short, to be considered
ignoramuses in the field of classical medicine because we desire to
explore human reality in a new direction? After all, most of us,
starting with FREUD, have been through the contemporary school of
medicine, and are trained physicians. An advance-guard never enjoys
the privilege of living through its age in the ignorance which can be
blissfully basked in by those who from their frame of reference declare
our methods of interpreting findings to be nonsensical and absurd.

In a general survey of the basic methods and principles of psychosomatic studies I cannot discuss in detail the special problems which
confront the analyst in this field. There are, however, a few which I
should like to mention in order to draw attention to some of the
problems which face us in our clinic at the present time. There is,
for instance, the question of which somatic symptoms arise directly
from an attempt to secure relief from an unconscious instinctual
conflict, and which arise after preparation during a preliminary
psychoneurotic phase with its symptomatology. The resemblance to
conversion symptoms and character symptoms is plain. FRANZ
ALEXANDER (3, 4) was the first clearly to formulate the difference
between two groups of symptoms in psychosomatic medicine: (i)
those which should be classified with hysterical conversion symptoms,
i.e. stand directly for an instinctual drive, a part being substituted for
the whole, and the place of one organ physiologically intended for
providing gratification being taken by another; and (ii) those which

originate from an individual's failure to adapt himself to his id wishes and hence also to his social environment. Thus unsatisfied instinctual needs lie at the root of these illnesses too. But their first outcome is a way of behaviour, an attitude of the self to its own emotions, which is significant for the person's whole character. This way of behaviour both in relation to the id within and the world without can be maintained only at the expense of excessive stress; there thus arises the vicious circle of anxiety and rigidity of behaviour, and the stress may have somatic consequences which in themselves do not directly express anything. ALEXANDER's classification is clear and helpful, but further careful observation is required. In particular—and this is a point to which I shall return—there is a series of symptoms the direct expressive function of which is denied commonly but nevertheless seem to us to have that function—diabetes mellitus, for instance.

Another interesting question which has so far scarcely been considered is this. When an individual finds himself compelled to give up libido objects and turns the cathected instinctual energy against himself, what symptom formations correspond to what abandoned libido objects? Here the pathological reaction seems to extend from the symptomatology of conversion hysteria to forms of illness reached by way of many intermediary stages of mental dynamics. To this category there belong questions such as that of symptom choice made under the conditions of early imposed reaction formations, the "anal character" described by FREUD (5), for instance; or that made under the conditions of "role diffusion" as attributed by ERIC H. ERIKSON (6) to different stages of individual development.

Days and hours of careful discussion would really be needed for all this. The few examples quoted are intended only to indicate the field in which psycho-analytic research takes place in the psychosomatic clinic.

At the present moment, when we in this conference make great efforts of mutual understanding between investigators who use different methods, I should like to draw attention to a few points which illustrate the present state of psycho-analytic theory in relation to our empirical experiences in the psychosomatic field.

1. We have moved further and further away from thinking in terms of *disease-entities* as the latter have developed in the classical clinic. The attempt to take over this clinical classification into our pathological scheme of things has failed. The doctrine of character-profiles which were said to be associated with individual organic

diseases has turned out on more detailed investigation to be untenable. The presence of any particular symptom tells us nothing whatever about any definite unconscious conflict in the patient. We should not forget FREUD's remark on the symptoms being the most alien contents of mind with which the Ego has to deal («das Ich-Fremdeste, das sich in der Seele vorfindet») (7).

2. That does not mean that the theory of the specificity of *conflicts* which lead to psychosomatic illness has been abandoned. All that has become clear is that relatively similar conflicts lead to relatively similar symptom formation. That is the typical conflict situations in ALEXANDER's terminology. But the conflict can make its appearance in very different character contexts. Frustrated oral satisfactions, for instance, can certainly have the pathological effect of producing a stomach ulcer. But in one case this may be the expression of a passive oral clinging dependency, while in another the id may be seeking to enforce such oral satisfaction against a total personality which regards such dependency as intolerable and fights against it by making increased demands on itself. Thus the question of specificity can be stated only in the context of the whole character structure.

3. From this it follows that *diagnosis* cannot be based on the physical symptom presented by the patient, but only on the structure of his unconscious conflict taken in relation to his conscious attitude. FREUD gave the following definition: "The symptom is indicator as well as substitute for an instinctual gratification which did not take place; it is the result of a repressive process. Repression starts from the Ego that—perhaps in the service of the Super-Ego—declines to take part in an instinctual activity incented by the Id." (8)

Connected with this is the position which the symptom occupies in the patient's experience. We refer to this under the concept of "*symptom pressure*". To what extent, that is to say, does the compromise reached in the symptom satisfy the id on the one hand and the ego and super-ego on the other? Furthermore, the prognosis depends to a large extent on the secondary gain from the illness; the greater the latter, the worse the former. In this connection it must again be pointed out that a high degree of pain and suffering and physical incapacity and impoverishment of life do not exclude a high degree of gain for the unconscious. In these difficult conditions the conscious part of the personality has to accept the fact that by means of a symptom the instinctual needs of the id have been blunted. In certain states the importance of blunting an unconscious conflict can override the worsening of the patient's mental and social plight that is the consequence of his illness. I am again quoting FREUD: "It does happen that the defensive struggle against unwelcome drives is terminated by the formation of the symptom. As far as we can see this is most easily achieved with the help of hysterical conversion. As a rule we find another pattern. The first repressive step is followed by a long-lasting or even unterminable afterlude, and the struggle against the instinctual drive is replaced by the struggle against the symptom". In due course the symptom is closely tied up with the Ego, becoming more and more indispensible. The secondary gain from the illness, in interaction with the Ego's efforts to integrate the symptom, will reinforce the fixation. "Whenever we try to lend analytic aid in the Ego's struggle against the symptom, we are faced with the fact that some sort of conciliatory alliance between the Ego and the symptom is active on the side of the patient's resistance." (9)

It follows from this that the secondary gain from illness is by no means an easy thing to discover; on the contrary, it reveals itself only in the context of the failure in adaptation, both internal and external, of the total personality.

(4) Treatment is thus concerned, not just with bringing about a disappearance of the symptom, but more essentially with dealing as far as possible with the failure in adaptation. Only when the place of the symptom has been taken by a less harmful solution of the conflict, that is to say, when the instinctual energies which went into the forma-tion of the symptom can be applied to purposes acceptable to the ego and productive to the ego and the environment, can we speak of an ideal *cure*. The figures for successful cures normally offered us in the clinic tell us nothing so long as it is not shown that the cure is ac-companied by a strengthening of the ego which on the one hand is accompanied by an increased capacity for tolerating frustrations and on the other enables the id impulses to be useful to the total personality.

(5) A diagnosis is, of course, complete only when it permits us insight into *pathogenesis*. In physical medicine diagnosis is based on physical tests, and the pathogenesis is deduced from theoretical models of the course of an illness. A test shows what stage has been reached.

In psycho-analysis the situation is very different. Here too the patient is of course at a particular stage of his illness. But the illness is regarded as an inter-action process of conscious and unconscious, of the cathexis of an organ function with instinctual energies which cannot be satisfactorily discharged through that organ. The pathophysiological reaction is the expression of the natural defense reactions at the disposal of the organ. In any individual case all this excludes diagnosis in terms of a theoretical model in which only physical reactions are taken into account.

The psycho-analyst has, however, one advantage which is denied to others. He is able to observe the curative process *in statu nascendi* with incomparable accuracy, to watch all its advances and retreats, and to adapt his therapy accordingly. In comparison with this, clinical tests are a rather crude instrument.

(6) One of the greatest difficulties of psycho-analytic diagnosis is the fact that we have learnt that every symptom is over-determined, i.e., expresses several often contradictory conflicts. The durability of a cure depends very largely on the *over-determination* being cleared up. At least the ambivalence present in the symptom must be understood and modified. This is a reflection of the two primary drives described under the concepts of libido and destrudo.

(7) It has certainly become clear that in psycho-analysis diagnosis is a process indissolubly bound up with the therapeutic process. In view of the complexity of events in the therapy, no experiments in the ordinary sense of the word can be carried out, apart from the fact that at this level of communication they are humanly out of the question. The consequence is that the only possible criterion of the *correctness* of an interpretation of the psycho-dynamics of a psychosomatic symptom is a cure. More particularly, to satisfy us the analysis must (a) show which interpretations contributed to a strengthening of the ego, enabling it to accept the split-off, unconscious conflict; (b) enable us to see what has happened to the instinctual drives which were fixated in the conflict and to follow them into their new destiny; (c) show us that these instinctual drives have found release in a manner more acceptable to the ego; or alternatively that an alteration has taken place in the ego making it possible for them to be integrated.

By the enumeration of these few points I have tried to give some indication of the psycho-analytic method in the investigation of psychosomatic disorders. What I have said could be amplified in many respects, but for that there is no time. In conclusion I should like to return to and amplify what I said early about purism of method. Though I do not believe that fruitful results are to be expected from automatically taking over findings resulting from a different methodology, I do believe that an *over-all view of discoveries* over as wide a front as possible must have a healthy and stimulating influence on the

observer, whatever his standpoint. I agree with GRINKER and ROBBINS
(10) when they say: "No one frame of reference implicit in any of the
theoretical systems is broad enough to encompass the entire psychosomatic field and cannot, therefore, satisfactorily explain any single
state of health or illness." If we take seriously the limitation of our
findings, we should not adopt a monistic philosophy incompatible
with that limitation. In this connection I shall briefly quote two theoretical assumptions which have been made. The first generalises from
the particular, the other attempts to regard homogeneously in a new
frame of reference findings which today we still regard as heterogeneous, namely as either mental or physical. The former is an
example of methodological eclecticism, the latter of an attempt to
arrive at a new understanding of organic symptoms by a theory which
does away with the dualism of mental and physical, but seems to us
still imperfect in many reasons.

I have selected the first hypothesis from a large number of similar
hypotheses with which you will have become familiar in the course of
years, because of the simplicity with which it can be stated. Its author,
IVES HENDRICK (11), first states the fundamental problem of the dualism
with which we are confronted. "The ultimate problem of psychosomatic medicine", he says, "is that of selection of organ systems in
the resolution of emotional conflicts by alteration of normal physiological function." He draws attention to the insufficiency of previous
attempts to find an answer. He mentions for example "that the locale
of disease is determined by the symbolic meaning of the organ, that
organ is fixated by coincidence of systemic disease and emotional
conflict during infancy, that each organ activity satisfies specific forms
of active or passive emotional needs." But all these things, he says,
"seem to me pertinent to special cases but do not provide an acceptable generalisation." For the purposes of this last he puts forward a
hypothesis according to which the organ choice is the result of
"physiologic infantilism, or immaturity of homeostatic processes in an
organ system." His hypothesis is "that psychosomatic diseases are
based upon a physiologic lability of the autonomic nervous system
normally found at immature development levels." The result is a
tendency "to discharge conflict in those organs where the physiologic
lability of normal immaturity has been retained or can be established."

I mention this hypothesis because on the one hand the return of
an old idea can be observed in it, namely ADLER's "organ inferiority",
and on the other hand because the phrase "or can be established"

tacitly assumes that a mature organ is capable of reverting to the state of lability of an immature organ. Assuming that that is possible, the question arises of what it is that causes the organ to behave in that way. In other words, HENDRICK's criticism of the hypothesis of others applies also to his own, for it fails to explain how every case of psychosomatic illness arises. We recently had in our clinic a woman aged thirty-six who for years had suffered from chronic inflammation of the gums and the vaginal mucous membrane. Investigation disclosed that the inflammation at both the oral and genital poles was an attempt at a compromise solution of an unconscious conflict powerful enough to resist any purely symptomatic local therapy. But what led to the inflammation? Does the idea of "physiologic infantilism" help in any way?

I see nowhere any theory which can show link by link the chain of cause and effect leading from the unconscious phantasy and the instinctual conflict associated with it to the inflammation of the gums and the vaginal mucous membrane. Now and again we are able to throw light on some small part of the chain of events, but most of it remains in the dark.

I think that the fact that after so much effort we have failed to establish a general psychosomatic theory is not without good reason. This is that psychosomatic ideas as a whole are artificial; that is, they are the outcome of the long period during which physical medicine ingrained in us the habit of thinking of the processes of life purely and simply as physically observable processes. What is now happening is purely an addition of the previously shrivelled mental area which is only at the surface amenable to any experimental observation. And along that path we seem able to get no further.

I believe that that was seen very plainly forty years ago by GEORG GRODDECK (12), who drew very bold consequences from it, so bold that, because they did not fit into the tradition, they have long been dismissed as wild phantasies and speculations, to my mind very unjustly. GRODDECK – and this is the second hypothesis of which I wish to speak – abandons differentiation between mental and organic in the pathogenetic process. For him the *operative entity* is the id, for which no difference between mental and organic exists. He says: "When I use the words body and mind, I understand by them different manifestations, if you like functions, of the id." He believes that, "if it is at all possible to analyse the id, it must be simultaneously possible to treat organic illness." GRODDECK possessed a probably unsurpassed

intuitive capacity for understanding the id in its normal and pathological manifestations in the individual as modeled by its own culture.

I do not know whether or to what extent it will be possible to
eliminate the dichotomy between physical and mental from our medical thinking, but efforts in that direction can in my opinion only help
psychosomatic medicine forward. That we have much resistance in
ourselves to overcome in the process I should like to illustrate from
an incident during the treatment of a tuberculous patient of mine
many years ago, a highly gifted, aesthetically cultivated young man of
twenty-two. His tuberculosis was disclosed by a haemoptomy shortly
before he came to me. There was a big infraclavicular cavern on the
right. Analysis quickly revealed a conflict situation which can be described as an inverted Oedipus complex. The young man's relationship
with his mother was one of intense, hate-filled jealousy, and at the
same time his whole character was impregnated with a far-reaching
identification with her. He idealised his father and hero-worshipped
him. At one session he produced a memory of a visit to a natural
history museum with his class, when he saw a human foetus for the
first time. The sight filled him with revulsion. In this context I interpreted his passive homosexuality and the cavern as an attempt to bear
his father a child. During the night after this session the patient vom-
ited several times and had a severe vasomotor collapse. Eight days
later an X-ray examination showed that the cavern had disappeared,
and 4 weeks later the patient was well enough to be discharged from
the clinic. You will appreciate that the reason for my hesitation before
communicating this episode was not just the sensational nature of the
disappearance of such a symptom, but much more the impossibility
of giving more than a brief glimpse of it. I cannot here describe
especially the whole transference and analytical situation which technically justified such a direct interpretation of an unconscious content.
Without taking the transference situation into account such an interpretation could, of course, only too easily be an example of "wild"
analysis. The reason of mentioning this case is my wish to stress the
power of id-processes in organic diseases. If we maintain the scheme
of thinking in terms of either organic or psychological, we will never
understand the definite message of the id in an organic symptom.

Since then I have not had many opportunities of dealing with
tuberculous cases but, even if I had had many such, I doubt whether
I should ever have been justified in suggesting as a tenable theory
that tuberculous caverns represented attempts to satisfy homosexual

pregnancy wishes. What I do not doubt, as a result of the whole course of treatment from which I have quoted this episode, is that in this case my interpretation of the symptom hit on the unconscious wish and had a corrective and therefore curative effect.

In this case a young man's pregnancy phantasy was causally connected with a tuberculous cavern. Not the slightest warrant for such a thing exists in our physiology of the human organism, our clinical idea of the pathogenesis of tuberculosis of the lungs. I may as well confess that my thorough training in physiological thinking made me almost ashamed of this and similar successful cures. In the ten years that have since elapsed I have made serious efforts to find a theory for my analytic successes and failures which would reconcile them with the traditional models of pathophysiology. Now I regard these efforts as having failed. I have increasingly come to see that GRODDECK was right in his idea that the pathogenetic prime motive force is to be sought in the id and its attempt to defend itself against the ego. From this the discovery follows that the plasticity of physiological functions as a means of communication for unconscious trends is far greater than we are ready to admit. I know of no plausible theory to explain why apatient with pseudocyesis gets fat, and of course I know of none to explain the coming and going of a tuberculous cavern. And again, of course, the hypothesis that "body" and "mind" are *fields of function* of our own unconscious organisation fails to cover the whole field. But a great challenge seems to me to be implicit in the indifference manifested by this psychosomatic theory to the material, causal analysis which dominates medicine. Moreover, forty years after the work of GRODDECK, we have in psycho-analysis an instrument which has been greatly refined since his time, and thus to a large extent protects us from scattering about "wild" and provocative interpretations. I should like therefore to conclude by reiterating that the psycho-analytic treatment of severe organic illness requires a large amount of previous knowledge, theoretical and practical, *i.e.*, that this method of treatment can be risked only after careful training; I look forward now to a good deal of violent disagreement in the discussion.

Bibliography

1. GRINKER, ROY, R.: Some current trends and hypotheses of psychosomatic research, in FELIX DEUTSCH: The psychosomatic concept in psychoanalysis. p. 37 ff. (Int. Universities Press Inc., New York 1953).
2. GRODDECK, GEORG: Das Buch vom Es. p. 124 (Int. Psychoanalyt. Verlag, Leipzig/Wien 1923).
3. ALEXANDER, FRANZ: Psychosomatische Medizin (Walter de Gruyter & Co., Berlin 1951).
4. ALEXANDER, FRANZ and FRENCH, TH. M.: Studies in Psychosomatic Medicine (The Ronald Press Co., New York 1948).
5. FREUD, SIGMUND: Charakter und Analerotik. Ges. Werke, Bd. VII (Imago Publ. Co., Inc., London 1942).
6. ERIKSON, ERIK, H.: Wachstum und Krisen der gesunden Persönlichkeit (Ernst Klett Verlag, Stuttgart 1953).
7. FREUD, SIGMUND: Ges. Werke, Bd. XV, p. 62 (Imago Publ. Co., Ltd., London 1940).
8. FREUD, SIGMUND: Ges. Werke, Bd. XIV, p. 118 (Imago Publ. Co., Ltd., London 1940).
9. FREUD, SIGMUND: Ges. Werke, Bd. XIV, p. 125–127 (Imago Publ. Co., Ltd., London 1940).
10. GRINKER, ROY R. and ROBBINS, FRED P.: Psychosomatic Case Book. p. 32 (The Blakiston Company, Inc., New York/Toronto 1954).
11. HENDRICK, IVES, in F. DEUTSCH: The psychosomatic concept in psychoanalysis. p. 139 (Int. Universities Press Inc., New York 1953).
12. GRODDECK, GEORG: Das Buch vom Es. p. 134 (Int. Psychoanalyt. Verlag, Leipzig/Wien 1923).

Author's address: PROF. DR. A. MITSCHERLICH, Psychosomatische Klinik der Universität *Heidelberg* (Germany).

From the Second Medical Service, Wilhelmina Gasthuis, Amsterdam, The Netherlands, and the Department of Medicine A, Hebrew University Hadassah Medical School and Hospital, Jerusalem, Israel

Methodology of Psychosomatic Research

J. J. Groen*

In this paper we will limit ourselves to the methodological problems of psychosomatic research within a scientific framework. We wish to stress that this methodology does not claim any superiority over the phenomenological approach; neither, however, does it accept to be inferior to the philosophical or purely psychological views on man and his diseases.

Psychiatric Studies

When the psychosomatic research group in the Wilhelmina Hospital in Amsterdam was founded in 1947, the problem of its methodology came up immediately (1). Its first steps certainly differed in no way from the psychiatric approach as used elsewhere. Results of interviews with patients were interpreted by the psychiatrist BASTIAANS with the help of psychoanalytical concepts and hypotheses were formulated. The physician, the author of the present paper, introduced the method of *biographical anamnesis*, in an attempt to objectify the psychiatric method, but he was fully aware that he was still using a method with a large subjective error. As a result of this largely psychiatric approach, the first communications of the research group offered little more than hypotheses about psychosomatic relationships in ulcerative colitis,

* Part of the work on which this paper is based was carried out with support of the Rockefeller Foundation.

peptic ulcer, bronchial asthma, hypertension etc. (2) (3). These hypotheses were perhaps formulated in more simple language coming from
a department of medicine, but they were fundamentally not different
from the hypotheses of Murray, Alexander, Flanders Dunbar and
others.

In this state of affairs two steps were taken which subsequently
proved to be a real help in the building up of a more systematic
methodology for psychosomatic research.

Psychological Studies

The first step came through the work of the psychologist BAREN-
DREGT, who pointed out that many psychological tests especially those
that require a subjective interpretation by the psychologist, are suffering from the same drawback as the psychiatric method itself, namely
a high and unknown degree of subjectivity. Against this the following
principle was adopted:

We divided our psychiatrical hypotheses into those which we
termed fruitful and (at least for the time being), not fruitful. Under
fruitful we understand a hypothesis which

1) is formulated in terms that can be understood and used by
workers from different fields, and

2) allows the hypothesis to be tested by the application of a method,
independent of the one by which it was arrived at. By this we meant
that a psychiatric hypothesis, to be fruitful, would have to lend itself
to be tested either by an independent psychological or a physiological
method, and vice versa.

It was in the testing of these fruitful hypotheses by independent
and validated tests that the psychologist found his main task.

Of the work which was done along those lines we mention
BARENDREGT's testing of the hypothesis of the psychosomatic etiology
of some disorders. In some of their earlier papers BASTIAANS and the
author had formulated the hypothesis that psychosomatic patients
were actually neurotics, who differed from the "openly complaining"
psychoneurotic patients proper by a strong tendency to inhibit the
neurotic behaviour patterns like compulsions complaining about
anxiety, crying, shouting, asking for help or putting excessive demand
on the doctors' time and patience. BARENDREGT deduced from this
hypothesis that if a number of psychosomatic patients from the department of medicine (and he chose for this purpose patients with

peptic ulcer and asthma), a number of psychoneurotic individuals from the department of psychiatry, and a healthy control group were given the MAUDSLEY test for neuroticism, there should be no significant statistical difference between the neuroticism score of the psychosomatic and the psychoneurotic patients, who would however both differ significantly from the score of the normals. On the other hand, when the same three groups were given a test for "sociability" it was predicted that the psychosomatic patients – because of their strong tendency to behave like normals – would not significantly differ from the healthy group, whereas the other group would. (For this last test a modification of EYSENCK's test for extraversion-intraversion was chosen.) The results confirmed all predictions with a high degree of statistical significance, and thus a psychiatric hypothesis based on biographical anamnesis and on a few psychoanalysed cases was supported (4).

It is obvious that a large field opens up here for clinical psychology in which this science (provided it can make its validated methods truly independent) can play a large role by putting our knowledge about man's mental processes in health or disease on a scientifically firmer basis, by supporting some psychiatric hypotheses and by not supporting, or rejecting others.

Physiological Studies

The second important contribution towards an objectivization of our researches came from the contact with HAROLD G. WOLFF, STEWART WOLF and their group in New York. Their work on Tom, the man with the gastric fistula, demonstrated that the stomach reacted to emotional stresses in a similar way as it did to local chemical and physical stimulation (5). This work however, was not only important by providing valuable support for the hypothesis of the psychogenic etiology of peptic ulcer, it meant also a tremendous step ahead in the methodology of psychosomatic research in general. WOLFF's method was based on the assumption that a hypothesis about the psychogenicity of a disease can be supported by physiological observations, if the reproduction of an emotional situation under controlled laboratory circumstances, produces similar bodily changes in the acute experiment as are chronically present in the diseased individual.

This physiological approach to the study of psychosomatic disorders has already borne rich fruits. During the following years WOLFF and his associates systematically applied the method to the study of the behaviour of the colon, the mucous membrane of the nose, the urinary bladder, the blood pressure and the blood sugar and ketone bodies, under the influence of experimentally induced emotional conflicts (6). In Amsterdam VAN DER VALK has similarly studied by continuous registration the behaviour of the electrical resistance of the skin, the sweat secretion, the skin temperature, the blood pressure, and of some other variables during emotional interviews and during what we designated as experimental self-control. This was achieved by bringing the individual into for him unknown surroundings (the laboratory) and there asking him not to speak and not to move while the physiological registrations were carried out (7) (8).

In another study carried out with DEKKER, a situation was reproduced in the laboratory which, according to the patient's history, had induced asthmatic attacks in him. In this way it was shown that asthmatic attacks can occur in situations which have a stressful meaning to the patient and where allergic influences could be excluded with practically complete certainty (9).

The physiological method, however, is not only a valuable means for putting certain psychiatric hypotheses to the test. It enables us to study the physiology of emotion as such and to deduce from this study physiological hypotheses. Thus HAROLD WOLFF's and our group independently, formulated the hypothesis that many so-called psychosomatic disorders are the result of reaction patterns like a rise in blood pressure, in blood sugar, in secretion of gastric juice, in intestinal motility, etc. which are regularly observed in normal individuals and therefore must be regarded as belonging to the natural behaviour of the organism in certain situations. These, in themselves normal patterns however, become disease-producing mechanisms when they occur in abnormal duration and intensity. This hypothesis has prompted further research into the question why some individuals, even if they are "qualitatively" normal, react in this quantitatively exaggerated way (6) (10) (11) (12).

Animal Studies

The clinical investigator, often derives great benefit for the elucidation of human disease from the study of animals. Animals can be bred in such a way that they become genetically almost identical, they are available in large numbers, and the investigator is less limited in the scope of his experimentation than in the case of human individuals where the ethical code of his profession forbids him to carry out an experiment which might do harm to the wellbeing of a patient. It is obvious therefore, that much useful knowledge could be obtained if we could produce and study psychosomatic disorders in animals. Two factors have held back progress in this field until recently. The first factor was the attitude of many psychiatrists that the human psyche is a unique phenomenon, which is fundamentally different from what is studied in so-called animal "psychology", so that results obtained in animals will never be applicable to the understanding of the psyche of man. The second objection maintained that it would never be possible to produce in animals the same complicated feelings of rivalry, humiliation, love loss, etc. that seem to play a role in the etiology of some psychosomatic disorders in man.

As far as the first objection goes, we seem to be dealing with a preconceived axioma rather than with an objective statement of fact. Even if one does not deny that religious experience, rational reasoning and linguistic expression are specifically human, it would be hard to prove that higher organised animals, although they cannot experience religion and cannot express themselves in language, are also unable to experience something comparable to certain of the more simple human feeling states. The reaction of animals following frustration in their food seeking, territorial or sexual behaviour is often strikingly similar to that of man. Thus for the pragmatic approach of the investigator, there is no reason why he should not at least try to use animals for psychosomatic ("neuro-visceral") studies. As far as the second objection goes, it is of course, obvious that one has to choose an environmental situation like that which has been supposed to be psychogenic in humans. For this purpose we have now two ways at our disposal.

A first approach is furnished by an increasing number of observations that animals which have been rendered experimentally neurotic by the technique developed by PAVLOV in dogs and which has been applied succesfully by MASSERMAN to cats and monkeys (13) not only show neurotic behaviour patterns like apathy, or unexpected and inadequate flight or fight reactions, but also exhibit disturbances in the autonomic sphere like food refusal, involuntary micturition or defecation, vomiting, tachycardia, and disturbances of respiration, which like in the dog NICKY, described by GANTT (14), are very similar to asthma. NOELPP and NOELPP (15) (16) have produced asthma-like attacks in guinea pigs by conditioning in a way very much resembling DEKKER's experiments in humans (18). Consequent application of these techniques might yield further interesting results, as it has already done in the elucidation of the "pure" neuroses.

Another experimental approach is based on the observations of the ethologists, that frustrations occur regularly in the life of almost every animal living in its natural surroundings. In the case of animals living, like man, in social groups, these frustrations are most often caused by conflicts with other members of the group. The animals can react to these frustrations by outwardly directed neuromuscular behaviour like fight or flight; occasionally neurotic patterns seem to appear but more often we observe patterns of so-called displacement. Up till now the ethologists have been mostly interested in the outwardly visible reaction patterns of their subjects, so that their studies of behaviour have been mostly restricted to the visible movements of the animal. However, as pointed out elsewhere (19), if one defines ethology as the study of the behaviour of the organism as a whole, there is no reason to exclude changes in movement of smooth musculature, of heart and blood vessel function, or of glandular secretion from these studies. Thus it has been shown in an interesting study that if new wild rats are introduced into an established colony they are attacked by the most aggressive male member of the group and almost always die as a result. The interesting finding in this connection was that the animal hardly ever dies from outwardly visible wounds, but from a state of exhaustion whiah may have its substrate in a depletion of the adrenal cortex of lipid material (20). We may also refer here to SCHUNK's work who has shown an increase in blood pressure leading to hypertrophy of the left ventricle in cats that were regularly exposed to barking dogs, without being able to flee or fight (21) (22). We have described elsewhere vomiting in female dogs as a result of conflicting emotions serving as a useful purpose for the feeding of the young (23). Lately, we have observed abortion in pregnant hamsters that were kept with so many in a small cage that there was no opportunity for them to build a nest. Thus, the study of naturally or experimentally induced frustrations in animals seems to offer an independant approach to the experimental study of psychosomatic disturbances.

Sociological Studies

If we return to the concept that psychosomatic disturbances are exaggerations of in essence normal patterns, which all individuals exhibit in reaction to frustration in their interhuman contact, another independent method of approach becomes possible, viz. by the application of sociological studies. Modern sociology is largely based on the concept that the behaviour of individuals in groups is determined by laws which can be deduced from systematic observations. Social behaviour can be measured; it can be subjected to a test by predicting the behaviour of a group under certain circumstances. The most important research tool for the sociologist therefore is the statistical evaluation of measurable phenomena, observed in comparable groups. In modern psychiatry this sociological-statistical approach is already in extensive use. That psychosomatic medicine can also derive benefit from the application of sociological methods is, amongst others, indicated by the fact that the prevalence of many of these disorders varies so markedly in different countries and even among different social groups within the same population. Thus ulcer of the stomach and duodenum was shown by KOUWENAAR in Indonesia to be fairly common among a group of Europeans and Chinese but to be practically absent in the Javanese (24). The prevalence of ulcer also differed markedly among the workers of different branches of industry in Greater London as established by AVERY JONES and DOLL (25) and by VERTIN, VAN ALPHEN DE VEER and their associates (26) among the workers of the Philips factory in Holland. The possibility that nutritional or "constitutional" factors are responsible for these differences cannot be excluded. However, it is equally possible (and indeed this was admitted by the patients themselves), that the strains and stresses associated with their work situation may have contributed to the origin of the ulcers in one group more than in another. VON UEXKÜLL ET AL, have also drawn attention to certain interhuman factors in the etiology of peptic ulcer (27). We might derive interesting knowledge if the sociologists could elucidate more about the exact nature of the pertinent strains and stresses.

Another example may be taken from a study of the psychogenic factors contributing to the causation of coronary thrombosis. Based on clinical observations and a number of biographies, we formulated a hypothesis which included, amongst others, that one of the precipitating events in this disease could be a marital conflict in which the patient felt disappointed and ununderstood by his marriage partner who, instead of giving him the submissive love which he expected, confronted him with dominance, indifference, nagging or preference for others. In many cases this conflict was felt as a situation of love loss and frustration.

At first sight it seems as if such a purely psychiatric formulation does not lend itself to be tested either by a physiological or even by a psychological independent method. However, we deduced from this hypothesis the prediction that such a situation must have occurred significantly more frequently in the lives of divorced than of married men, whereas it might also be anticipated that the love loss caused by the death of a marriage partner will be experienced in a similar way. We therefore predicted that if mortality and morbidity figures for coronary occlusion would show a higher incidence among divorced than among married men of the same age group, the hypothesis would be supported, thus using a sociological method, viz., biostatistics, to test a psychiatric hypothesis. Indeed it was found that in the American mortality statistics, there was a great excess of mortality of coronary occlusion among divorced men who had in all age groups more than 1.5 times as many deaths as the married men; also among the widowers there was a considerable excess (28).

Controlled Therapeutic Trials

If the concept is correct that certain somatic disorders have a psychogenic etiology, it can be expected that methods of psychotherapy, if properly chosen and applied, must have a therapeutic effect in these conditions. Here again, is a fruitful testable prediction. Unfortunately, whereas the literature abounds with reports on the reputedly successful psychotherapy of patients with psychosomatic disorders, only very few of these relate to properly controlled studies.

A few examples may be given. GROEN and BASTIAANS (29), GRACE and WOLF (30) and PAULLEY (31) have reported on the treatment of series of patients with ulcerative colitis with psychotherapy. They had no control groups so that they had to compare their results with the figures from the literature on patients with ulcerative colitis treated by medical and surgical means. They concluded that the effect of psychotherapy was about the same as claimed for medical and surgical treatment and suggested that this indicated that medical and surgical methods of treatment might work through their concomitant psychological influence. It is obvious that the lack of a comparable control group makes these conclusions tentative rather than conclusive.

SELTZ and his associates (32) have compared the results in two groups of ulcer patients, one being treated by conventional methods of bed rest and diet, the other by group psychotherapy. The results were not worse and even somewhat better in the group treated with psychotherapy.

Two investigations have recently been carried out on the effect of group therapy on bronchial asthma. SCLARE and CROCKET (33) in Glasgow reported no significant difference in improvement of the asthmatic symptomatology between sixteen female patients under group psychotherapy and those from the control groups. However in GROEN and PELSER's therapeutic experiment a statistically significant difference between the treated and the control group was noted (34).

As a last example a case of severe malignant hypertension may be quoted, described by GROEN, VAN DER VALK and BASTIAANS. This patient improved to an extent of almost complete clinical cure after frontal leucotomy and psychotherapy (35). Although this observation concerns only one case, the fact that a patient who, according to all experience, should have been dead within one or two years, is healthy and at work 10 years after the operation, supports the hypothesis that the disease is of central nervous origin.

From these examples it may be clear how much there still can be done in this direction. Up till now the psychosomatic hypotheses have received relatively little support from the results of psychotherapy, not so much because psychotherapy has not been tried in these cases but because the psychotherapy was not planned for this purpose. It is hoped that those investigators who occupy themselves with the psycho-therapy of psychosomatic disorders will realize more than so far that their work can serve a double purpose: the treatment or support of patients and the scientific testing of a theory. The use of tranquilizing or psychomimetic drugs in psychosomatic patients offers similar possibilities.

Summary

The author, in discussing the methodology of psychosomatic research advocates the formulation of fruitful hypotheses which lend themselves to be tested by independent validated methods. As such he reviews the contribution of psychiatrical, psychological, physio-logical, experimental biological and sociological methods of investi-gation and the evaluation of the results of properly controlled psycho-therapeutic trials.

Bibliography

1. GROEN, J.: Origin and development of the psychosomatic researchgroup in the Wilhelmina Gasthuis. J. Psychosom. Res. *2*: 82 (1957).
2. GROEN, J.: Publications from the Psychosomatic Research Unit, Amsterdam. J. Psychosom. Res. *2*: 147 (1957).
3. GROEN, J.: Emotional factors in the etiology of internal diseases. J. Mt. Sinai Hosp. *18*: 71 (1951).
4. BARENDREGT, J.T.: Lijders aan psychosomatische kwalen als sociaal aangepaste neurotici. Ned. T. v. Geneesk. *102*: 2045 (1958).
5. WOLFF, H.G. and WOLF, S.: Human gastric function (Oxford University Press, New York, 1943).
6. WOLFF, H.G. ET AL.: Life Stress and Bodily Disease. Proc. of the 29th Annual Meeting of the Ass. for Research in Nerv. Ment. (Diss., 1950).
7. VAN DER VALK, J.M. and GROEN, J.: Electrical resistance of the Skin during induced emotional stress. Psychosom. Med. *12*: 303 (1950).
8. VAN DER VALK, J.M.: De electrische huidweerstand (Diss., Amsterdam 1958).
9. DEKKER, E., and GROEN, J.: Reproducible psychogenic attacks of asthma. J. Psychosom. Res. *1*: 58 (1956).
10. WOLFF, H.G.: Stress and Disease (Thomas, Springfield 1951)
11. GROEN, J.; PRICK, J.J.G., en FABER, H.: Psychosomatiek, Geneeskunde en Menschbeschouwing (Scheltema & Holkema, Amsterdam 1953).
12. GROEN, J.; PRICK, J.J.G., en FABER, H.: Psychosomatic disturbances as a form of substituted behaviour. J. Psychosom. Res. *2*: 85 (1957).
13. MASSERMANN, J.H., and PECHTEL, C.: Neurosis in monkeys. Annals N. York Academy Sciences *56*: 253 (1953).
14. GANTT, W.H.: Experimental Basis for Neurotic Behaviour (Hoeber, New York 1944).
15. NOELPP, B., and NOELPP-ESCHEN LAGEN, I.: Die Rolle bedingter Reflexe beim Asthma Bronchiale. Helv. Med. Acta *18*: 142 (1951).
16. NOELPP, B., and NOELPP-ESCHEN LAGEN, I.: Das experimentelle Asthma bronchische des Meerschweinchens. Int. Arch. Allergy *2*: 308, 321 (1952). Ibid. *3*: 108, 207 (1952).
17. DEKKER, E.; PELSER, H.E. and GROEN, J.: Conditionning as a cause of asthmatic attacks. J. Psychosom. Res. *2*: 97 (1957).
18. GROEN, J.: The physiological basis of psychosomatic disturbances. Acta Physiol. Pharmacol. Neerl. *7*: 58 (1958).
19. BARNETT, S.A.: Physiological effect of "Social Stress" in wild rats—The adrenal cortex. J. Psychosom. Res. *3*: 1 (1958).
20. SCHUNK, J.: Emotionelle Faktoren in der Pathogenese des essentiellen Hochdrucks. Z. Klin. Med. *152*: 251 (1954).
21. SCHUNK, J.: Nierenfunktion und Psyche. Z. Psychosom. Med. *2*: 255 (1955).
22. GROEN, J.: De mens als psychosomatische totaliteit van reactiepatronen. Ned. T. Psychol. *10*: 187 (1955).
23. KOUWENAER, C.: Ulcus ventriculi et duodeni onder verschillende bevolkingsgroepen in Nederlandsch Oost Indië. Ned. T. v. Geneesk. *82*: 2042 (1938).
24. DOLL, R., and AVERY JONES, F.: Peptic Ulcer in Industry. Medical Research Council. Spec. Report Series No. 276, London 1951.

25. VERTIN, C.: Ulcus ventriculi et duodeni onder arbeiders (Diss., Groningen, 1954).
26. PFLANZ, M.; ROSENSTEIN, E., and VON UEXKÜLL, TH.: Socio psychological aspects of peptic ulcer. J. Psychosom. Res. *1*: 21 (1956).
27. PERETZ, M., and GROEN, J.: Marital status and disease (in preparation).
28. GROEN, J., and BASTIAANS, J.: Psychotherapy of Ulcerative colitis. Gastroenterology *17*: 344 (1951).
29. GRACE, W.J.; WOLF, S., and WOLFF, H.G.: The human colon (Hoeber, New York 1951).
30. PAULLEY, J.W.: Psychotherapy of Ulcerative colitis. Lancet *2*: 215 (1956).
31. ZETZEL, L, and SLESNICK, S.: Results of Group psychotherapy in patients with peptic ulcer. Gastroenterology *3*: 47 (1944), id. *14*: 364 (1950).
32. SCLARC, A.B.,en CROCKET, J.A.: Group psychotherapy in bronchial asthma. J. Psychosom. Res. *2*: 157 (1957).
33. GROEN, J., and PELSER, H.E.: Ervaringen en resultaten van groepspsychotherapie bij asthma bronchiale. Ned. T. v. Geneesk. *103*: 65 (1959).
34. GROEN, J.; VAN DER VALK, J.M., and BASTIAANS, J.: A case of malignant hypertension treated with prefrontal leucotomy and psychotherapy. J. Psychosom. Res. *2*: 120 (1957).

Author's address: PROF. DR. J.J. GROEN, Department of Medicine A, Hebrew University Hadassah Medical School and Hospital, *Jerusalem* (Israel).

Methodological Considerations on Psychosomatic Research

F. ASKEVOLD, Oslo

Every definition within the sphere of medicine which is concerned with diagnosis and limitations of the pictures of illnesses, is based on abstractions from collocation of symptoms and thus a product of subjective interpretation. It has no existence per se independent of the human thought. The general world-wide agreement on diagnosis and description of symptoms must therefore be based upon a mutuality in thinking. This interindividual agreement of thinking originates in generally accepted principles within the natural sciences-principles which are accepted across the borders of differences in other fields—cultural, socio-economic, in ways of living and in ways of thinking. It is then quite natural that when other fields of experience which are more coloured by tradition and way of living—are taken into consideration with regard to medicine—differences in opinion are more apt to occur.

The so-called psychosomatic medicine is an example of a concep where the definitions are determined by a wider variety of fields of experience than the more traditional medicine which is fixed in the thinking lines of the natural sciences. Within psychosomatic medicine one will find concepts with references to different, often mutually quite independent, scientific orientations.

In order to simplify matters I will consider psycho-somatic medicine from two main aspects which are rather dominating today. One regards theory where I want to present a point of view and the other is a proposal for research.

The point of view—the rediscovering and defining of the holistic concept—namely that it is the total human being who is ill, not a part of him, has given impetus to the beginning of a change in our attitude at the hospital bedside, in the general doctor-patient relationship, and in humanizing the laboratory-fixed and over-specialized medicine today.

This change is certainly very valuable, but in its consequences all medicine thus becomes psychosomatic. This appears as a correct statement but on the other hand it makes the field so vast that it is impossible to handle, at least with the small training in holistic thinking which we have at present.

As a trend of research, psychosomatic medicine today is to a certain extent, clouded by a conglomerate of hypotheses and theories—often incompatible—and coloured by the fact that these theories belong to other fields, and which are then applied to psychosomatic medicine.

It seems as though it has often been considered more important to try to make psychosomatic medicine correspond to one existing theory or an other, rather than to develope new theories of its own. In my opinion there are at least two reasons for this—one is the lack of a specified starting point regarding basic consepts—and the other the lack of adequate research methods.

As an attempt to limit the field with which we have to deal it is useful to start with what I consider as not belonging to psychosomatic medicine proper, as an research area. I hope you will agree that the study of the individual's adjustment to an illness, an interesting problem in itself, belongs rather to the field of psychology. When we turn to the problem of functional and structural changes, their classification as diseases and the influence of psychic processes on the development and course of disease, the opinions are more controversial.

Some will consider functional disturbances, without any evidence of structural alterations, as neurotic manifestations. Other will look upon them as organic components of emotional reactions and still other see the functional disturbances as forerunners to organic disease, without having any real evidence to bridge the gap between the functional disturbance and the structural change classifing the latter as disease with eventual secondary changes in function. In my opinion psychosomatic disorders are something different from a neurotic manifestation, even if we today have few possibilities of conceptualizing this difference.

The attempts of limiting the field in my opinion only have a practical and no principal purpose. If we take our starting point in a rather narrow area the opportunities of obtaining better defined concepts are increased.

In accordance with this line I propose that we regard the well defined diseases with objective signs of structural changes as our starting point and then try to study the role of the psychic processes in the development and course of these diseases.

The basic question which then remains may thus be formulated: Can psychic processes cause structural alterations in the body tissues resulting in what we up till now in somatic medical terms have called illness?

The methods used in psychosomatic research fall into 6 main trends: Clinical, physiological, genetical, epidemiological, more or less combined psychological and philosophical.

Clinical publications, which consist mostly of well-prepared case reports, have the defect that they, based on simultaneous occurence of symptom-formation and the traumatic situation, regard the basic question as having been answered in the affirmative—and on this postulate build a series of theories and hypotheses, again based upon the theoretical orientation of the investigator. A few examples of this kind are: DUNBAR's (1948) theory on flight-fight reaction in relation to personality profiles, ALEXANDER's (1952) on reception-expulsion as basic conflict and with reaction formation either located as con-

version in the sensoro-motoric area or phenotypical in the autonomous
nervous system, WISDOM's (1957) theory on internalization of tactile
and kinastethic sensations which can not be experienced as visual
images, and projection of guilt, and KARDINER's (1941) frustrated
action-syndrome.

I regard such theories as highly valuable and even very probable,
but they all lack scientific validity as answers to the basic question. The
neurophysiological theories based upon SELYES (1946) general adaptation syndrome, especially WOLFF's (1952) extensive work, or the
PAVLOVIAN concept of conditioned reflexes, stick more to the experimental methods, but I am tempted to cite the Danish PROFESSOR
JÖRGENSEN: "BOHR has, for example, mentioned the fact that a
really exhaustive analysis of a live organism must result in the death
of the organism, so that an atomic or microphysical description of
such an organism seems to be outside the realms of possibility; it
seems then to be impossible to draw a sharp line between the micro-
physical elements of a live organism and those belonging to its
surroundings, its exterior and interior environment—this, of course,
makes it impossible to arrive at a microphysical definition of the
concept, an animate being. It would be absurd to attribute to the
parts features that can only be observed and defined as features of the
whole...

We are confronted with a fundamental limit to biological analysis, and we should have to use either a macro-physical biological
description or a micro-physical physio-chemical description, but we
should, in principle, be precluded from combining these descriptions
to constitute a physico-chemical theory of vital phenomena."

With regard to the physiological methods, the research situation
itself influences that which is to be observed and the basic question
cannot be *answered* with the methods available.

Genetic investigations are almost totally lacking but newer
epidemiological ones, such as HINKLE's (1957) seem to be very
promising. Here we meet the concept of stress in the frame of the
individual's perception and related to his conscience. This field—
which is more psychological is, in this respect, only on the threshold
of elucidating the concept which may lead to a more holistic vew of
the psychosomatic disorders. It is worth noting that even this word
includes exactly the dichotomy which we try to avoid: There are no
pure somatic or psychic processes.—The central point is the brain
and every thought and every somatic reaction have, as their basis,

neurophysiological reactions. What we lack are adequate methods for measuring and, perhaps even still more pertinent at the moment, well-defined concepts regarding consciousness and perceptive psychology.

It seems to follow from what I have said above as if the basic question is a too ambitious one to answer with the methods at hand. We have to develop new methods, which is a long-lasting and arduous enterprise. In the meantime it would perhaps be advantageous to commit ourselves to a simpler and less pretentious task.

It is often said by the adherents of psychosomatic medicine that the patients with structural, organic diseases will profit by the simultaneous application of psychological and somatic methods in the investigation and treatment of the disease. When the problem is stated in this way it becomes easier to handle scientifically. I will therefore consider this statement as my starting point.

There are allready a vast number of publications on this matter, but very few are done as controlled experiments. Such studies are also difficult to compare as they are formulated according to the different orientations of the investigators and are mostly limited to a small number of patients.

A research which could avoid these pitfalls ought to be based on large numbers of patients—which are more than difficult to obtain. This is especially the case with regard to therapy, because to be complete it must include time-consuming psychoanalysis.

Furthermore, it must be founded on precise criteria both in sampling, in investigations and in methods of treatment. It is impossible to satisfy such ideal claims, especially in research on humans but it ought to be possible to come nearer than we are at the moment. I have, therefore, in the following, dared to sketch out a plan of research. It may, at first glance, seem utopic but I hope that it will be discussed seriously because I believe that it should be possible to carry it through. The basic principles are correct but the project is a big task, perhaps too big.

One single center, occupied with psychosomatic medicine, will, for many reasons, not be able to give an answer which is complete. My idea is to do this in cooperation with different centers in different countries. By this we would not only be able to give a more complete answer but we would also obtain possibilities of evaluating influences from the differences in cultural aspects.

This is a side line, but also an example of the additional results which would be made available by such a study. I return to my sketch of the practical planning.

In each of the centers the team should consist of internists, psychiatrists, psychologists, psychoanalysts, physiologists and sociologists. The first step would be to agree on general criteria for the sampling and for the further procedure, and to come to conclusively defined variables to be used.

In order to clarify the matter I will put forward the further procedure as a concrete plan. If one certain disease is chosen as a starting point—e.g. duodenal ulcer—one must agree on the somatic criteria such as length of history of illness, hæmatemesis or not, number of medical cures and exclude any complicating diseases. For example, patients with radiologically observable duodenal ulcer, with a history of illness of 3–5 years duration without hæmatemesis, and who previously have had 2 medical cures—and so on. Alcoholic patients are excluded.

Within this group are then chosen one sex, and a certain interval of age, and this composes the group, to be investigated unless we wish to make it even more homogenous by including only a certain socio-economic and vocational level.

The group is studied from as many angles as one considers desirable—somatic; physiological, constitutional, eugenic and psychological; behavioural, experiential and intrapsychic.

Especially in this field it is pertinent to reach mutual agreement on the criteria to be used and a lot of preliminary work is necessary, with regard to choice of tests and concepts of personality factors for example.

When the group has gone through all the investigations it should again be divided at random into different groups—one of which is to be treated solely by the internist and serve as the somatic control group. The internist on the team ought, perhaps, to be a stubborn somatist.

The other different groups would undergo, different types of psychotherapy—for example, one orthodox psychoanalysis, another modified analytical therapy, and again another group-psychotherapy.

As a sideline we will then be able to do a comparative study of different therapies. The therapies must be well defined and conscientious therapy reports must be given. The patients have to undergo a somatic control once a year and a total investigation at the end of the project, which will last perhaps 5 years or more.

Further details will have to be considered by those interested in the project. The financial side is a big problem but it should be possible to solve it if enough people are interested and willing to go in for the project and to go through with it, especially with regard to the common principles and definition of variables.

From what I previously have said it might seem as if I look upon all earlier psychosomatic research as beeing without scientific value.

This is by no means my intention. I have been concerned with the clinical field, where I find the big obstacle seem to be the lack of comparability. My statements have not been concerned with the experimental research. My aim has been not to discuss the theories but more to emphasize on our present methods and which in my opinion do not fulfil strict scientific requirements. On this basis I have dared to propose a research project with a more modest aim than the final answering of the basic question. I feel that if the project could be effectuated it might be a step forward in the direction of a better understanding of the psychosomatic processes and also of testing the validity of existing theories.

Bibliography

ALEXANDER, F.: Psychosomatic Medicine (Allen & Unwin, London 1952).

DUNBAR, F.: Psychosomatic Diagnosis. 4th ed. (Paul B. Hoeber Inc., New York 1948).

HINKLE, L.E., JR.; PLUMMER, N. ET AL.: Studies in Human Ecology. Amer. J. Psychiat. *114*: 212–220 (1957).

JORGENSEN, J., cit. GEERT-JORGENSEN: On the Concepts Psychogenesis and Psychosomatics. Acta psychiat. scand. Suppl. *108*: 135–149 (1957).

KARDINER, A.: The traumatic neuroses of war. Psychosom. Med. Monogr. Suppl. *1*: 169–171 (1941).

SELYE, H.: The general adaptation syndrome and the diseases of adaptation. J. clin. Endocrin. *6*: 117–230 (1946).

WISDOM, J.: On mechanisms and purpose in psychosomatic disorder. Paper read to the British Psycho-analytical Society, London 1957 (unpublished).

WOLFF, H.G.: Stress and disease (Thomas, Springfield 1952).

Author's address: DR. F. ASKEVOLD, Ulleval Sykehus, *Oslo* (Norway).

The Place of Animal Psychology
in the Development of Psychosomatic Research

P. L. Broadhurst, London

Two main purposes will be evident in this paper. The first is to assess the relevance to our understanding of psychosomatic problems of the work done on experimental neuroses in animals, and the second is to suggest the most fruitful lines of approach at present available to us in advancing towards a solution of such problems.

The work on experimental neuroses in animals is doubtless familiar to you, and was pioneered by Pavlov in Russia before the first world war, though it did not become widely known in the West until the 1920's (1). It was then actively taken up in America. If I draw more heavily for examples upon this later American work, it is principally because the language difficulty with the earlier work makes it necessary to place reliance upon reviews and abstracts, which is not a satisfactory substitute for studying the original research data.

The first important point to be decided is whether or not it is possible to regard the disturbed behaviour produced by the Pavlovian conditioning procedure as truly abnormal. This depends very largely on the view that one adopts regarding human abnormality. Firstly, there is the older view of human neurosis (and psychosis, for that matter) as disease entities, qualitatively different from the normal, or secondly, one may prefer to regard the abnormal as the extreme manifestation of behaviour on a continuum, or set of continua, which range from the normal through to the extremes we term abnormal. Let us consider the first view. In this case it is clearly necessary to have some criterion by which to decide if the behaviour observed in the animal is really a "neurosis", and so having relevance to our understanding of similar behaviour in humans. Unfortunately, this is difficult to do in the absence of speech in the animal. Most comparative work using animals has to face a similar problem of interpretation, and it is especially difficult in this case, for it is evident that what a patient reports plays a large part in the psychiatrist's diagnosis of neurotic disorders. No doubt it would be possible to make a diagnosis of neurosis without communicating with the patient through the medium of language, though I think that most psychiatrists would probably prefer not to do so. Yet this is exactly what has been attempted in the cases of so-called abnormal behaviour in animals. Worse than that, the interpretation is frequently made on subjective grounds, dependent on the personal opinion of the experimenter concerned—an essentially unscientific procedure.

There is, however, a way out of this difficulty, which has been pointed out by HEBB (2). He has defined human neurosis in behavioural terms—that is, without recourse to language. The criteria of human neurosis he arrived at can then be applied to animal behaviour. In HEBB's view, there are at least six necessary conditions to be fulfilled before abnormal behaviour observed in humans, and consequently in animals, can properly be described as neurosis. Briefly, they are as follows. The behaviour must be abnormal in both of the two senses of the word. That is, not only must it be abnormal in the sense of being undesirable from a biological point of view, either for the individual or for the species, but it must also be abnormal in the sense of being statistically rare. It must be persistent, that is, chronic and not limited to one or two occasions, and it must be generalised, that is, seen in different ways and especially in different situations. In addition, it must involve emotional arousal of one sort or another, and, finally, and obviously, it must not have a definite physical causation. We have in HEBB's formulation a powerful tool to assist in assessing the validity of the claims of the work on experimental neurosis to represent an animal equivalent of human neurosis.

How does the large body of American work stand up to such an assessment? For the purposes of a recent review (3), the available literature was examined in the light of HEBB's criteria, and the conclusion was reached that no case of experimental neurosis reported in the literature can be unequivocally accepted as such. This may appear somewhat harsh, but is, it seems, inescapable. Also it is important to make the point that the search for the experimental neurosis has not yielded, and probably will never yield, a solution to problems in the human sphere, partly because of the intractability of these problems themselves, and partly because it is clear that we do not have, in the cases of experimental neurosis reported, the animal analogue of the human disorder.

What, then, are we left with as a result of all this work? Noteworthy, for our present purposes are some of the observations of three groups of workers, headed by LIDDELL (4), GANTT (5), and MASSERMAN (6) who worked on the sheep, the dog and the cat respectively. LIDDELL, one of the pioneers of the conditioning methology in the United States, reports disorders of respiration and cardiac functioning in some of his so-called neurotic sheep. The disturbed breathing was especially associated with the laboratory, and so may well have been learned as a conditioned response to the stimuli associated with the laboratory setting. In any case the observations are not sufficiently precise to be sure of the etiology. A curious inversion of the T wave was observed on the cardiogram of some sheep, but, since it was observed in sheep designated normal as well as neurotic, the significance of this finding is hard to assess.

GANTT (5) reports more convincing examples of possible psychosomatic disorder, especially in his admirable long-term study of the dog "Nick". The striking functional disturbances found in this animal are well known—they involved the respiratory and the urinogenital system. Nick is reported as habitually adopting a loud and raucous breathing when being brought to the laboratory for experimentation and also whenever he encountered people associated with the experimental work, even away from the laboratory. Here again it is more than probable that what we are dealing with is a conditioned emotional reaction. The whole experimental procedure gave rise to fear responses which included disturbed breathing, these generalised to the experimental setting, including the people concerned in it, which thus became conditioned stimuli for it. The other disturbance shown by Nick is more interesting. He showed pollakuria in and near the experimental room, and sexual erection and even ejaculation in the conditioning harness. These phenomena have been widely cited as evidence of the generalisation of disturbances established by conditioned reflex procedures to involve systems other than those employed in the (in this case) alimentary response to an auditory signal. Further, the implication has been drawn that a psychological conflict engendered by the conditioning procedures has in some way spread and has emerged in seemingly anomalous sexual responses. But the following has not before been stressed, I believe. These signs did not arise spontaneously. They occurred after the introduction of a bitch in oestrus into the experimental situation for therapeutic purposes, following the earlier manifestations of experimental neurosis. The pollakuria and sexual erections noted in this dog may in fact have been conditioned responses to the experimental situation, the female acting as the original unconditioned stimulus giving rise to the normal innate responses of sexual excitement. It is worth noting that the transient abnormalities of sexual function GANTT reports in another dog followed attempts to develop actual sexual conditioned responses in the experimental setting.

MASSERMAN (6) developed apparent anorexia in his cats. His theoretical interpretation of abnormal behaviour need not concern us here except to note that the basis upon which he designed his experiments was to produce "conflict" between one drive and another. What he did was this. He trained hungry cats to respond to a sensory signal by opening a food box to obtain food. Then he subjected them to a noxious stimulus, a blast of air, or electric shock, just at the moment of feeding. Changes in behaviour resulted—the animals showed fear of the situation and of the experimenter, and refused to feed further—even to the point of starvation. But certain deficiencies in the design of his experiments make it impossible to draw any satisfactory conclusions from them. Thus WOLPE (7) repeated part of MASSERMAN's work using the essential control group which MASSERMAN had omitted—that is, he gave the cats the noxious stimulus alone, without any "conflict" between the fear motivation thus induced, and the hunger which, in MASSERMAN's animals, operated as well— and found that the same behaviour occurred. They refused to feed in the experimental box. It hardly needs to be said that a fear response to a threatening stimulus is not abnormal even when it is so strong as to prevent feeding, and it seems that here is yet another example of a conditioned emotional response being developed. In this case its effects were particularly seen in suppressing another activity, feeding.

What then are we to conclude from these examples of psychosomatic disorder in animals, culled from the literature on experimental neurosis? In each case it seems that, as far as the frequently imperfect design of the experiments and inadequate nature of most of the data allow, it is permissible to conclude that the behaviour observed was based on learned responses to some definite aspect of the experimental procedure, and certainly not involving abnormal reactions. How much better, then, to recognise this probability, and to set up one's experiments in such a way that enables these aspects to be quantified and controlled satisfactorily. To take MASSERMAN's work as an example: the conditioned emotional response (CER—8) can be studied by its effect on a learned feeding response, pressing a lever to obtain a food reward, usually using rats or monkeys as subjects. With this technique to study the CER, its growth, intensity, and the effect of drugs and other experimental procedures, can be observed in an absolutely objective and quantified way merely by seeing how much the bar pressing is decreased.

Let us now consider the second view of the contribution which animal psychology has to make to problems relating to psychosomatic research in humans. If we take the view previously referred to, that is, that in human neurotic behaviour we see the extreme manifestations of normal behaviour, and that such extremes may be regarded as the manifestation of faulty learned responses, determined in part by environmental conditions and in part by the individuals' inherited predisposition to such learning (9), then the potential contribution of the discipline of animal psychology, by way of carefully controlled laboratory experiments yielding quantitative data, is indeed considerable. The sort of experiments which may be valuable will not necessarily be concerned with the demonstration of overt signs of abnormality as such. For the reasons given above it is held that the search for complete animal analogues of human abnormalities of behaviour is likely to be fruitless, and is probably best avoided. Rather, such experimentation may be concerned with the study of one limited aspect of a psychosomatic function thought to be involved, in its extreme form, in human abnormal behaviour. As we have seen, the work on experimental neurosis already done is useless for this purpose primarily since the work was not orientated in this direction from the start, and secondly because much of it was neither adequately designed or quantified. Furthermore, with the advances in the field now available, the most promising approach seems to lie in the application of learning theory to human abnormal behaviour, especially to what EYSENCK (10) has called "behaviour therapy". From the time of PAVLOV onwards, much of modern learning theory has been elaborated on the basis of animal experiments, and there seems no reason to doubt that they will play their part in new applications and extensions. Many probably complementary approaches are available—the conditioned emotional response technique already mentioned, the experimental production of gastric ulcers in the monkey (11) and in the rat (12), and the study of emotional reactivity, also in the rat (13). However, some other work from our own Laboratory perhaps illustrates the point better. This has direct relevance to one example of the methods of behaviour therapy already elaborated, that which has been used in the treatment of tics in humans. These have been treated by making the patient practice the tic voluntarily under standard conditions, usually of massed practice, which favour the growth of what is termed in HULL's learning theory "conditioned inhibition". Under these favourable circumstances this conditioned inhibition may grow to such an extent that two things begin to happen. Firstly, the patient has difficulty in making the response voluntarily during the practice sessions, and secondly, the generalisation effect takes place and the frequency of the involuntary tics outside the therapeutic sessions begins to decrease, even to the point of disappearance. But our understanding of the theoretical construct "conditioned inhibition", which is regarded as an important element in this method, is not complete, and this is where animal experimentation helps, as may be seen in the work of KENDRICK (14). If you place a thirsty rat at one end of a simple straight runway with water at the other, the animal will soon learn to run to the water and drink. But it is possible to arrange such intense practice of this response on so many successive days that the rat no longer runs to the water, despite the fact that it is still thirsty and is not exhausted. It is thought that conditioned inhibition is operating in this situation also, and preventing the occurrence of the response, in the same way as in the patient practising a tic. In the laboratory and using animal subjects it is easier to control many of the relevant variables in a way which is not possible in the therapeutic situation, and to make systematic study of other variables which may influence the growth and the decay of the conditioned inhibition. It is in such ways as these, it is believed, that animal psychologists can make the maximum contribution to the development of psychosomatic research.

Bibliography

1. PAVLOV, I.P.: Lectures on conditioned reflexes: Vol. II. Conditioned reflexes and psychiatry (Lawrence and Wishart, London 1941).
2. HEBB, D.O.: Spontaneous neurosis in chimpanzees: theoretical relations with clinical and experimental phenomena. Psychosom. Med. 9: 3–16 (1947).
3. BROADHURST, P.L.: Abnormal animal behaviour. In: EYSENCK, H.J. (Ed.): Handbook of Abnormal Psychology. Pitman, London (in press).

4. ANDERSON, O.D., and PARMENTER, R.: A long-term study of the experimental neurosis in the sheep and dog. Psychosom. Med. Monogr. *2*: 3 and 4, 1–150 (1941).

5. GANTT, W.H.: Experimental basis for neurotic behaviour—origin and development of artifically produced disturbances of behaviour in dogs. Psychosom. Med. Monogr. *3*: 3 and 4, 1–211 (1944). Also published: Hoeber, New York 1944.

6. MASSERMAN, J.H.: Behavior and neurosis: an experimental psychoanalytic approach to psychobiologic principles (University Press, Chicago 1943).

7. WOLPE, J.: Experimental neurosis as learned behaviour. Brit. J. Psychol. *43*: 243–268 (1952).

8. BRADY, J.V., and HUNT, H.F.: An experimental approach to the analysis of emotional behavior. J. Psychol. *40*: 313–324 (1955).

9. BROADHURST, P.L.: Studies in psychogenetics: Applications of biometrical genetics to the inheritance of behaviour. In: EYSENCK, H.J. (Ed.): Experiments in Personality. Routledge & Kegan Paul, London (in press).

10. EYSENCK, H.J. (Ed.): Behaviour Therapy and the Neuroses. Pergamon Press, London (in press).

11. PORTER, R.W.; BRADY, J.V.; CONRAD, D.; MASON, J.W.; GALAMBOS, R., and RIOCH, D.McK.: Some experimental observations on gastrointestinal lesions in behaviorally conditioned monkeys. Psychosom. Med. *20*: 379–394 (1958).

12. SAWREY, W.L., and WEISZ, J.D.: An experimental method of producing gastric ulcers. J. comp. physiol. Psychol. *49*: 269–270 (1956).

13. BROADHURST, P.L.: Determinants of emotionality in the rat: I. Situational factors. Brit. J. Psychol. *48*: 1–12 (1957).

14. KENDRICK, D.C.: Inhibition with reinforcement (conditioned inhibition). J. exp. Psychol. *56*: 313–318 (1958).

Author's address: DR. P.L. BROADHURST, Institute of Psychiatry, Maudsley Hospital *London S.E. 5* (England).

About Methods for an Initial Psychosomatic Investigation of Clinical Syndromes
(Exemplified by a Research on the So-Called Idiopathic Hirsutism)

A. E. MEYER and D. v. ZERSSEN, Hamburg

First Part

D. v. ZERSSEN

The scientific value of any investigation and of the theories derived from it depends mainly on the methods used for collecting empirical data and for their theoretical interpretation. We shall point out here the methodological considerations that seem most important to us in the field of psychosomatic research and exemplify their application in a concrete study, namely the first steps of a psychosomatic approach to idiopathic hirsutism.

First of all, the subject of a study should be well-defined in terms common enough to make the results comparable with those of other investigations of the same subject. Precise diagnostic criteria have to be applied. If possible, they should be objective or even measurable.

The material studied may consist of individual cases or of statistical data from case-histories, health-statistics and the like. The advantage of case studies lies in the concreteness of their results, the disadvantage is the impossibility to draw general conclusions regarding the diagnostic category as a whole. The advantage of mere statistical studies lies in the survey one gains on correlations within the group under consideration in comparison to the normal population and/or other diagnostic groups. Here disadvantages arise from the impossibility to ascertain the causes of these correlations in general and the varying roles they play in the individual case. The most satisfactory way, therefore, seems to be a thorough investigation of a certain number of cases that—according to important variables—can be regarded as representative for all cases in the diagnostic category investigated; moreover the number must be great enough to obtain data for statistical analyses.

After the problem per se has been delineated the question about the investigator arises. As a single person can hardly survey the complex field of psychosomatic relations and be trained in the different physical and psychological techniques of investigation, usually a team of specialists has to be composed. It should contain clinicians and technical specialists in the somatic sector and psychiatrists, psychoanalysts and clinical psychologists—or at least one specialist of these kinds—in the psychological sphere.

The techniques employed in an initial approach must have been proved effective in previous investigations. Standardized methods should always be included to make data available for statistical analyses and an exact comparison with the results of control-studies.

As to the procedure of investigating the individual case, the application of the different techniques should be restricted to a short interval of time and relatively constant external conditions so as to minimize the influence of spontaneous development in and accidental external factors on the personality and his or her disease. This, usually, makes an inpatient-study inevitable.

Having gathered the empirical data, the results gained by different techniques should be evaluated separately. This allows a rating of their specific findings within the study and a comparison with the results of control-studies, in which the same or similar techniques might be used. The next step then would be the integration of all the findings. Hypotheses on the nature of connections between the findings have to be developed step by step from the empirical basis of the study. This means that the hypotheses should be restricted to what was actually investigated and not expanded on aspects for which there is insufficient data in the own material. They must, however, also take regard of what has already been found by others in the field of the study.

Let us turn to the example of a concrete study on idiopathic hirsutism and see how the principles of methodology were applied to it.

The subject was specified according to the well-known definition given by PRADER in LABHART's textbook on clinical endocrinology.

A comprehensive case-study was planned on as many cases as

could be gathered during half a year from the case-material of our (medical) clinic. A series of 42 cases covering the diagnostic criteria implied in the definition were found among the total number of patients studied at our clinic during the last 6 years. Out of this series we were able to collect a group of 15 volunteers for the study. Our sample could be demonstrated to be representative of the whole series in respect to most of the biological and social variables that could be drawn from the case-histories (such as age, educational level, marital status and so forth). The number of cases was great enough to allow statistical analyses of some of our findings.

The physical status of each patient was clarified by members of the clinical and technical staff of the clinic. Psychological examination was done by DR. MEYER as a psychoanalytically trained psychiatrist and myself as a clinical psychologist.

Physical examination included medical, gynecologic and anthropologic studies, x-ray-studies of the skeleton and biochemic assay of urinary steroids.

DR. MEYER explored the patients emphasizing biographical data and actual interpersonal dynamics during the interviews, and I gave a battery of tests. This consisted of psychometric measurements on the one hand (HAWIE = *H*amburg-*W*echsler *I*ntelligenztest für *E*rwachsene and questionnaires), which enabled us to compare our findings with normal standards; on the other hand projective techniques were employed to gain a deeper insight into the dynamic structure, the self-picture and the themes of fears and desires of the individual case (among others the picture-frustration-study, the Rorschach-test, drawing-tests and the TAT were used).

Each patient was examined physically in an inpatient-study of about 3 weeks length. During this period the patients were interviewed daily for at least one week and afterwards tested psychologically for usually the same length of time.

The results of every single examination and of every single technique were then figured out separately and only afterwards compared with each other.

DR. MEYER will tell you now about the process of integrating the different findings of the psychological part of this initial investigation and finally about the search for adequate hypotheses that seem to fit best the empirical data thus far obtained by us and others in this field.

Author's address: DR. D. v. ZERSSEN, II. Medizinische Universitätsklinik *Hamburg-Eppendorf* (Germany).

Second Part

A. E. MEYER

To exemplify the process of synopsis of data accumulated by the separate members of a psychosomatic research-team, I will give some illustrations.

Let me skip the simple and easy problem of the rating of intelligence, by stressing that the clinical impression should always be corroborated by tests. You know that the first studies on KLINEFELTER-Syndromes, omitting intelligence-tests, missed the important fact of a significantly lowered intelligence.

Our clinical impression is, that all our hirsute patients are psychologically disturbed; the aspects and structures of these disturbances fit well in the picture of neurosis but not of psychosis or of endocrine psychosyndrome.

The structures of the respective neuroses, that is to say of the different personalities, are highly dissimilar; they cover practically the whole diagnostic field: hysteric personality-structures, hysterias with conversions, with anxiety, with acting out, compulsive characters, compulsive neuroses, narcissistic structures, and so on.

Within this wide field of different personalities, however, two findings are very frequent: one is an underlying insecurity of sex-identification—when and where present it was in most cases deeply unconscious. Judging from behaviour, clothing and social adaptation all our patients impressed as thoroughly feminine.

The other constant finding is a very special symptom-pattern, that most of our 15 patients show with monotonous congruity. It consists of an intensive shyness to expose themselves, a withdrawal from personal relations and a constant anxiety of being found out and ridiculed. One could call it intraversion or autism or "inhibition of exhibition".

The degree of neurotic disturbance would—by our standards—have justified analytic treatment of everyone of our patients, provided the other necessary indications, e.g. insight and willingness, suitable age and so on, had been present, what, of course, often was not the case. Now, all these are subjective criteria, liable to possible doubts. Thanks to the tests we can corroborate, even prove, our findings.

Beginning with the results of the two questionnaires: MMQ and PIT (illustration 1): the MMQ on the left demonstrates that all the patients whose lie points are low enough to make their responses

Illustration 1 *

Neurotische Züge im MMQ und P-I-T

Namen der Patientinnen	MMQ		P-I-T		
	Lügenwert	neurot. Tendenz	Selbst-kritik	neurotisch	nicht neurotisch
	normal 3–9	normal 0–14	normal +	normal 4–8	normal 12–16
M. T.	4	36	+	13	7
H. S.	6	20	+	6	14
B. R.	7	20	+	4	11
B. G.	7 (2)	31 (27)	+	13	5
M. B.	8	17	+	9	11
U. G.	8	16	+	12	8
M. H.	9	25	—	12	7
D. S.	9 (11)	27 (21)	—	12	7
C. S.	11	29	+	10	10
E. K.	12	26	+	11	8
H. M.	10 (11)	26 (24)	—	7	13
E. W.	12	27			
G. G.	16	14	—	8	12
M. O.	16	8	— !	—	20
Gruppen-Querschnitt	135:14≈10	322:14=23	+:—=8:5	117:13= 9	133:13≈10

Erläuterungen

MMQ		P-I-T
Lügenwert	Testergebnis	Selbstkritik +: —A < 6,08
		+A > 8,52
0– 2	zweifelhaft interpretierbar	
3– 9	interpretierbar	
10–12	zweifelhaft interpretierbar	Selbstkritik —: —A > 6,08
darüber	nicht interpretierbar	+A < 8,52
Testwert		
0–14	normal	neurotisch:
15–20	Normalität zweifelhaft	normal 3,97–7,69 (≈4–8)
21–26	abnorm	nicht neurotisch:
darüber	schwerwiegend abnorm	normal 11,65–15,51 (≈12–16)

interpretable have a score of neurotic tendencies that is higher than normal. The only two patients who seem to be definitely non-disturbed have too many lie-points.

---

* Text of illustration is given in the original German version.

Illustration 2 *

			+	
nde Selbstkritik	-|A		+|A	Selbstkritik
ale Einstellung	-|B		+|B	soziale Einstellung
rsion	-|C		+|C	Extraversion
sch	-|D		+|D	nicht neurotisch
:ch	-|E		+|E	nicht manisch
siv	-|F		+|F	nicht depressiv
d	-|G		+|G	nicht schizoid
-id	-|H		+|H	nicht paranoid
liv labil	-|I		±|I	vegetativ stabil
ben	-|O		+|O	Landleben
			P	handwerklich
			Q	wissenschaftlich
			R	Verrechn., Verwaltg.
			S	Umgang mit Menschen in Gesch. und Wirtsch
			T	bildende Kunst
			U	sprachlich, literarisch
			V	musikalisch
			W	soziale Berufe

Linke Wellenlinie männlich, rechte Wellenlinie weiblich

P–I–T

Kombinierter Persönlichkeits- und Interessen-Test
nach Mittenecker und Toman

(Durchschnittswerte der 7 sicher auswertbaren Einzeltests)

The group-average in neurotic tendencies, 23, is almost identical with the mean value of EYSENCK's group of neurotics, 22,56. The right half of the table showing PIT data gives a similar picture.

PIT, personality-interest-test, is an Austrian questionnaire, the personality part of which is derived from the Minnesota multiphasic personality inventory. We show the group profile of all the patients whose objectivity (Selbstkritik) is sufficient to allow a reliable interpretation (illustration 2). The manifest common deviations are under the headings of neurotic traits, depressive traits and vegetative lability. Common tendencies lie in the direction of introversion and schizoid features. In the profile of interests there is only one common deviation: relations to fellow—humans are reduced.

PIT also confirms our clinical impression: the neurotic personality traits revealed in the interviews show themselves as neurotic tendencies, vegetative lability and depressive traits in the tests, the withdrawal from human contact is reflected in the interest part and in the tendencies to schizoid and introversive features.

Rorschach tests on the other hand with their highly structured and individual pictures have few features in common, namely a restricted number of responses, a tendency to introversion and non adapted narcissistic emotions. Again the clinical findings are con-

* Text of illustration is given in the original German version.

firmed: personal traits are so different, that they annihilate each other, only the common tendency to withdrawal remains.

Thematic Rorschach interpretations and other projective tests allow us to corroborate the insecurity of sex-identification.

The final and crowning step of course is the integration of all the somatic and psychological findings: time of onset, degree and progress of hirsutism, endocrine data, body-build, biography, dynamic personality structure and conflicts synchronous to the beginning of hirsutism.

A discussion of methods is not the adequate occasion to present the highly complex evaluation of etiology, especially concerning eventual psychogenetic factors. However let me repeat, what DR. V. ZERSSEN has stressed, that the evaluation of etiology must by no means leave the framework of shown or proven facts, e.g. in our case, that the basis of hirsutism is an excess of androgens.

We found four cases with impressive mental conflicts slightly preceding the development of hirsutism. Regardless of the fact that this is a minority in our group, the idea of psychogenesis for these cases is very tempting. Nevertheless we must stress, that a definite statement concerning psychogenesis is illegitimate, as long as we do not know anything about what emotions have what influence on androgen production. This must be the next step in research.

Psychoanalysis might be very enlightening if the androgen-production can be measured in certain critical phases. But psycho-analysis is and must be a primarily therapeutic venture.

Let me illustrate our opinion with a short case-history: The patient was twenty when she began to enact a magic ceremonial with the conscious purpose of becoming a man. Synchronously—under the pressure of her family—she began a very ambivalent relationship with a man. Every night she lay on her bed for hours and concentrated on the idea of already being a man, feeling in spells of depersonalisation her body changing and becoming stiff, while she herself was outside of it. During the day-time, with her boy-friend, she submitted to the usual courtship. Half a year later hairs began to grow on her face.

Rorschach revealed a schizoid personality with strong depressive features, suspect of an inclination to psychotic break-down.

You will agree that this spectacular biography suggests psychogenesis in a very pointed way. Taken as an example of hirsutism as a group the case would be entirely misleading; we have mentioned that this is not the rule but an exception.

In this case we have begun psychoanalysis, not to learn something about hirsutism but to help the patient with her feelings of isolation, her spells of anxiety, and her depersonalisation. If in the process of therapy we learn nothing about hirsutism we will not be disappointed, if we do learn something, we are fortunate.

Bibliography

MEYER, E. A. and v. ZERSSEN, D.: A psychological investigation in women with so-called indiopathic hirsutism. J. psychosom. Res. (in press).

v. ZERSSEN, D.: Die Objektivierbarkeit in der klinischen Psychologie (To be published).

v. ZERSSEN, D., MEYER, A. E. und AHRENS, D.: Klinische, biochemische und psychologische Untersuchungen an Patientinnen mit gewöhnlichem Hirsutismus. Dtsch. Arch. klin. Med. (To be published).

From the Psychosomatic Research Unit, Wilhelmina Gasthuis, Amsterdam

Author's address: DR. A. E. MEYER, II. Medizinische Universitätsklinik, *Hamburg-Eppendorf* (Germany).

Personal Factors in Sterility

H. BLIJHAM, Groningen

At the request of the Congress Committee and in view of the time available, our purpose here is to explain the methods used, rather than to deal in detail with the psychosomatic aspects of sterile marriage.

Experience gained as a general practitioner and later as a psychiatrist and especially in consulting functions in gynaecological departments has led me to the conclusion that in a considerable number of cases human sterility should be regarded as a syndrome and as a manifestation of the total personality. This total personality is essentially an inseparable structural entity with somatic, psychical and social aspects. A study of the literature gave the same impression.

It seemed worth while to carry out a systematic investigation into the personal factors of sterile individuals, in order to gain a firmer basis for these impressions. Neither causality nor specific relationships were assumed a priori. The principal object of this study was to demonstrate that in sterile marriages not only the somatic aspects, which receive due attention in a modern sterility clinic, but also mental and social factors are often important. Neglect of these factors may have untoward results for the couple concerned.

The case material was a successive series of sterile married couples, viz. all the couples who in 1955 and 1956 came for the first time to the sterility clinic of the Gynaecological and Obstetrical Department of the Academisch Ziekenhuis (Head: PROFESSOR DR. B. S. TEN BERGE). Their number was 192. For all these couples the data obtained on somatic examination of both husband and wife at the sterility clinic were evaluated. A list was made in which short note about the somatic and gynaecological state of the partners was added for each couple. In 65 couples there was uncertainty on account of incomplete examination. These couples were, therefore, not called up for psychosomatic examination. The rest of the couples were invited by letter as follows, to attend such an examination, this letter being so worded as not to offend mental hygiene.

In relation to the sterility-examination performed in the Gynaecologic Department in 1955 I ask you, also in the name of PROF. TEN BERGE, to come another time, together, in order to have a talk and a completing examination. Also in the case you want no further examination yourself or in the case pregnancy arose already, we should estimate it, if you would accept this invitation.

We expect you, together,

on . . . . day

at . . . . hour

Each couple was called only once.

To facilitate evaluation of the series, the couples were numbered in alphabetical order. For each couple the following facts were ascertained:

1. whether pregnancy had developed after the first examination at the clinic;

2. whether sperm anomalies had been found;

3. whether there were somatic abnormalities in the woman;

4. whether sexual disturbances had been found at examination at the sterility clinic;

5. whether complete examination of husband and wife had revealed any somatic changes;

6. whether somatic treatment had been instituted.

In the various tables and surveys which follow, these six possibilities are indicated by V, VI, VII, VIII, IX, X, respectively. This notation was maintained throughout the further course of the investigation. Various couples were, of course, classified in more than one of the groups V-X.

I will now show you a table with a survey of the whole series of couples. This shows that the group of 192 couples can be subdivided into those not invited, those who did not appear (subdivided into those who answered and those who did not answer), and those who came. We see also that some of the couples were referred to me and other to a colleaguegynaecologist. The arrows indicate that I personally subjected 32 couples to a detailed psychosomatic examination.

It will be noted from this table that 12 couples with sexual disturbances were not called up on account of incomplete somatic examination; in many cases the existence of psychosexual disorders was a contraindication for somatic examination on psychological grounds.

Another notable fact is that the development of pregnancy was the reason why many couples did not respond to our invitation for psychosomatic examination.

The table also shows what proportion of the couples of groups V-X appeared for psychosomatic examination, the figures being mutually comparable. The further study deals with these 32 couples.

Before telling you about this I will show you a second table, which likewise concerns all the 192 couples. In this table the mutual correlations between groups V, VI, VII, VIII, IX and X, and also group I (the couples not invited) are demonstrated.

I would like to draw your attention to the following points in this table. A high percentage of the couples with sexual disturbances show sperm anomalies, and vice versa.

Pregnancy occurs in a high percentage of marriages with sperm anomalies. A high percentage of the group without somatic changes shows sexual disorders. I shall now discuss in more detail the 32 couples whom I examined psychosomatically.

These 32 couples were examined for the presence or absence of correlations between certain personal factors and their classification in groups V-X. This was done to get an insight into the suspected possibility of a rôle of psychogenic factors in human sterility. For the study of personal factors, a question form was used. The questions asked were partly derived from KELLY AND FISKE's "The prediction of performance in clinical psychology" and partly from the technique of taking down a psychiatric and biographical history while other questions were concerned with the sterility as such.

When answering the questions asked personally, the patient was invited to choose from 2 to 5 possibilities, which were verbally repeated after every question.

The method was, thus, a psychiatric interrogation method, using questions with a choice of answers.

There were 80 questions. It was considered important to examine the partners of each couple separately immediately after one another, so that they could not discuss the questions between examinations. In all case, the wife was examined before the husband.

The questionnary was not handed to the patients; the questions were asked them orally and one by one.

For the sake of evaluation, the questionnary was coded as far as the answers were concerned, and the coded answers were tabulated. A brief diagnosis from the sterility clinic was added for each couple. In this way it was possible to survey the entire answer material, as will be shown by the following table.

This table can be worked out in the following 3 ways to achieve the desired purpose.

1. Horizontal evaluation. The frequencies with which the possible answers to each question chosen can be assessed for each of the group V–X.

In this way a table can be made for each question. They permit an immediate conclusion as to whether there are correlations, for the question concerned in the table, and if so, to what degree. I shall now show you a number of these tables.

The study of this $\pm$ 160 tables permits the following conclusions, Numerous personal factors, partly showing in the direction of neurotisation, have been found, in the females generally somewhat more frequent than in the males. The frequencies of these factors were generally higher in the groups VIII and IX, than following group VI and finally VII. This holds for the factors referring the home situation in the youth (broken homes, unhappiness of parents, patterns of education, feelings of guilt). In the females was found a dominating mother and a fatherbinding. In all the individuals was a total lack of sexeducation. Masturbation was not found in the females and in the males, 10 had never practised masturbation and 8 had masturbation-problems, which were correlated with the group IX. In one female out of the group IX and one male out of the group VI there was manifest homosexual behavior. In more than 50% of the females frigidity was found; this was correlated with group IX. In group IX there was more contraception practised than in the other groups. The females in group IX and the males in group VI had in generally appreciated pregnancy less than the other groups. The females of group IX were very active in society. Many females and males chose religion as to be the main factor concerning the succes of a marriage.

In a number of individuals the desired number of children was overcharged. There was found in sterile individuals a correlation with allergic diseases, with nervousness especially in females of group IX and males of group VI, with abdominal complaints especially in females of group VI. There was a very striking correlation with headache of the migraine type in about 50% of all the males and females. Finally many of the examined individuals indicated themselves as to be not well-balanced, melancholic and agitated.

2. Vertical evaluation of the survey table.

40 of the questions deal in particular with the possibility of neurotic development in the individuals.

In the following table these question are underlined and also underlined are those answers that can be regarded as exceptional or possibly indicative of a neurotic state of the individual concerned. The scores of these answers given by each wife, husband or couple can be established by counting.

I show you these scores in 4 tables. The scores indicate the degree of neurotisation. The conclusion may be made that in generally the disturbance in neurotic direction is most clear in the group VIII and IX, than follows groups VI and the group VII is disturbed least.

3. In the general survey table of the answers the possibility of mutual correlations between the answers can be studied. An instance of this is demonstrated.

The value and significance of this method lie principally in the fact that it provides a utilizable working hypothesis for further research, e.g. clinical-psychological studies. The correlations shown are not claimed to be statistically significant, and have not been checked for that purpose. For this reason, no definite conclusions can be reached with this technique. However, it is of essential importance that psychosomatic research should have methods available which can yield working hypotheses, and that is the reason why this report has been made.

Author's address: DR. H. BLIJHAM, Psychiatric Department University Hospital, *Groningen* (Netherlands).

Psycho-Social Factors in Industrial Absenteeism by Illness

R. PIERLOOT, L. GELISSEN and M. REYNDERS, Louvain

In clinical psychosomatic research we try to understand the meaning of a symptom or a syndrom in the framework of the psychological attitudes and behavioural patterns of the patients. The goal of our research is always to obtain information about the different forms of expression of the psychological life of the patients and to compare these with the reaction patterns of other people, forming control groups.

The different sources of information about psychological attitudes determine the different forms of methodological approach in the research work. Thus we can obtain our information from direct statements of the patients or by analysing their behaviour in the transference situation of psychotherapy or by registering their reaction patterns in experimental psychological or physiological test situations.

But the psychological life, considered as a communication between the individual and his environment, finds an expression in different facts and realizations of social relations, considered in a narrower sense (family and relatives) and broader sense.

Social factors, as school and vocational formation, choice of profession, changes of profession, nature of work and change of work, marriage and divorce, number of children, financial status, and hobbies are all influenced in their form and course by many biological and social factors. But to a certain degree they are also dependent on psychological attitudes. In these social facts we find a certain crystallization of the psychological life of the individual. We call "psycho-social investigation" the study of these social facts, considered as crystallized expressions of behaviour patterns. Considered in this way, the knowledge of these facts gained by the study of larger groups and compared with control groups, can help us to improve our insight into certain psychosomatic phenomena.

We have applied this method to the problem of psychological influences in industrial absenteeism by illness. A number of patients with different somatic symptoms have in common as their most prominent complaint the inability to perform their work. Moreover, since the existence of health insurance, they make claim for compensation from this source.

The ability to work is a psychosomatic phenomenon and can be approached from different points of view. Schematically, we can distinguish three main starting-points: the anatomical, considering the somatic equipment necessary to perform the work; the physiological, considering the supply and distribution of energy, required for the activities; the psychological, considering the stimulus driving and activating the man to work.

Factors diminishing or annihilating the ability can be considered in the same framework: a broken or paralysed arm is an anatomical defect, rendering impossible certain forms of work; infectious, metabolic, circulatory diseases influence the energy available for the work; but the ability to work depends also upon the attitude of the person towards his work, of the place taken by the work in the whole of the psychical life of the worker.

While anatomical defects can be judged by direct observation, it is not so easy to evaluate the exact repercussion of an internal disease in its effect of diminishing the energy available for work. Still more complicated is the problem of psychological influences on the inability to work. It is commonplace to group all patients, complaining of inability to work, without physical basis, under the term "neurosis". But starting from this qualification, we still have to get an insight into the structure of the neurotic personality and the significance of the inability to work in this structure. Moreover, many neurotics work very hard and do not easily neglect their work.

Using the method of psycho-social investigation, we have tried to approach the problem of psychological aspects in the inability to work. Trying to isolate the factor "psychological influences", we have studied a group of 35 labourers, presenting an inability to work, complaining of different somatic symptoms, but having in common the absence of organic lesions. The diagnoses were: general asthenia

(8 cases), cardiac neurosis (10 cases), functional gastro-intestinal troubles (8 cases), and colonneurosis (9 cases).

For the composition of a control group we wanted labourers, being in the same situation of inability to work, but on an absolutely evident physical basis. Therefore we chose men suffering from anatomical defects. The diagnoses were: blindness (4 cases), operation for intervertebral disc (3 cases), spastic paraplegia (4 cases), fractured leg (3 cases), osteomyelitis of tibia (2 cases), operation for ruptured meniscus of the knee (5 cases), amputation of foot (1 case), fracture of humerus (1 case), fracture of radius (3 cases), arthrotic ankylosis of ankle (4 cases), osteomyelitis of handbones (2 cases), rupture of muscle (2 cases), operation for bursitis of right elbow (1 case). We would formulate the difference between the 2 groups in this way: in the studied group the absenteeism was the meaning-giving symptom; in the control group it was a secundary effect.

We wanted to exclude the cases of short absenteeism, which are mostly occasioned by very chance factors, and therefore we took only persons being at least 30 days absent from their work. Furthermore, it seems impossible, for the judging of their social setting, to mix unmarried persons with heads of a family; and so we have limited our study to persons belonging to the last category.

The age distribution in the group was: Fig. 1.

Fig. 1. Age-distribution in the group.

Years	Studied group	Control group
≤ 25 y.	3	4
26–35 y.	11	11
36–45 y.	12	10
46–60 y.	9	10

Both groups were gathered by random choice from a health insurance office in Brussels, and consisted of labourers, resident and working in Brussels and suburbs.

The information was gained by direct inquiry of the patient, supplemented by official data (e.g. days of absenteeism and financial status). Our purpose was to limit our information to objective facts. A personal judgment was asked only concerning the degree of satisfaction in relation to the factors intervening in the working situation. This information was classified in very simple categories as satisfaction, indifference and dissatisfaction.

Starting from an actual absenteeism by illness, a first point we can examine is the former history of the patient in this respect. So, concerning the absenteeism by illness in the last five years, we took into account the number of periods, the number of days and the variation of symptoms, justifying the absenteeism. Figures 2, 3 and 4 give the results.

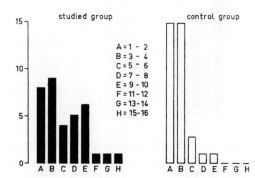

Fig. 2. Number of periods of absenteeism.

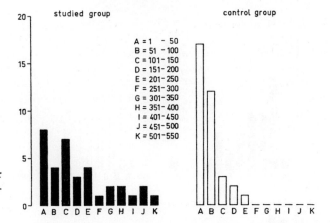

Fig. 3. Number of days of absenteeism.

For the periods, we have a X^2 of 11, corresponding to a significance at the 0.01 pt. For the days, the X^2 is 14.04; significance is at the 0.05 pt. For the variation X^2 is 5.96, significance at the 0.05 pt.

The findings suggest that the psychological factors are not just chance, but exercise a more steady influence, provoking more than average absenteeism, justified by pronounced varying symptoms.

To the popular mind, the most important stimulus to work is

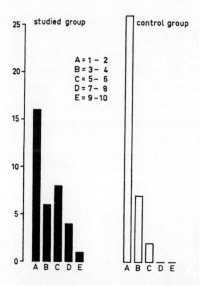

Fig. 4. Variation in symptoms justifying the absenteeism.

the financial gain involved. Thus we studied the financial status of the patients and the diminution of total income when the head of the family was ill (figs. 5, 6, and 7).

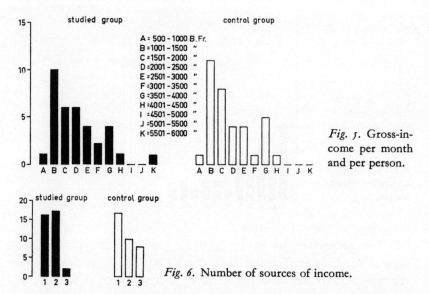

Fig. 5. Gross-income per month and per person.

Fig. 6. Number of sources of income.

In none of the studied factors do we find any difference. So our findings do not give support to the idea that the resuming of work is especially influenced by the importance of financial loss, since in our studied group financial loss is not in the least less important than in the control group. It is possible that these findings are influenced by the fact that we studied people with at least 30 days of absenteeism.

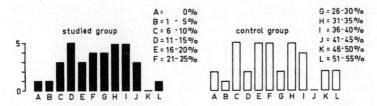

A =   0%
B = 1 - 5%
C = 6 -10%
D = 11-15%
E = 16-20%
F = 21- 25%

G = 26-30%
H = 31-35%
I = 36-40%
J = 41-45%
K = 46-50%
L = 51- 55%

studied group   control group

Fig. 7. Diminution of total income because of sickness of the head of the family.

Perhaps for shorter periods the financial factor would play a greater part.

When we analyse the degree of satisfaction in relation to the factors intervening in the working situation, we find striking differences. A survey of the results is given in fig. 8.

Fig. 8. Analysis of the degree of satisfaction in relation to the factors intervening in the working situation.

	studied group	control group
Contact with the foreman	+ 7	+ 19
Contact with the fellow workers	+ 3	+ 26
Possibilities of promotion	— 24	— 11
Possibilities of periodical pay increase	— 7	— 20
Freedom of movement in working situation	— 14	— 9
Nature of working conditions	+ 1	+ 7
Working system (divisions and time of work)	+ 3	+ 8
Distance from and possibilities of transportation to work	+ 4	+ 26
Degree of interest of work	— 16	+ 12
Wage scale	— 5	— 1
Wage system	+ 8	+ 16
Sum	— 40	+ 73

Satisfied	= + 1
Indifferent	= 0
Unsatisfied	= — 1

The results of these comparisons were the subject of a special study by analysis of variance, and the conclusions indicate significant differences.

In the same way argues the study of the previous working-history of our patients. First we have considered the number of trades exercised, and we find a X^2 of 12.69, corresponding to a significance at the 0.01 pt (fig. 9).

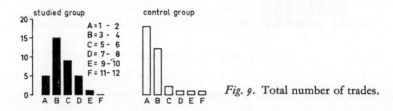

Fig. 9. Total number of trades.

The change of trade can be motivated by positive factors (e.g. more possibilities of promotion), by indifferent factors (closing of a business), or by negative factors (dissatisfaction, conflicts with boss). In fig. 10 we see that here also significant differences are found. The X^2 is 10.629; significance at the 0.01 pt.

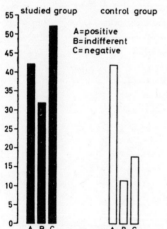

Fig. 10. Motivation of change of trade.

The total number of changes of trade is 127 in our studied group, against 72 in the control group. On the other hand, the total number of changes of work in the same groups is not very different: 128 in our studied group, against 109 in the control group. So the negative attitude towards the work seems to be deep-rooted, resulting in change of trade more than in change of work in the same trade.

Concerning the unemployment during the last five years up to the actual absenteeism, we find no significant differences in the number of periods (X^2 is 3.44); but for the number of days the X^2 is 7.02, giving a significance at the 0.05 pt. (fig. 11 and 12).

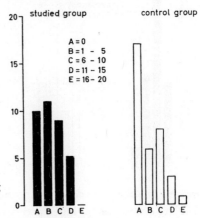

Fig. *11*. Periods of unemployment during the last 5 years up to actual absenteeism.

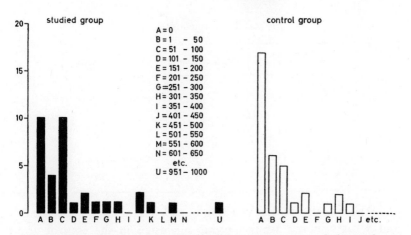

Fig. *12*. Days of unemployment during the last years to actual absenteeism.

The free-time occupation (fig. 13), where we distinguish an occupation by chance, passive occupation (e.g. football or cinema-going), against personal or social active occupations, shows also significant differences. X^2 is 13.2 with a significance at the 0.01 pt.

Further, we have considered the life-history in its narrower and

broader social aspects. First, the trade category of the father. For
classification of trade-categories we have used the classification of the
Dutch Ministry of Social and Public Health, ranging the trades in

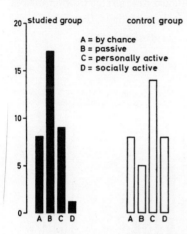

Fig. 13. Free-time occupation.

seven gradients, according to the required level of ability or skill.
Fig. 14 shows no significant differences (X^2 is 1.4).

Fig. 14. Trade-category of father.

level	studied group	control group
1	3	1
2	6	3
3	11	10
4	8	6
5	6	13
6	1	1
7	0	0

As far as the mother working outside the home is concerned, we
find 8 cases in our studied group against 6 in the control group,
which is not significant (X^2 is 0.4). But as regards disorders in the
family milieu during childhood or adolescence (death of parent or
separation), we find 19 cases against 5 in the control group, which is
significant at the 0.01 pt. (X^2 is 12.42).

For the number of children of the parents (fig. 15), we find no
significant difference (X^2 is 0.52), nor for the rank in birth (X^2 is 5.3)
(fig. 16).

Fig. 15. Number of children of parents.

	studied group	control group
1	3	6
2–3	16	10
4–6	8	6
> 6	8	13

Fig. 16. Rank in birth.

	studied group	control group
only child	3	6
oldest	13	5
youngest	10	11
in between	9	13

The comparison with the trade level of brothers and sisters shows that in our studied group more persons are either on the highest or on the lowest level of their family (fig. 17). The significance is at the 0.05 pt.; X^2 is 6.41.

Fig. 17. Comparison of trade-level of brothers and sisters.

	studied group	control group
only child	3	6
highest level	15	10
in between	2	9
lowest level	15	10

The school and vocational training is given in fig. 18, and the difference is not significant (X^2 is 5.51).

Fig. 18. School and vocational training.

	studied group	control group
Grammar school not finished	11	4
Grammar school finished	19	20
Vocational training not finished	3	5
Vocational training finished	2	6

The age of family formation (fig. 19) shows no significant differences (X^2 is 3.716).

Fig. 19. Age of family formation.

years	studied group	control group
18–20 y.	2	7
21–25 y.	15	18
26–35 y.	12	10
36–45 y.	6	0

The social adaptation of the family life (fig. 20) is less in our studied group, expressing itself in more asocial forms (concubinage, living with another). X^2 is 6.2, significant at the 0.05 pt.

Fig. 20. Social adaptation of family life.

	studied group	control group
married	27	34
legal divorce, not remarried or legally remarried	1	1
legally divorced and living with another	2	0
concubinage	2	0
living with another	3	0

In our studied group, in 20 cases the spouse works outside the home, against 12 in the control group, which is not significant. X^2 is 2.83.

The number of children of the patients (fig. 21) is not a significant difference (X^2 is 0.65), nor is the mode of residence (fig. 22). X^2 equals 0.38.

Fig. 21. Number of children.

	studied group	control group
0–1	20	17
2–3	9	12
4–6	5	3
> 6	1	3

Fig. 22. Mode of residence.

	studied group	control group
ownership	3	4
still to pay		
(installments)	2	3
renting	30	28

In our studied group we find in 8 cases important past events in family or social relations preceding the actual absenteeism, against 2 cases in the control group. The difference is not significant (X^2 is 4.2).

When we compare the actual trade of the patients to the trade of the father (fig. 23), and to their own original choice (fig. 24), regarding decline, equality or rise, we find no significant differences with the control group. For the first comparison, the X^2 is 1.9, and for the second, 0.486.

Fig. 23. Comparison of actual trade with trade of father.

		studied group	control group
decline	4 cat.	1	1
	3 cat.	6	4
	2 cat.	5	5
	1 cat.	5	7
equal		4	8
rise	1 cat.	8	4
	2 cat.	4	2
	3 cat.	2	4

Fig. 24. Comparison of actual trade with original choice.

	studied group	control group
rise	11	9
equal	14	14
decline	10	9

Conclusions

We have compared a series of psycho-social factors in a group of 35 labourers presenting an absenteeism by illness in absence of organic lesions, with a group presenting evident anatomical defects justifying their inability to work.

The most prominent finding is a preponderance of a negative attitude towards work in our studied group. Already suggested by a higher number of recidives in the absenteeism, justified by pronounced varying symptoms, this finding is confirmed by direct statements about different factors intervening in the working-situation, a higher frequency of change of trade, provoked mostly by negative factors, and also a higher number of days of unemployment.

But we find also significant differences in the free-time occupations, showing for the studied group a preponderance of chance or passive forms of occupation. Concerning the family life, the social adaptation is less in our studied group, expressing itself in more asocial forms of family life (concubinage, living with another).

These findings suggest that the influence of psychological factors in absenteeism by illness seems to be connected to a more general difficulty of adaptation to psycho-social stress, approaching in this way the concept of "social neurosis" described by Von Weizsäcker.

As regards the relations of the parental milieu, we find in our studied group a higher frequency of disorders (death of one of the parents or separation) in the childhood or adolescence. In the choice of their profession, the differences between the patients and their brothers and sisters are more pronounced, the patients being either on the highest or the lowest level. For other factors (tradelevel of father, mother working, rank in birth, etc.) we could not find significant differences.

Regarding financial factors, the studied group was not in the least different from the control group.

Acknowledgments:—We are grateful to the medical direction of both the Christian Health Insurance Co. (Dr. Hellemans), and of the St. Michael Federation (Dr. Swennen) for the opportunities provided for our studies.

Bibliography

Brown, J.A.C.: The Social Psychology of Industry (Penguin Books, Harmondsworth 1954).

Classificatie van de beroepen naar hun onderlinge verwantschap. Ministerie van Sociale zaken en Volksgezondheid, Staatsdrukkerij en Uitgeverijbedrijf ('s Gravenhage 1952).

Hogewind, F.J.E.: De Mens en zijn Werk (Stenfert Kroese, Leiden 1954).

Smith, H.C.: Psychology of Industrial Behaviour (McGraw-Hill Book Co., New York 1955).

Waterink, J.: De Mens in het Bedrijf (Zomer en Keunings, Wageningen).

Weizsäcker, V. von: Soziale Krankheit und Soziale Gesundung (Vandenhoek & Rupprecht, Göttingen 1955).

Authors' addresses: Dr. R. Pierloot, Drs. L. Gelissen and Mr. M. Reynders, 146, Boulevard de Namur, *Louvain* (Belgium).

Psychosomatic Methods of Investigation in the Recognition of Organic Disease

S. Barton Hall, Liverpool

One of the most welcome general trends in psychiatry to-day is the movement towards integration with general medicine. The middle of the nineteenth century saw the creation of a clinical science; and the rapid advance of the physical sciences, the emphasis on morbid anatomy and the cellular theory adumbrated by Virchow and others inevitably directed attention to tissues, objective features and physical signs, the aim in view being a more inductive and, it was hoped, "scientific" attitude towards diagnosis. In this context it was tempting to regard the organism as a machine composed of several assemblies of parts, the systematic examination of which should lead to detection of the fault or the cause of disorder. By the turn of the century this process had become so elaborate that the erstwhile human being, the patient, was in a fair way to becoming an interesting, if rather unpredictable, vehicle for test findings.

The psychiatry of the past forty years has helped to restore a more balanced viewpoint. At a moment when it was beginning to be thought that the vein of clinical observation had been fully worked out, the bare outline of the patient's medical history, as previous generations knew it, has been reinforced by a biological, phenomenological and sociological approach. Furthermore, to objective assessment has been added the subjective method with its psychodynamic undertones. This return to a holistic conception has enabled physician and psychiatrist to co-operate in evolving psychosomatic means of investigation which, it is submitted, could provide a diagnostic instrument of great delicacy not only in the elucidation of stress disorders but in the recognition of subacute and chronic organic disease.

Until comparatively recent times, and in the diagnosis of organic disease—say, of the central nervous system—the physician was restricted to the results of careful clinical examination. Only when physical signs were present could he feel satisfied that the presence of organic disease was established; and by that time such disease was often relatively far advanced. Special studies—biochemical tests, contrast media, air studies, electroencephalography—have added refinements of approach, but not all these are applicable as a routine: some may be justifiable only when the results of clinical examination have suggested their use.

Two important reasons why comprehensive psychosomatic investigation may in certain cases assist in the recognition of organic disease at an earlier stage are first, the fact that mental changes may precede the appearance of physical signs by a considerable interval of time and, second, that a biographical anamnesis, interviews with relatives of the patient, the application of psychometric tests and, above all, the subjective rapport established with the patient himself may uncover some detail of information which does not fit in with any purely psychiatric diagnosis but which, in a moment may reveal that the case is in the organic field.

Let there be no misunderstanding. This paper is not a plea for the negative policy of regarding all patients who complain of psychological symptoms with suspicion, and subjecting them to exhaustive investigation, often with adverse effect for the person concerned. The aim is the positive one of trying to discern what psychological symptoms and personality changes may be regarded as pointing to organic disease, and employing this knowledge in a planned diagnostic approach.

Clinical Aspects

Of patients referred to the psychiatric department of a general hospital, both from within the hospital and from outside by their family doctors, a proportion, though presenting with mental symptoms, prove to be suffering from organic disease of which those symptoms may be found to have been the first sign. In 1000 consecutive cases studied by the writer in 1936 6.7% came into this category. Among the ailments brought to light in this way, disease primarily affecting the nervous system—multiple and combined sclerosis, neoplasms, extrapyramidal syndromes—accounts for a proportion, but a variety of other pathological conditions, such as hypothyroidism, are encountered. From the standpoint of social medicine it is significant that of recent years pulmonary neoplasm has had to be added to the list, two such cases presenting at our clinic during the past twelve months. Time forbids detailed description of more than one clinical example:—

An electrician, aet. 54, was referred to our clinic by his doctor on 11 February, 1957. He complained of soreness of the tongue, difficulty in swallowing, anorexia, pruritus ani, progressive asthenia, dryness of the mouth and disturbance of taste. He had been in good health until 1952 when he first noticed soreness of the tongue. In 1953 he had begun to suffer from phases of depression for which, in 1955, he was treated by E.C.T. in a psychiatric hospital. By the Spring of 1955 he was attending for treatment of his pruritus ani by a dermatologist, who referred him to a general physician. Apart from marked emphysema and chronic bronchitis no physical abnormality was found, but the patient was described as being "very talkative, almost hypomanic". His tongue symptoms were considered to be of psychogenic origin.

When seen at our clinic his symptoms were considered suspicious of organic disease, but it is fair to say that the complaints of dysphagia and disturbance of taste could not be substantiated objectively. On the other hand, there was no doubt that the patient's tongue was acutely tender, he had a slurring dysarthria and a nasal intonation. Two subjective observations were regarded as being significant: he volunteered that he could no longer wrestle with his son, who was now able to push him around at will; and the patient's wife described how, during the previous five years, he had completely changed in personality. Before, he had always been helpful, sociable, fond of going out, but he had gradually become irritable and bad-tempered with wife and workmates.

At this point the patient was referred to a neurologist. At first, the result of clinical examination was inconclusive, but on 4th May, 1957, the blood picture was described as "very suggestive of pernicious anaemia", and he was admitted to hospital. By 14th October 1957, he had made a complete physical and mental recovery. The blood count and picture had returned to normal following administration of high dosage intramuscular vitamin B complex, excluding vitamin B_{12}: the haemoglobin was 113%. In fact, however, the diagnosis proved to be not pernicious anaemia but early pellagra.

The point of this illustration is not that the case is in any way remarkable, but that mental symptoms preceded an accurate diagnosis by six years, and that the subjective physical complaints were attributed to psychogenic cause.

Psychological Symptomatology

In designating psychological symptoms which represent an expression of organic disease, it would seem advisable to employ a distinguishing term. Previously the word "psychopathological" has been used (BLEULER, 1951), but it is considered that this adjective is more appropriately applied to mental processes that are primarily of psychogenic origin—the sense in which it has most commonly been employed hitherto. Accordingly, the term "pathopsychological" is suggested, since it is felt that this might convey an emphasis on *pathology*, as used in the commonly accepted sense. Psychological symptoms might thus be grouped as follows:—

1. Psycho-pathological   Of psychogenic origin
2. Psycho-somatic   Of an actual bodily disorder
   contributed to
   aggravated or
   precipitated by psychogenic factors
3. Somato-psychic   Arising from, and secondary to, the patient's *reaction to* having a bodily disease
4. Patho-psychological   Of organic origin and, therefore, an *expression of* bodily disease

It may be seen that it is to the fourth category that this paper refers.

Patho-psychological Symptoms

It seems important to emphasise that the diagnosis of affective disorders, such as psychoneurosis, is not properly made by a process of exclusion. Negative findings on physical examination, and even of more detailed studies, do not exclude the presence of organic disease. Certain positive requirements are essential: in their absence a presumption in favour of organic disease should remain.

It is not proposed here to detail these positive requirements, nor to refer to those three classical groups of symptoms—clouding of consciousness, the dysmnesis syndrome, and dementia. Neither will reference be made to those objective methods and tests specially devised for the examination of patients suffering from organic cerebral disease, and covering such conditions as aphasia, sensory and perceptual anomalies, disturbance of body scheme and the like. Although all these may be of assistance in diagnosis, they may not afford very early indication of organic disease, somatic evidence of which may already be apparent. For the finer points we must rely upon those more subtle clues which the more total methods of psychosomatic investigation may supply.

Among these I should include a patient's urge to find a purely psychological explanation for his illness. Unconsciously sensing its real nature, he attempts to belittle any physical disability and to prove that his symptoms are due to lack of confidence or to connect them with some emotional experience. This tendency is in marked contrast to the psychoneurotic who is on the defensive against any such explanation and who frequently clings to one of physical disease. Again, any reported change of personality, irritability of temper in one previously stable, and actions that are out of keeping with former character traits must arouse suspicion. Thirdly, it may be one clinical feature only, as instance gain in weight where we should have expected decrease, that does not accord with a clear psychiatric diagnosis, but one the importance of which outweighs all the others.

In numerous instances it has been found helpful to have the patient give a specimen of his handwriting. His total response to this request, which should of course be for something more than his name and address, may be very revealing. Apart from the calligraphy itself being possibly indicative of organic disease, the patient, although having successfully complied with the requirements of the examination up to that point, may, when he is asked to write, show certain peculiarities of response or, indeed, prove quite unequal to the task.

It is again emphasised that it is on subjective, as distinct from objective, observations that we are often dependent for our clues. These may consist of spontaneous remarks—which, incidentally, it is useful to record verbatim—let fall by patients or relatives, or their responses to specific questions, even leading questions, by the examiner.

Another fertile field for psychosomatic investigation is that of bladder function. Too often, patients who have difficulty in managing their bladders, and in whom no organic explanation has been found, are not regarded seriously. The complaint of frequency is apt to be attributed to anxiety, that of retention to hysteria, while an episode of diurnal enuresis, particularly if it coincides with an experience of emotional stress, may be ascribed to mere lack of self-control. But we know that control of visceral function is laid down early in life, and becomes deeply rooted in the development of personality and self-esteem: consequently, any departure from complete continence, particularly in an adult, must be suspect of organic involvement. The wife of a patient aged 49 who, though he made no complaint on his own account and did not himself seek medical aid, was described as having changed in various ways, was asked whether her husband had ever lost control of his bladder. "No" she replied, and then, after a brief pause, "only once" (two weeks previously). The subsequent diagnosis was one of cerebral neoplasm.

Not to be overlooked is the inappropriate or facetious remark. A serious-minded middle-aged man of irreproachable morals and way of life, who was asked during physical examination if he had ever had any venereal infection, replied "No—not yet", thereby indicating at once the organic nature of his illness.

To do justice to this theme would require numerous clinical examples and detailed case descriptions: nevertheless, it is hoped that this short paper may have indicated the possibilities provided by psychosomatic methods of investigation in the earlier recognition of organic disease, and its importance for the initiation of appropriate treatment and, hence, for prognosis.

My thanks are due to the Editor of The Practitioner for permission to include certain material which appears in this paper.

Author's address: Dr. S. Barton Hall, 41 Rodney Street, *Liverpool* (England).

II

Concept of Constitution in Psychosomatic Medicine

From the II. Medizin. Univ.-Klinik und Poliklinik Hamburg-Eppendorf
(Direktor: PROF. DR. A. JORES)

The Concept of Constitution in Psychosomatic Medicine

(Introduction)

H. FREYBERGER

As a rule in physical medicine the term constitution covers all those qualities of an individuum which are determined by his genotype (6). Seen from the angle of organic medicine in the case of many diseases the eventual manifestation is largely based on the patient's constitution. In the majority of cases it is primarily the physical aspect that is decisive when forming an opinion on the constitution.

When speaking of constitution in psychosomatic medicine, the psychological aspects have also to be considered. If we start from the principle that it is the ultimate task of psychosomatic medicine to examine in how far psychic processes have harmful effects on the body, the importance of constitutional factors in psychosomatic medicine may be demonstrated by the following two points, namely:

1. Whether apart from peristatic factors likewise genotypic influences are of any importance with regard to the final manifestation of pathological and psycho-physical phenomena.

and 2. whether in case of evident peristatic—psychic disturbances the resulting organic symptoms can be explained exclusively on account of psychological processes, or whether it has to be assumed that a somatic constitution has existed from the beginning. This fact is directly to related to certain aspects of the problem of which organs will be affected.

In German-speaking countries this problematic question is reflected in rather contradictory manner in two theories which are widely discussed at the moment. On the one hand the psycho-physical system by KRETSCHMER, and the concept of psychoanalytic-ally orientated psychosomatic medicine on the other hand (2, 7).

KRETSCHMER is of the opinion that all psychic and physical phenomena including psychosomatic symptoms are lastly determined by the genotype. One day, however, the pathological effects of the latter will become apparent in which case the influences of environ-ment are only of indirect nature. Among others this point of view is based on the study of the body build, above all on that of the lepto-some, athletic and pyknic types, which are considered to be the morphological expression of the constitution. In all these types, although without any detailed psychological examination of the unconscious, KRETSCHMER did not only succeed in proving different traits but also a particular correlation between certain diseases and certain types. As for example a relationship between the pyknic type and hypertonia and the leptosome type and gastric ulcer. Furthermore bronchial asthma chiefly affecting the athletic type, as was found by own observations (4). From this point of view, according to KRETSCH-MER such diseases are constitutional. Accordingly, without employing any psychoanalytical methods his psychotherapeutical approach is based on the solution of the actual conflict as well as on the patient's recog-nition that psycho-physical disposition is closely related to his consti-tution.

Particularly with regard to the subject of constitution and psycho-somatic diseases, the conception of psycho-analytically orientated psychosomatic medicine is strongly opposed to KRETSCHMER's posi-tion.

Let me simplify the matter by giving you the example of a psychoanalytic interpretation of gastric ulcer. Apart from anorexia nervosa, this disease, in my opinion, may be regarded as the most closely studied psychosomatic disease.

Based on FREUD's doctrines, as early as during the first five years of a child's life the relationship of body and soul plays an important part, as the organic functions, owing to the early process of impulse and need—based on a mother—child relationship—are closely linked. During the first year, for example, the oral phase i.e. the gastric function, and during the second year the anal phase i.e. defecation and urination. During the oral phase the psycho-physical relationship of the child to its environment is determined by the satisfaction of hunger. Hunger, in this case has to be understood in the psycho-physical sense i.e. not only for food but also for love. In case of a harmonious mother-child relation all physical functions connected with ingestion run smoothly. In case of an inharmonious mother-child relationship an irritation of the gastric functions may occur resulting from insufficient nutrition. Similar to the clinical experience that hunger, in the psycho-physical sense may lead to a stimulation of peristalsis and the secretion of hydrochloric acid.

These disturbances of the human relationship which appear during the oral phase as well as the closely correlated organic functions may well influence the child's future life. These symptoms may reveal themselves when overcoming conflicts in early life or may become apparent in future critical stages, the so-called stage of temptation and frustration (FREUD). Several authors (11) unanimously demonstrated in more than 300 cases of ulcer that the wish for being fed and loved—which had never been fulfilled in the patient's early life—remained alive in the latter's subconscience throughout his life. Although this desire was concealed and compensated by an intensified wish for achievement and independence, it was stimulated again in moments of specific and an immediate frustration. Owing to the patients inability to solve this problem consciously, it led to a considerable stimulus of peristalsis and secretion thus manifesting the existence of ulcer.

By means of such psychoanalytical interpretation of ulcer it is possible to demonstrate the continuity in the psychosomatic development. Being emotionally controlled the latter is characterized by frustrations which —in the sense of simultaneity—affect the gastric functions as the origin of this psychosomatic development has to be sought in the oral phase. Eventually, as a result of an intensification of the contrast between conscious and unconscious desires such a development leads to ulcer.

Under this psycho-analytical aspect the assumption of genotypical factors, which determine psychological constitution as well as the choice of the afflicted organ are to a large extent of minor importance.

R. SPITZ (10) to whom we are indebted for many informative examinations on the relationship towards external objects, is of the opinion that compared to the complex aspects of environment the innate factors are composed as follows:

1. interuterine influences during pregnancy.
2. influences becoming effective during the process of birth.
3. inherited disposition, by which SPITZ nothing but the natural process of maturity in the somatic and psychological spheres e.g. the interaction or uninterrupted sequence of oral, anal, and phallic phases.

Thus it follows that, for SPITZ, it is only the sequence of phases "as such" that is constitutional, however not the final result of such phases e.g. the oral and the anal characters.

In view of these two extreme positions namely KRETSCHMER's typology and the psychoanalytical conception, the question arises whether, psychosomatically speaking, it is possible to define clearly between genotypical and peristatic-psychic elements in view of their importance with regard to the manifestation of a psychosomatic disease.

Such an experiment proves to be rather difficult. One of the chief arguments of experts on constitution, namely that the existence of identical symptoms in successive generations point at heredity have caused objections.

There are psychoanalytical observations according to which in the course of the process of identification during early childhood, the human being may adopt unconsciously a symptom from one or both his parents. This process is called "Symptom tradition" by MIT-SCHERLICH. Another way of identification may be possible in that one parent tries to create those reactions in the child that had gained importance during the parents childhood. The same symptoms may then be responsible for the child's disease because the latter must develop his personality under the identical circumstances as his parent.

By means of analytical studies made with patients suffering from ulcer, SCHWIDDER thinks that certain importance may be attributed to the genotypical factors only if psychological examinations of the unconscious prove the existence of normal and comparatively undisturbed developmental conditions during early childhood. Systematic examinations in this direction, however, are unknown to me.

Finally, a further possibility of objectifying genotypical factors in case of psychosomatic diseases is the correlation of physical structure and disease. As mentioned at the beginning, according to KRETSCHMER and a number of other authors (9) statistically significant positive correlations between the type of structure and a certain disease are supposed to be proof of the constitutional determination of such a disease. In fact, this seems to be a criterium, which may possibly give certain indications for genotypical tendencies (the so-called psychosomatic basic structure as interpreted by JORES). It is from this point of view, too, that we have to consider the fact that the correlation between gastric ulcer as standard example of a psychosomatic disease on the one hand, and the pyknic type on the other hand is negative, whereas it is highly positive in the case of a leptosome-athletic type. Such a possible genotypic aspect, however, in no way affects the great importance of peristatic causes, found on account of analytic methods. It will ultimately depend on the latter, whether certain genotypical tendencies will have a chance of developing or not.

Further examinations will show whether on the other hand the statement may be made that in case of a pyknic type who is suffering from ulcer, a predominance of peristatic-psychic factors is to be assumed.

Summing up I should like to point out expressly that in this case the definition of genotypical constitution was applied. This, as a matter of fact, is the original definition of the constitution, especially when discussing the question of "environment and disposition" in psychosomatic diseases, and, in my opinion, it is the most suitable one. The above mentioned definition, however, was lately modified by several authors of organic medicine, in that they assert that the constitution may also imply qualities that have been acquired (3). Other authors of organic medicine consider the actual phenotype and constitution to be identical (1). Apparently these modifications of the original concept of "constitution" have partly been supported by psychological thoughts on the significance of neurosis in medicine. In this context is has to be added that an identification of phenotype and constitution can only be conclusive when including psycho-analytical principles, too. This necessity may be demonstrated by the continuous psycho-somatic development as exemplified by means of gastric ulcer.

From this point of view, the concept of constitution with regard to genotype and phenotype are not only of great scientific interest in psychosomatic medicine, but on the other hand modern psychosomatic results may contribute towards a considerable widening of the concept of constitution in physical medicine.

Bibliography

1. BAUER, K.H.: Chirurg Vererbg.-Konstit.lehre; Hb (KIRSCHNER-NORDMANN 1939).
2. CREMERIUS, J.: Freud als Begründer der psychosomatischen Medizin. Acta Psychotherapeutica *IV*: 252–265 (1956).
3. CURTIUS, F.: Klin. Konstit.lehre (Springer, Berlin 1954).
4. FREYBERGER, H.: Körperbau und Asthma bronchiale. Asthma u. Allergie *4*: 332 (1958).
5. JORES, A.: Der Mensch und seine Krankheit (Klett, Stuttgart 1957).
6. KRETSCHMER, E.: Körperbau und Charakter (Springer, Berlin 1955).
7. MITSCHERLICH, A.: Über die Reichweite psychosomatischen Denkens in der Medizin. Psyche *III*: 342–358 (1950).
8. SCHWIDDER, W.: Die Bedeutung psychischer Faktoren in der Aetiologie der Ulcuskrankheit. Psyche *IV*: 561–575 (1951).
9. SELBERG, W.: Die morphologischen Korrelationen der inneren Organe bei den verschiedenen Körperbauformen und ihre funktionalen Beziehungen. Z. menschl. Vererb.- u. Konstit. Lehre *33*: 283–300 (1956).
10. SPITZ, R.: Die Entstehg. d. ersten Objektbeziehungen (Klett, Stuttgart 1957).
11. STINE AND IRUY: cit. n. MITSCHERLICH, A.: Med. Klin. *53*: 165 (1958).

Author's address: DR. H. FREYBERGER, Medizinische Universitätsklinik und Poliklinik, *Hamburg-Eppendorf* (Germany).

Constitution and Neurosis

L. REES, London

Definition

The term constitution is used in a variety of meanings. I propose to use the term in it's wider connotation according to the following definition. "Human constitution is the totality of those morphological, physiological, psychological and immunological characteristics of the individual which are mainly determined by heredity but influenced, in varying degrees, by environmental factors".

Physique lends itself more readily to exact measurement than other constitutional attributes and provides a convenient starting point for the study of correlations between different aspects of human constitution. There are a large number of morphological features that can be chosen for this purpose, ranging from individual anthropometric measurements, body size, the configuration of the body as a whole or of it's constituent parts, to the relative development of physical dimensions or of different tissues in various parts of the body. Morphological attributes which show marked variability between individuals and relative constancy within the individual are more likely to be useful for human constitutional research. The concept of human constitution thus connotes predominant genetic determination and the relative constancy of constitutional attributes within the individual.

The present status of constitutional research can best be considered against the background of it's historical development.

Historical perspective

The study of possible associations between physical and mental attributes has the respectable virtue of being rooted in antiquity. The teachings of Hippocrates and Galen paid great importance to relationships between bodily habitus on the one hand and temperamental disposition and susceptibility to disease on the other. Detailed descriptions of different temperamental types, allegedly due to various humoural admixtures and characterized by specific physical features were given by Galen. The humoural theories of Hippocrates and Galen werenot only doctrines of disease causation but also attempted to explain individual differences in behaviour.

Very little progress was made in knowledge of human constitution, during ensuing, 2000 years, not until the late 19th century, when Beneke (1878) described relationships between physical type, the morphology of internal organs and different diseases and Di Giovanni, the founder of clinical anthropometry, described investigations into physique in the Italian population and went to the extreme of trying to prove that the morbidity of an organ resided in it's morphological characteristics (Giovanni, 1919). The work of the Italian school has continued by Viola (1932), who extensively investigated the physical characteristics of the population of Northern Italy and considered that there was a reciprocal relationship between the development of the trunk and the development of the limbs. By means of a rather cumbersome index derived from eight measurements, he differentiated three types: 1. the megalosplanchnic, characterized by large trunk and short limbs, 2. the microsplanchnic, characterized by long limbs and small trunk and 3. the normasplanchnic which is midway between 1. and 2., having a harmonious relationship between trunk and limbs. BOLDRINI (1925), an eminent statistician, substituted VIOLA's unwieldy index with a more simple index consisting of the ratio $\dfrac{\text{chest circumference.}}{\text{stature}}$ BOLDRINI's system was statistically strong but anatomically weak in contrast to VIOLA's system which was strong anatomically but weak statistically.

The work of the Italian school together with that of the German school founded by BENEKE (1898) and continued by KRETSCHMER (1921) provided the foundation for the modern development of knowledge in somatology.

A very great impetus to constitutional research was given by the publication by KRETSCHMER in 1921 of his book «Körperbau und Charakter». KRETSCHMER (1921) described his now classical physical types viz the asthenic (leptosomatic) type; the athletic type; the pyknic type and a number of dysplastic physiques. His description of correlations between physical type and normal personality types as well types of psychosis brought interest on human constitution al research to the forefront after having been relegated to the background for many years and overshadowed by the spectacular rise of knowledge in pathology and bacteriology.

One of the difficulties confronting workers in constitutional research was that the variations in physique in the normal population were not known and that the various typological classifications which had been proposed were largely based on unverified hypotheses. What was clearly needed was an inductive method for ascertaining the nature of the variations in physique in the normal population and how these could be most effectively and economically described.

The following methods have contributed most to our understanding of the nature of constitutional variations in recent years.

1. Factorial analysis and related statistical techniques
2. SHELDON's system of somatotyping
3. LINDEGARD's system
4. A variety of miscellaneous techniques e.g., a) tissue component analysis, including assessment of fat, muscularity, water content, etc.

and their relationship to skeletal development, b) the assessment of disharmonious growth between different parts and between different components of the body (dysplasia), c) the measurement of bodily disproportions, d) the assessment of relative masculinity and femininity (Androgyny, Gynandromorphy).

Factorial analysis of human body build

Factorial analysis provided a relatively objective and inductive method of elucidating the variation of physique in the normal population and their description in an economical and effective way. Factorial analysis achieves the resolution of a set of variables into terms involving a smaller number of categories or factors which account for the correlations. It has a special advantage for the study of human constitution as it provides a holistic representation of human physique which is far more comprehensive than that given by anthropometric measurements alone.

The steps required for employing factorial analysis of body build in this way are as follows:

First of all a random and representative sample of the normal population is selected and a comprehensive series of anthropometric measurements, covering all parts and dimensions of the body is taken on the sample. Each measurement is then correlated with all the other measurements for the total group, which gives a matrix of correlations between the anthropometric measurements. One of the primary assumptions in factorial analysis is that when any two variables are correlated there must be a common factor. The next step is to determine the factors underlying the correlations or covariations in the matrix and removing the effect of each factor from the matrix before extracting the next factor, this process being repeated until the residual correlations are statistically insignificant. Factorial techniques may extract factors which are independent (is uncorrelated or orthogonal factors). Other techniques involve rotation of factors in an attempt to get a better descriptions of groups of correlations and produce correlated (oblique) factors. The most common procedure used is the extraction of a general factor first, then group factors relating to the shape of the body as a whole or of it's constituent parts.

Factorial techniques thus provide a means of classifying the variations in body build with the smallest number of anthropometric measurements. The results of factorial analysis of physique also tell which measurements are likely to be most effective for discriminating physical types. Such measurements may be combined to form indices of body build, either in the form of suitably constructive ratios or as regression equations of weighted measurements. Factorial analysis may also be used in another way for studying physical types viz the factorial analysis of persons instead of anthropometric measurements. This method determines how true an individual is to a particular type and involves the specification of the type in question by a set of representative measurements expressed in standard measure. The correlation of a given individual with the standard pattern indicates how closely he approximates to a perfect representation of the type.

To illustrate the application of factorial methods for analyzing physique I will describe briefly the results of factorial analysis which I carried out on a group of 200 adult men and a group of 200 adult women.

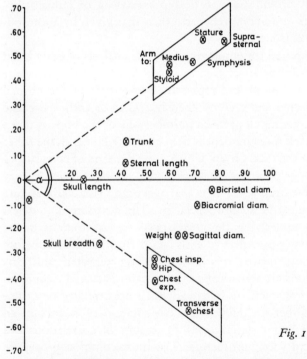

Fig. 1

Some eighteen variables were intercorrelated and factorized. In both men and women it was found that all the correlation coefficients between physical measurements were positive indicating the existence of a general factor. This general factor was first extracted and found to contribute 34 per cent of the variance. The second factor extracted was bipolar having positive saturations with length measurements and negative saturations with breadth and circumferential measurements. These two factors were found in both the male and female groups. The second factor clearly differentiated the linear type of physique at one extreme preponderating in length measurements in relation to breadth and circumference, from the broad type at the other extreme, preponderating in breath, width and circumferential measurements relative to length. The factor saturations of body measurements for the male and female groups are shown in Figures 1 and 2 respectively. In the male group two measurements having the highest correlations with the type factor were stature and transverse chest diameter which were combined to form a body build index as follows:

$$\frac{\text{Stature} \times 100}{\text{Transverse chest diameter} \times 6}$$

In the female group there were four measurements with high correlations with the type factor, namely stature, symphysis height,

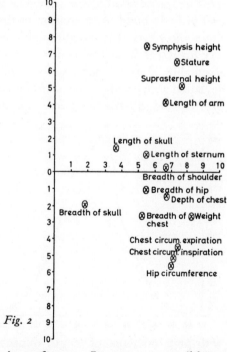

Fig. 2

hip circumference and chest circumference. It was not possible to construct a simple index as for men and a new female body build index was devised consisting of a regression equation of these measurements (expressed in standard measure) as follows. Female body build index = + 0.59 stature + 0.47 symphysis weight — 0.31 chest circumference — 0.64 hip circumference.

The REES-EYSENCK index of male body build was calculated on a group of 1000 neurotic soldiers the frequency distribution curve of which is shown in Figure 3. The REES female body build index was an calculated on 400 female neurosis patients serving in the Armed Forces, the frequency distribution curve is shown in Figure 4. Figures 3 and 4 show that body build both in men and women is distributed along a unimodal frequency distribution curve approximating the normal frequency curve. There is no evidence of multimodality or bimodality, which would be the case if physical types existed in the sense of mutually exclusive descrete categories. What is in fact found is continuous variation in physique from one extreme to the other with the extremes of the curve, only, impressing us as well marked types. The body build index for men and the female body build index measure the position of the individual in a normal frequency distribution of body build. Any division of the continuous variation in physique into physical types, although convenient and sometimes necessary for research, will be arbitrary. It was considered that statistically acceptable abitrary demarcation points would be one standard deviation above and one standard deviation below the mean, dividing the frequency distribution curve into three classes viz ,1. leptomorphs,

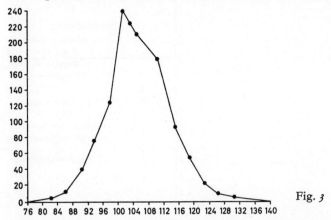

Fig. 3

with preponderance of length dimensions, compared with breadth, width and circumference, 2. eurymorphs, with large circumferential breadth measurements in comparison to length, 3. mesomorphs, with an intermediate relationship between lateral and circumferential on the one hand and linera measurements on the other. These categories of physique are not in any way intended to convey the impression that they are disparate types. They are in fact ranges of body build

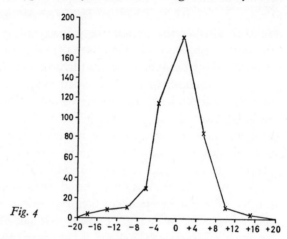

Fig. 4

objectively measured by new indices of physique and demarcated by statistical criteria for purposes of description and research.

SHELDON's *classification of varieties of physique*

SHELDON's (1940) system was originally based on the inspection of standardized photographs of a large number of individuals. He considered that there were three components in physique, designated endomorphy, mesomorphy and ectomorphy, which he considered consisted of tissues derived from the three germinal layers, the endoderm, mesoderm and ectoderm. Each individual was rated by inspection, for each component, on a 7-point scale. A 711 rating would represent an extreme endomorph, with preponderence in breadth and circumferential measurements; a 171 rating is the extreme in mesomorphy, with marked bone and muscle development, broad shoulders, muscular limbs; a 117 is an extreme ectomorph, characterized by linearity and relative poor development of breadth, width and circumferential measurements. SHELDON's method is an advance over those previous typologies which tended to regard physical types as disparate and mutually exclusive categories. The method has been criticized because of it's subjectivity and because there is evidence that the somatotype, as claimed by SHELDON, is not necessarily constant in an individual. LASKER (1947) found that a somatotype significantly changed with changes in nutrition and NEWMAN (1952) found significant somatotype changes with increase in age. SHELDON's hypothesis that his three components are derived from the three primary germinal layers has not been scientifically verified. It is also doubtful whether the number of primary components described by SHELDON (1940) is valid. HUMPHREYS (1957), for example, found that the correlations between endomorphy, mesomorphy and ectomorphy given by SHELDON, in fact, provided evidence for the existence of only two independent (but not necessarily valid) types of physique. Similarly, HOWELLS (1952) using factorial analysis of persons in a group of individuals who were markedly dominant in one of the three components, found that the factors or scale arrangements of persons extracted, did not correspond to SHELDON's (1940) three components. His findings suggested that ectomorphy and endomorphy were not independent factors, but were opposite manifestations of one factor being opposite extrems of a continuum. The researches of EKMAN (1951) and SILLS (1950) also indicated that two components fitted the data rather than three.

Physique, temperament and neurosis

Although a much greater volume of research has been devoted to the study of relationships between physical type and psychotic type, various schools of constitutional typology have also carried out investigations into physique and it's temperamental and neurotic correlates. NACARATI (1924) of the Italian school, using VIOLA's index classified neurotic subjects into microsplanchnic, normosplanchnic and nacrosplanchnic types. He found that the neurotic groups had a higher proportion of extreme physical types than a normal control group. He also found that neurasthenic patients were more microsplanchnic whereas those whom he designated emotional neuroses were more macrosplanchnic. His classification of neurosis and lack of statistical treatment make acceptance of his findings difficult.

GREENWOOD and SMITH (1934) following the work of BOLDRINI (1925), and using his index of $\dfrac{\text{chest circumference}}{\text{stature}}$ instead of VIOLA's index, found correlations to the order of $+ .23$ between the index and anxiety and obsessional symptoms.

Followers of the Kretschmerian school carried out a great deal of research into the temperamental and personality correlates of

KRETSCHMER's physical types (REES, 1959). More recently BRATGARD (1950) investigated the relationship between personality attitude and body build in a series of 1000 patients attending a psychiatric clinic. This investigation is particularly interesting because ratings of personality attitude had been made some time before body build had been assessed by means of STROMGREN's (1937) index. It was found that syntonic attitudes were associated with a pyknic physique, whereas psychasthenic attitudes were associated with leptosomatic body build.

Factorial studies

BURT (1938), in a factorial analysis of a group of schoolchildren found low correlations between stoutness and cheerful emotions on the one hand and between thinness and inhibitive and repressive tendencies on the other.

Using body build indices derived from factorial analysis of physique for the study of relationships between physical type, personality and neurosis, REES and EYSENCK (1942) investigated 1000 soldiers and REES (1950a) a similar study on 400 women serving in the Armed Forces and suffering from neurosis using the regression equation already described. In both men and women it was found that leptomorphs tended towards dysthymic symptoms and traits, whereas eurymorphs tended towards hysterical traits and symptoms. Leptomorphs had a greater tendency to introversion and schizothymic, tendencies, whereas eurymorphs tended to be more extrovert and cyclothymic, thus confirming KRETSCHMER's hypothesis. The leptomorph also had a higher incidence of somatic manifestations of emotional tension and autonomic dysfunction. This is in conformity with the study of SANFORD (1943) on normal children and REES (1945) who found that patients suffering from effort syndrome tended to be more leptomorphic, in physique than the normal population and that leptomorphic patients in the group tended to have a lifelong history of symptoms of autonomic dysfunction in contrast to the smaller number of eurymorphic effort syndrome patients, in whom exogenous rather than constitutional factors were more important in the aetiology.

Studies using SHELDON's somatotypes

SHELDON (1942) described very high correlations between his physical components, and three components of temperament described by him: namely between endomorphy and viscerotonia +.79, between mesomorphy and somatotonia +.82, between ectomorphy and cerebrotonia +.83 per cent.

HUMPHRIES (1957) severely criticizes SHELDON's methods and states that the evidence provided by SHELDON supports the existence of not more than two independent (but necessarily valid) types of temperament and he applied similar criticisms to the three-fold component classification of physique.

The investigation of FISK (1944) and TANNER (1956) provided little to support SHELDON's claims for high correlations between somatotype and temperament.

DAVIDSON, McINNIS and PARNELL (1957) studied 100 school children and found that anxiety was associated with ectomorphy but that the correlations between somatotype and psychological attributes were of a low order.

Studies based on LINDEGARD's method

LINDEGARD and NYMAN (1956) found that the muscle factor correlated with the SJÖBRING's personality trait-validity (relating to expansivity and self-confidence versus unobtrusiveness) both muscle and fat factors were negatively correlated with "stability" (emotional warmth versus coolness).

The temperamental and neurotic correlates of body size

From the results of factorial analysis already described, a body build index was devised consisting of the product of stature and transverse chest diameter. The frequency distribution curve of this index approached the normal type with some positive skewness. Using demarcation points of one standard deviation above and below the mean, the group was divided into three classes

    1. those of small size, microsomatics,

    2. those of medium size or mesosomatics, and

    3. those of large size or macrosomatics.

The results are presented in detail by REES (1950), who concluded that the general picture emerging from the study was, that neurotics of large body size tend to be more active, to have more stable personalities, better musculature, even a higher intellectual level and a better prognosis for return to military duties. There was little to suggest that the small person who developed a neurotic illness had shown evidence of overcompensation of an agressiv or dominating behaviour. Instead they showed a high incidence of weak, dependent and timid personalities and of anxiety and hypochondriacal personality traits. It is interesting to note that the psychological correlates of body size are different from those associated with body type and that whereas the eurymorph and eptomorph tend to be associated with hysterical and anxiety reactions respectively the latter showed no significant differences between the groups classified according to body size.

Bodily disproportions

Seltzer (1946) investigated a group of students by means of anthropometric measurements and he calculated a large number of body build indices. If a patient had an index value which diverged markedly from the mean, it was designated disproportion which was not intended to indicate abnormality but rather a normal deviate from the mean of the group as a whole. He found that disproportions were more frequent among individuals with unstable autonomic nervous systems. Linear patients were twice as frequent in disproportions. Disproportions were least common in marked endomorphs and marked mesomorphs.

Conclusions

We may summarize by stating that the available evidence shows that the study of associations between a large number of different physical attributes with temperamental characteristics and neurotic illnesses although frequently revealing statistically significant correlations, these were usually small and in the region of 2 to 3 and, are not great enough to supplant the more direct methods of assessing personality, or neurosis or to serve the needs of diagnosis.

If future research using new methods and techniques provides evidence of a greater correlation between physical attributes and personality and susceptibility to psychiatric disorders there will still be the question of the precise nature of the factors responsible for these associations.

Two main hypotheses may be postulated:

1. that the associations are an outcome of the person's life experiences arising conditioning processes linking certain psychological attributes to particular physical traits.

2. As Rees (1959) points out a more probable explanation is that they are integrated biological relations between different constitu-

tional aspects and that the association may prove to be genetic with the genes responsible for body build exerting a modifying influence on the manifestation of inherited aspects of personality and the genetically determined psychiatric illnesses.

There is an urgent need for further genetic research in this field particularly in combination with longitudinal growth studies which should provide scientifically valid data for the elucidation of relationships between physique, personality and disease.

Bibliography

BENEKE, F.W.: Die anatomischen Grundlagen der Konstitutionsanomalien des Menschen (Marburg 1898).

BOLDRINI, M.: Sivluppo corporeo e predisposizioni morbose, Vita e Pensiero (Milan 1925).

BOLDRINI, M., and MENGARELLI, C.: Comit. Ital Stud. Prob. Pripol. Atti Roma *195*: 3-27 (1933).

BRATTGARD, S.O.: Personality attitude and physical make-up. Acta Psychial. Neurol. scand. *354*: 339-354 (1950).

BURT, C.: The analysis of temperament. Brit. J. Med. Psychol. *17*: 518 (1938).

COPPEN, A.J.: Psychosomatic aspects of pre-eclamptic toxaemia. J. Psychosom. Res. *2*, (1957).

DAVIDSON, M.A.; McINNES, R.G., and PARNELL, R.W.: The distribution of personality traits in seven-year-old children. Brit. J. Educ. Psychol. *27*: 48-61 (1957).

EKMAN, G.: On typological and dimensional systems of reference in describing personality. Acta. Psychol. *8*: 1-24 (1951).

FISKE, D.W.: A study of relationship to somatotype. J. Appl. Psychol. *28*: 504 (1944).

GIOVANNI, DI.A.: Clinical Commentaries deduced from the morphology of the body. Tr. by Eyre, London and New York 1919.

GREENWOOD, M., and SMITH, M.: Brit. J. Med. Psychol. *14* (1934).

HOWELLS, W.W.: A factorial study of constitutional type. Amer. J. Physiol. Anthropol. *10*: 91-118 (1952).

HUMPHREYS, L.G.: Characteristics of type concepts with special reference to Sheldon's typology. Psychol. Bull. *54*: 218-228 (1957).

KRETSCHMER, E.: Körperbau und Charakter (Springer, Berlin 1921).

LASKER, G.W.: The effects of partial starvation on somatotype. Amer. J. Physiol. Anthropol. *5*: 323-341 (1947).

LINDEGARD, B.: Variations in Human Body Build (Copenhagen, Munksgaard (1953).

LINDEGARD, B., and NYMAN, E.G.: Male sex characters in relation to body build, endocrine activity and personality. Body Build, Body Function and Personality (Ed. B. LINDEGARD 1956).

NACCARATI, S.: The morphological basis of the psychoneuroses. Am. J. Psychot. *3*: 527 (1924).

NEWMAN, R.W.: Age changes in body build. Amer. J. Phys. Anthropol. *10*: *75* (1952).

PARNELL, R.W.: Physique and performance. Brit. Med. J. *2*: 491 (1954a).

PARNELL, R.W.: The relationship of masculine and feminine physical traits .. academie and athletic performance. Brit. J. Med. Psychol. *28*: 247 (1954b).

REES, L.: Physical constitution in relation to effort syndrome, neurotic and psychotic types. M.D. Thesis, Univ. Wales (1943).

REES, L.: Physique and Effort syndrome. J. ment. Sci. *9*: 89 (1945).

REES, L., and EYSENCK, H.J.: A factorial study of some morphological and psychological aspects of human constitution. J. ment. Sci. *91*: 8 (1945).

REES, L.: Physical and psychological apsects of constitution. Eugen. Rev. *37*: 635–638 (1945).

REES, L.: Body size, personality and neurosis. J. ment. Sci. *96*: 168 (1950a).

REES, L.: A factorial study of physical constitution in women. J. ment. Sci. *96*: 620–632 (1950b).

REES, L.: Body build, personality and neurosis in women. J. ment. Sci. *96*: 426–434 (1950c).

REES, L.: Chapter on constitution and abnormal behavior in text book of Abnormal Psychology, ed. by H.J. EYSENCK, in the press, 1959.

REYNOLDS, E.L.: The fat/bone index as a sex differentiating character in man. Human. Biol. *21*: 199–204 (1949).

REYNOLDS, E.L., and ASAKAWA, T.: A comparison of certain aspects of body structure and body shape in 200 adults. Amer. J. Physiol. Anthropol. *8*: 343–365 (1950).

SANFORD, R.N.; ADKINS, M.M.; MILLER, R.B., and COBB, E.A.: Physique, personality and scholarship. Washington Soc. Res. Child. Develpm. nat. Res. Council (1943).

SELTZER, C.C., and BROUHA, L.: The "masculine" component and physical fitness. Amer. J. Physiol. Anthrop. *1*: 95 (1943).

SELTZER, C.C., and BROUHA, L.: Body disproportions and dominant personality tracts. Psychosom. Med. *8*: 75 (1946).

SILLS, F.D.: A factor analysis of somatotypes and their relationship to achievements in motor skills. Res. Quart. *21*: 424–437 (1950).

SHELDON, W.H.; STEVENS, S.S., and TUCKER, W.B.: The Varieties of Human Physique (Harper & Bros., New York 1940).

SHELDON, W.H., and STEVENS, S.S.: The Varieties of Temperament (Harper & Bros., New York 1942).

STROMGREN, E.: Über anthropometrische Indices zur Unterscheidung von Körperbautypen. Z. ges. Neurol. Psychiat. *159*: 75–81 (1937).

STUART, H.C., and SOBEL, E.H.: The thickness of the skin and subcutaneous tissue by age and sex in childhood. J. Pediat. *26*: 637–647 (1946).

TANNER, J.M.: Current advances study of physique. Lancet *1*: 514 (1951).

TANNER, J.M.: Physique, character and disease. Lancet *2*: 635–637 (1956).

VIOLA, G.: La constituzione individuale. Copelli, Bologna 1937.

WRETMARK, G.: The peptic ulcer individual. Acta. Psychiat. et Neurol. Scand. Supp. 84 (Munksgaard, Copenhagen 1953).

Author's address: DR. L. REES, Maudsley Hospital, *London S.E.* 5 (England).

A Modern Psychosomatic View of the Theory of Organ Inferiority by Alfred Adler

H. Hoff and E. Ringel, Wien

It is now 50 years since Alfred Adler published his great work «Minderwertigkeit von Organen» (Organ Inferiority). In this study he discussed the matter of predisposition to disease, a question which is of major importance in the whole realm of medicine. On the basis of a large case-history volume, Adler formulated the premise that general hereditary influences are not so significant as familial constitutional predispositions relating to specific systems of organs. It is perhaps difficult for us today to realize how revolutionary such a concept was in Adler's own time, as we now accept his ideas as more or less self-evident truths.

Adler pointed out that his theories provided the only possible logical basis for many otherwise unexplained symptom-complexes, and for certain conclusions derived from experimental pathology. He was firmly convinced of the significance of his theories concerning organ-inferiority within the entire scope of the neuroses. The inferiority of specific organs in childhood, he believed, frequently established marked psychological patterns of self-debasement, anxiety and inhibition. Such symptoms, according to Adler's concept, eventually culminate either in total discouragement or in over-compensation. Adler did not live to know that his theories established him as one of the fathers of modern psychosomatic medicine. His ideas were unique in his own day. When we read his word today, that "even the course of infectious disorders may be influenced by organ-inferiority" we can appreciate even more fully the true significance of his contribution to modern psychosomatic medicine.

One factor of prime importance in ADLER's theories concerns the influences which determine the specificity of localization of organ-inferiority. It was significantly pointed out by STERN that "the tendency of psychotraumatic experiences to be manifested in somatic phenomena makes use of preparate possibilities within the individual human being for their realization". In such cases both congenital and acquired organ inferiorities play an obviously significant rôle. ADLER strongly emphasized this component of his original theory. Every human being, he taught, has an "Achilles Heel"—a deficiency—somewhere within his organic heritage. This weakness may be localized within the gastro-intestinal tract, the cardiovascular system or the uro-genital tract. It follows, ADLER taught, that released conflicts are localized within the gastrointestinal tract, the cardio-vascular system or the uro-genital tract. It follows, ADLER taught, that released conflicts are localized within deficient portion or portions of the individual's organ-system. In one individual a psycho-traumatic experience, for instance, may be manifested as diarrhea; in another it may result in a headache, in still another an uncontrollable urge to urinate, in yet another a cardiac disturbance. Regardless of the extent to which ADLER's ideas are at present accepted by the general public, the fact remains that they are considered of major importance by the orthodox FREUDIAN School, as KEMPER has emphasized. We are in hearty agreement with this, and firmly believe that ADLER's theories of organ-inferiority constitute an essential part of the entire structure of modern psychosomatic medicine.

In conducting our study we investigated 100 patients at random in our psychosomatic wards with special reference to possible familial predispositions to malfunction in specific organs or organ-systems. Thereby we searched not alone for hereditary predispositions to diseases as such, but for signs of specific organ-inferiority. We conducted this search by assembling data from the patients themselves, their siblings, their parents, grandparents, and the brothers and sisters of the parents. We used only proved, objective data. In some cases our data were assembled through direct interviews with the persons concerned. It is a matter of discussion whether a single familial stress situation (load) affecting a specific organ system is a true sign of an existing organ-inferiority. Our criterion for a "positive" finding was the discovery of several identical organ-inferiorities in members of a single family. In our series of 100 unselected patients we found that 54 fulfilled the requirements of our test criterion, demonstrating specific organ-inferiorities within individual families. This result, we felt, offered undeniable evidence in favour of ADLER's theories. But before interpreting our study in further detail we shall discuss briefly our psychosomatic concept as a whole.

Table 1. Etiology of psychosomatic diseases

---

1. Development of a neurotic conflict in early childhood (dermal, oral and anal phasis)
2. The neurotic conflict affects the organ system which at the time of onset is most emotionally involved
3. Development of psychosomatic pattern of reaction in the child
4. Re-appearance of the psychosomatic pattern of reaction established in childhood under the influence of a precipitating trauma

---

Psychosomatic disease

It is our belief that certain psychosomatic diseases demonstrate the basic characteristics of the neuroses in that the groundwork of both is laid in early childhood, and that after a variable latent period both become manifest following an experience of stress (we are speaking now only of neuroses which are capable of producing organic changes). In this connection we recall that the psychosomatic reaction patterns of childhood, are based, in psychoanalytic terms, upon areas of localization known as the dermal, the oral, the anal, the urethral and the genital. This terminology, of course, is utilized to express the usual areas of emotional preoccupation in the child. If a neurotic conflict arises, it becomes manifest in one or more of these areas of sensitivity. The nature of the area response to conflict is dependent upon two factors:

1. The type of conflict.
2. The age at which the conflict appears.

Concerning point 1 KÜHNEL and SCHWIDDER expressed the opinion that one cannot neglect the correlation between certain instinctual impulses (conscious or unconscious) and certain specific functions of organs. Referring to point 2 KEMPER states that "whether a child is subjected to psychological trauma at the age of 3 months, 9 months or 3 years is a matter of no small significance". We would like to add that on each and every occasion of psychic trauma a different area of sensitivity becomes the object of a psychosomatic pattern of reactions. We know that in all probability what we call today, psychosomatics such patterns are not predetermined in childhood: we differentiate, in the theory of neurosis, between true neurosis (originating in childhood) and neurotic reactions, which are caused by actual difficulties in the life situation. In the same way one must differentiate between true psychosomatic disease and psychosomatic reactions. In the case of certain psychosomatic disturbances we cannot determine, in the present stage of medical knowledge, to which category they belong. This is particularly understandable when one considers the difficulties attendant upon retrograds research into the problems of childhood.

Returning to the question of the true significance of ADLER's theories of organ inferiority, what is its relationship within the foregoing concept of psychosomatic medicine as a diagnostic and therapeutic entity? A more detailed differentiation of our case material with special reference to specific diseases will offer further information.

Our 100 cases are distributed among the following groups of diseases.

Table 2

Diseases		Familial organ-inferiority in:
of the gastro-intestinal tract (gastritis, ulcus, colitis, obstipation, cachexia nervos)	29	20
Cardio-vascular disorders (hypertonia, hypotonia, nervous tension)	21	15
Vegetative neurosis.........................	20	1
Disease of the skin (eczema, pruritus)	16	13
Bronchial asthma...........................	6	4
Spondyloarthrosis	4	0
of the urogenital tract (adnexia)	4	1
Total	100	54 cases

We recognize the limitations involved in our study, and we realize further that not all psychosomatic disorders have been considered, and in the case of some, the group under consideration has been small. On the other hand we believe that in view of the fact that our study involved a comprehensive and unselected group of patients, representing a true cross-section of our admissions, we are justified in rendering valid conclusions.

First one may say that the importance of organ-inferiority is not of the same degree in all psychosomatic diseases. Besides diseases in which the correlation with organ inferiority is high, we have observed cases in which such a relationship does not exist. We have observed over a period of years in cases other than those in our present series that our findings are more than merely incidental: invariably we have found that organ inferiority, especially in psychosomatic diseases related to the gastrointestinal tract and skin, are of much more significance than in other disturbances. If one seeks an explanation for this fact one must take into consideration that in the former psychosomatic disorders the organ inferiority plays a special rôle in which the psychosomatic pattern of reaction is already established in childhood. Now here may such an immature reaction—pattern be more commonly found than in diseases of the skin and in disturbances of the gastrointestinal tract. Less often we have found an immature reaction-pattern related to bronchial asthma, which also shows a relatively high correlation to an existing organ inferiority. This was clearly shown also in our Present series, especially in patients with diseases of the gastrointestinal tract and skin.

In all these cases the following two factors work together during childhood to bring into flower the symptoms of psychosomatic disease:

1. The development of a neurotic conflict (corresponding to the type of individual and his age at the time of onset) which leads to a certain psychosomatic pattern of reaction.

2. A specific organ-inferiority in the organ or organ-system in which the psychosomatic pattern of reaction is established.

When one examines these factors in proper perspective, important conclusions emerge:

a) It cannot be postulated that familial constitutional predispositions alone are responsible for the appearance of psychosomatic disease in specific organs or organ-systems. ADLER himself was well aware of this, emphasizing in his original study that inferior organs sometimes functioned perfectly throughout the life, failing to break down under stress as otherwise might have been expected. To explain this ADLER introduced his concept of "relative" organ inferiority, where in the inferiority of an organ becomes evident only during an attack of illness, or where overcompensation in the inferior organ provides the sole indication of such. But we believe that other factors, too, influence the appearance of disease in an inferior organ. ADLER prouped these together as the influence of "casual events". We believe this term to be a misnomer, as we do not recognize the existence of "casual" events. This leads us to our next conclusions:

b) In our opinion the idea that a psychosomatic pattern of reaction inevitably must develop in an inferior organ merely because it *is* inferior, is false. Actually, localization of the psychosomatic pattern is greatly dependent upon the type of neurotic conflict and its time of onset. If these factors happen to unite to localize the diesease in inferior organ, the probabilities are increased that a fixation will occur for the duration of the patient's life. On the other hand we have observed numerous instances in which early psychosomatic reactions faded and never again reappeared. In none of these cases, however, were we able to find evidence of organ-inferiority. We conclude from these observations that chronic psychosomatic disease develops only the genetic factors we have outlined combined with later stresses in a certain, specific proportion. We see an analogous situation in the genesis of psychosis. In our opinion a psychosis can be created by many complicated correlated factors acting in concert. When even one such factor in the multifactorial chain is suppressed and the inter-lationship correspondingly disturbed, a psychosis exists.

c) The earlier a psychosomatic disease occurs, the greater is the importance of organ-inferiority in its genesis. On the other hand in cases characterized by actual conflict, or "psychosomatic reaction", organ-inferiority seems to be relatively less significant. The genesis and course of neurosis originating from the autonomic nervous system including hyperthyroidism; rheumatic affections, spondylo-arthrosis and susceptibility to infections are primarily dependent upon actual events (specific conflicts, types of reactions, etc.). It is interesting in this connection to note the relatively slight significance of an organ inferiority in the selection of a specific organ or organ system in which a vegetative neurosis is already manifested.

The vegetative neurosis is seldom established in an inferiority organ system. This may be carefully explained by the fact that a vegetative neurosis seldom produces a long-lasting organ defect. KAUDERS describes this as a protective mechanism. The genesis, the therapy and the prognosis together thus constitute a different problem from that in true psychosomatic disease.

It was interesting to observe in our investigation a relatively high correlation of organ-inferiority to cardio-vascular disease, especially where hypertonia was associated. By analogy one can conclude that even in these diseases a reaction-pattern was developed in childhood, a theory which cannot readily be proved. The development of specific pattern of reactions in childhood culminating in this type of disorder is not easily proved, but in our opinion must exist. We believe that we have pointed out that the theory of organ-inferiority by ALFRED ADLER provides a valuable supplement to psychosomatic knowledge as a whole, and that through it organ fixation rather than organ selection has been given due emphasis. We use the term "supplement" advisedly, as we cannot ignore the contributions of psychoanalysis to this field—particularly those of the School of ALEXANDER, which emphasizes the specificity of certain conflicts for certain diseases. Thus, to achieve its proper perspective in a modern psychosomatic scheme ADLER's theory of organic inferiority requires not only psychoanalytic supplementation but psychoanalytical interpretation to render it valid.

ADLER himself pointed out that even the child is naturally inclined to concentrate on his inferior organ. What the child does not know is hat this parents are characterized by an identical organ-inferiority. An individual's whole destiny may be altered or at least influenced by this fact. The child not only has been endowed with a negative predisposition, so to speak, but he becomes aware of undue emphasis of the inferior organ on the part of the parents. From such situation neurotic "ceremonials" within the family frequently developed, particularly where diseases of the gastrointestinal tract, skin affections and migraine are concerned. Here the famous words of WAGNER-JAUREGG are so apt: "The defective forebear damaged his descendant in a double way: first he passes on a negative inheritance then he forces his descendant to live with him."

JORES has pointed out that "the mechanism of the identification (shown by psychoanalysis) through the inferior organ of itself compelled the child's attention as the focus of interest". Such forced attention over long period of time undoubtedly irritates the inferior organ and perhaps thereby increases its susceptibility to malfunction.

Finally, it should be emphasized that while organ-inferiority of itself may and often does influence the individual's whole mode of life, this influence may be modified by psychodynamic factors which affect the organ, such as incorrect dietary habits, faulty hygienic mode of life, overindulgence, etc. Such factors obviously can "tip the scale" and weaken still further an already inferior organ.

In summing up, one may say that psychosomatic medicine in its modern sense is no more reactivation of ancient medical ideas concerning the relationship between body and psyche. Far more than this, psychosomatic medicine today represents the introduction of complex psychological theories into the etiology of certain disease and a corresponding emphasis not only on the role of psychoanalysis but on that played by individual psychology.

The theory of organ-inferiority by ALFRED ADLER represents not alone a useful contribution but can be considered an indispensable adjunct in the management of psychosomatic disease.

Bibliography

ADLER, A.: Studie über Minderwertigkeit von Organen (Verlag Urban & Schwarzenberg, München 1907).

ALEXANDER, F.: Psychosomatische Medizin (Berlin 1951).

HOFF, H.: Zur Kritik des Begriffes der Manager-Krankheit. Acta Psychother. *III* (1955).

HOFF, H., und RINGEL, E.: Zur Therapie psycho-somatischer Erkrankungen. Z. Psychosomat. Med. *IV*: 1 (1957).

JORES, A.: Der Mensch und seine Krankheit (Klett-Verlag, Stuttgart 1956).

KAUDERS, O.: Vegetatives Nervensystem und Seele (Urban & Schwarzenberg, München 1946).

KEMPER, W.: Persönlichkeitsstruktur, Konfliktart, Organwahl und psychosomat. Medizin. Z. Psychosom. Med. *IV*: 3 (1958).

KÜHNEL, G., und SCHWIDDER, W.: Stellungnahme zum Problem der Spezifität der Persönlichkeitstypen. Z. Psychosom. Med. *IV*: 3 (1958).

SCHULTZ-HENKE, H.: Lehrbuch der analyt. Psychotherapie (Thieme, Stuttgart 1954).

STERN, E.: Zum Problem der Spezifität der Persönlichkeitstypen und der Konflikte in der psychosomat. Medizin. Z. Psychosom. Med. *IV*: 3 (1958).

WAGNER-JAUREGG, J.: Über erbliche Belastung (1902).

Authors' addresses: DR. H. HOFF and DR. E. RINGEL, Psychiatrische Universitätsklinik, *Wien* (Austria).

Über Psyche und Konstitution in analytischer Sicht

R. LAFORGUE, Paris

Diese Arbeit war ursprünglich als Beitrag zur Festschrift anlässlich des siebzigsten Geburtstages von PROFESSOR KRETSCHMER gedacht. Wir wissen, wie bahnbrechend KRETSCHMER mit seinen Arbeiten über den sensitiven Beziehungswahn sowie über Körperbau und Charakter geworden ist. Wir müssen trachten, auch dem Künstler in ihm gerecht zu werden, demjenigen der uns die richtige Sicht gewiesen hat. Mit sicherem Blick hat KRETSCHMER den Unterschied zwischen den Charakteren der Leptosomen, der Pykniker und der Displastiker erkannt, davon ausgehend die Mischformen der verschiedenen Typen dargestellt und die Konstitutionslehre ein gutes Stück weitergebracht. Was kann die Psychoanalyse uns auf diesem Wege bringen?

Der Psychoanalytiker kann feststellen, dass es ihm nie gelingen wird, aus dem Charakter eines Leptosomen den eines Pyknikers oder eines Athletikers herauszuarbeiten. Er kann nur dazu beitragen, die Konfliktsituationen, die sich für jeden Typus auf dem Gebiet seines Charakters und seiner Konstitution ergeben, so oder so bewältigen zu helfen.

Zwischen Charakter, Körperbau und Konstitution gibt es eine von der Natur geschaffene Beziehung, sei es eine ererbte oder eine durch das Milieu in jahrhundertelanger Anpassung oder durch Zuchtwahl geschaffene. Spanische Typenforscher und Psychiater haben schon ebenso wie wir auf das Vorherrschen des leptosomen «Wüstentypus» in der Sahara hingewiesen, eines Typus ebenso häufig zu beobachten bei Arabern wie bei Berbern, so wie es JOSÉ SOLÉ-SOGARRA in seinem Beitrag zu oben erwähnter Festschrift darlegt. Wenn man bedenkt, dass, so wie Solé-Sogarra es aussagt, «der schlanke und geschmeidige «Wüstentyp» das spanische Substrat bildet, das aus der langschädeligen, mediterran-afrikanischen oder der ibero-afrikanischen Gruppe besteht», so kann man dem Bedürfnis schwer standhalten versuchen zu wollen, sich ein Bild über die Milieubedingtheit dieses Types und der dazugehörigen Konstitution zu machen um zu begreifen, inwieweit der Charakter zur Schaffung einer Konstitution beiträgt und umgekehrt der Körperbau und die Konstitution zur Schaffung eines Charakters.

Nach Solé-Sogarra sind ca. 58% aller Spanier Leptosome. Ohne eine genaue Statistik gemacht zu haben, dürfen wir annehmen, dass ca. 50 bis 60% der Südfranzosen es ebenfalls sind und zu dieser Körperbaugruppe gehören. Was den Leptosomen-Charakter anbetrifft, so meint Solé-Sogarra, dass nach Angaben erfahrener Gerichtsärzte der Anteil der Pykniker an den Verbrechen niedriger ist als der Anteil an der Bevölkerung im allgemeinen, d. h. bei den Leptosomen, die danach den weitaus grössten Prozentsatz der Verbrecher stellen, und denen erst in zweiter Linie die Athletiker folgen. Schön weist Solé-Sogarra auf die Analogie hin zwischen dem Typus der Leptosomen und dem des Don Quichotte und jener zwischen dem der Pykniker und Sancho Pansa. Aber damit wäre für einen Psychoanalytiker, der Gelegenheit hatte, den leptosomen «Wüstentypus» in Nordafrika von nahem zu studieren, die Frage nicht befriedigend beantwortet. Man muss sich vorstellen, dass wir es da mit ca. 80% von Leptosomen zu tun haben, deren Konstitution wesentlich durch den Einfluss der Wüste und die dort entwickelte Mentalität markiert ist. Wir haben es in dieser Hinsicht dort mit einer Art von Reinkultur eines Menschentypes zu tun, und wir können bei dieser Gelegenheit deshalb da leichter die Beziehungen zwischen der Psyche und der Konstitution dieses Menschenschlages studieren als anderswo. Natürlich müssen wir uns vorläufig damit begnügen, die Wechselbeziehungen zwischen Umwelt, Psyche und leptosomer Konstitution zu beobachten, um an Hand der so gesammelten Erfahrungen jene zwischen Psyche und Wald, Berg oder Meer und anderen Konstitutionen besser beurteilen zu lernen.

Um sich ein richtiges Bild über die Formung der Psyche dieses «Wüstentypus» zu machen, müssen wir uns etwas mit deren Schaffung, d. h. mit der sie bildenden Volksmentalität, beschäftigen, jener die zur Formung dieser Psyche und der dazugehörigen Konstitution wesentlich beigetragen hat. Am leichtesten begreift man diese Mentalität da, wo sie sich nicht auf sozialem oder religiösem Gebiet sondern auf dem der Kunst ausgewirkt hat.

Tatsache ist, dass der Stil der Kunst des Islams auf der ganzen Bandbreite der Wüste – von Marokko über Arabien bis nach Indien hin – etwas in seinen Formen ganz typisch Einheitliches hat ebenso wie der dort verbreitete Menschentypus. Die Baukunst wurde ursprünglich den Arabern von Byzanz überliefert, und die ersten Moscheen in Kairo und auch in Jerusalem – von den Omeiaden erbaut – haben noch das Gepräge, das ihnen die byzantinischen Architekten und Künstler gegeben haben, so wie z. B. die Säulen mit dem Säulenkapitell, in das sich die griechischen Acantusblätter zart einschmiegen. Aber bald sind auch diese Acantusblätter verschwunden, denn die bildende Kunst durfte sich nur entwickeln mit einer durch geometrische Zeichen stereotyp charakterisierten Ornamentik, da der Islam, dem Charakter des «Wüstentypus» gemäss, die Abbildung von Mensch, Tier und Pflanze verbietet und auf dieser Basis die Ornamentik depersonalisiert in einer Weise, wie wir es in den Zeichnungen gewisser Schizophrener beobachten können. Einen besonderen Platz in dieser Ornamentik nimmt die Arabeske ein, d. h. die rhythmisch schwankende, schmiegsame Linie, so wie sie auch in der arabischen Schrift zum Ausdruck kommt, ebenso wie in der Tanzkunst, wo das Bestreben der Tänzerin nicht auf einen erotischen Exhibitionismus des Körpers und seiner Formen hinauszielt sondern hauptsächlich auf die rhythmische Darstellung der Arabeske, d. h. jener Linien, die in der Schrift mit ihrem Auf und Ab und auch in der Vokalisierung der Sprache mit ihrem eintönigen Näseln oder in der monophonen Musik ihr Spiegelbild finden. Die arabische Sprache ist eine Wurzelsprache und keine Assoziationssprache. Im Gegensatz zu letzterer werden ihre Elemente nicht affektiv durch Assoziationen aneinandergekettet, sondern sie verfügt über verhältnismässig wenig Sprachwurzeln (ungefähr 3000), die durch Töne charakterisiert sind, d. h. durch eine Vokalisierung, die je nach Tönen, dem Näseln, der Art der Vokale den Wurzeln erst ihren richtigen Sinn geben.

Um die Rolle der Arabeske in Kunst, Schrift und Psyche richtig verstehen zu können, muss man sich im klaren darüber sein, unter welch ganz besonderen Bedingungen sich die Volksmentalität der Araber gebildet hat. Grenzenlos, d. h. uneingeengt von natürlichen Schranken, zieht sich die Sandwüste, die der Sahara sowie der anderen, dahin und auch zeitenlos in dem Sinne, als es keine richtigen Jahreszeiten gibt sondern nur Tag oder Nacht, eine glühende Sonne oder einen endlosen, sternenklaren Himmel. In diesem Raum, wo alle künstlichen Schranken rasch durch Sand verdeckt werden, findet sich der Mensch vornehmlich durch seinen Gesichtssinn zurecht: Er ist zugeteilt und nicht zugehörig, zugeteilt wie die Individuen einer Herde, die allen sichtbar abgestempelt sind und nicht zugehörig zu einer im Boden harmonisch verwurzelten Natur wie Pflanzen und Bäume, die nicht nur auf das Auge sondern auch auf das Ohr wirken. So ist der Wüstenmensch hauptsächlich Nomade geworden, zum Teil Hirte, und nur in wenigen Gebieten, den Oasen, ist er Ackerbauer, d. h. an den Boden gebunden und an ein lebendes Bild der Natur.

Die Wüste mit ihren unerbittlichen klimatischen Verhältnissen ist eine harte Mutter, die nur spärlich ihre Kinder ernähren kann und nur unter der Bedingung, dass die Schwachen und am wenigsten Angepassten rücksichtslos ausgerottet werden, was eine ganz besondere Zuchtwahl bedingt.

Die Art, wie der Mensch sich diesen Lebensbedingungen angepasst hat, und wie er die Forderungen der ihn umgebenden Natur übernommen hat und verarbeitet, ist das für die Formung der Psyche des «Wüstentypus» Charakteristische und benötigt, dass wir etwas genauer darauf eingehen, umso mehr als es dem Europäer fast unmöglich ist, aus seinen eigenen Erfahrungen heraus sich ein richtiges Bild zu machen über die Natur des Wüstenmenschen. Erst wenn wir uns eine konkrete Vorstellung über die Formung dieser Psyche verschafft haben, können wir versuchen mit einigem Glück, uns ein Bild über ihren Einfluss auf Charakter und Konstitution zu schaffen.

Die Erfahrungen, die wir in Europa bei der Beobachtung unserer Frustrierten erworben haben, helfen uns beim Aufbau dieses konkreten Bildes. Unsere Frustrierten entwickeln eine ähnliche Struktur der Psyche wie jene des Wüstenmenschen mit dem Unterschied, dass sie unter ihrer Frustriertheit gewöhnlich leiden und dieselbe sie daran hindert, sich in das bei uns herrschende soziale Milieu zu gewöhnen, während im Gegenteil beim «Wüstentypus» wir selber eine persönliche Schwierigkeit haben, uns in das dort sich entfaltende soziale Leben zu integrieren, wobei gerade die Struktur der Psyche des «Wüstentypus» denselben ganz hervorragend dazu befähigt, sich den herrschenden sozialen und Naturzuständen anzupassen und eine ihnen adäquate Gesellschaftsordnung aufzubauen. Diese letztere hat mit der unsrigen in Wirklichkeit trotz äusserem Anschein sehr wenig gemeinsam. Aber es ist uns doch leichter, uns an die arabische Psyche zu assimilieren, als es dem Wüstenmenschen möglich ist mit seinem in Jahrtausenden durch Zuchtwahl kultivierten Rassetypus sich an das Europäische zu adaptieren. Mit anderen Worten: die arabische Psyche assimiliert in Nordafrika den Europäer und nicht der Europäer das Arabische, welche Illusionen man sich oft über diese Tatsachen machen kann, wenn man nur einen kolonialistischen Standpunkt einnimmt oder nur an die Werte der modernen Kultur glaubt und vermeint, durch Überzeugung und Beispiel den Wüstenmenschen zur Europäisierung bekehren zu können. Erst nördlich eines gewissen Breitengrades, wenn der Charakter der Wüste verschwindet, wird es anders so wie z. B. in Spanien und in Süditalien, wo aus den Mauren in Jahrhunderten Spanier mit ihren Leptosomen oder Süditaliener, d. h. Sizilianer und Kalabresen, geworden sind.

Was ist nun für die Struktur der Psyche des Wüstenmenschen ganz gesonders charakteristisch? Am besten ist es, wir gehen nicht nur vom Studium der Kunst des Islams aus, um dies Charakteristische zu verstehen, sondern auch von der psychoanalytischen Forschung über die Psyche der Frustrierten, d. h. über die mentalen Strukturen jener Ich-Gefüge, die wir seit langem analysiert haben in unseren Arbeiten über Schizonoia (seit 1926 in den Arbeiten der französischen psychoanalytischen Schule zusammen mit meinem leider verstorbenen Mitarbeiter PICHON, dem Schwiegersohn von JANET). Wir zeigten damals, wie das frustrierte Kind versucht, die Mutter, die ihm in Wirklichkeit fehlt, zu kompensieren, so dass es in seinem Ich einen besonderen Komplex entwickelt, welcher auf die weitere Ich-Entwicklung des Frustrierten einen ganz besonderen Einfluss hat. Dieser Vorstellungskomplex oder, wie wir analytisch sagen, diese vom Ich übernommene Identifizierung mit der Mutter ist in diesem Falle charakterisiert durch die Substitution der Idee an Stelle der Realität und weiterhin beim frustrierten Kind durch die Substitution der wärmespendenden Exkremente an Stelle der wärmenden Mutterbrust. Diese Substitution ist ein Folge einer narzisstischen Regression des Kindes, dessen affektive Valenzen, die nicht mehr an die Mutter gebunden sind, ihre Sättigung in Eigenbrödelei und bipolarer Ich-Struktur suchen, in gerade jener Struktur, die wir unter dem Namen Schizonoia trotz des Widerspruchs von FREUD vor über 30 Jahren beschrieben haben. In der Folge hatten wir das Glück feststellen zu können, dass FREUD seinen Standpunkt korrigiert hat, und dass Psychoanalytiker wie RENÉ SPITZ in ihren Forschungen über die Frustrierten unsere zuerst aufgestellten Hypothesen bestätigen konnten.

Wie wirkt sich weiterhin bei der Ich-Entwicklung des Frustrierten diese Kompensation der Mutter durch einen Ich-Anteil des Frustrierten aus, oder besser gesagt, wie entfaltet sich der Einfluss eines unter solchen Umständen entwickelten mütterlichen Über-Ichs?

Die Übernahme der Haltung der frustrierenden Mutter durch das Ich des Frustrierten ist besonders deutlich von SPITZ beschrieben worden. Er stellt fest, in wie hohem Grade die frustrierten Kinder wirklichkeitsabgewandt sind, in sich versunken hauptsächlich mit ihren Exkrementen spielend, mit Kot oder Urin genauso wie wir es bei schmierigen schizophrenen Patienten beobachten können. Diesen wärmespendenden Exkrementen unterschiebt das Ich des Frustrierten in der Folge die fixen Ideen der abstrakten Formeln, mit denen man spielt oder spekuliert, die glänzenden Steine oder auch die Metalle, wie Silber und Gold, die eine grosse Anziehungskraft entwickeln. Kurzum es ergibt sich so bei ihm eine besondere Fähigkeit für Abstraktion und Spekulation, um die Bindungen an von der Natur gegebene Werte durch Bindungen an leblose Objekte zu kompensieren, die Mutter und Natur ersetzen, was beim Frustrierten ein grosses Allmachtsgefühl entwickelt. Dies bedingt beim Individuum nicht nur eine Introversion sondern vor allen Dingen eine Inversion der Appetenzen. Das für uns Schöne und Anziehende wird bei ihm ersetzt durch harte oft abstossende Materie, durch abstrakte Formeln, durch Zwangsdenken, wobei alles Faulende, Stinkende und Hässliche als Gegenpol des Schönen und Lebendigen den Platz desselben auf dem Gebiet des Geschmacks, der Ästhetik und der Liebe einnimmt. Damit jedoch kommt es bei diesen Frustrierten zu keiner wirklichen Synthese des menschlichen Lebensbildes da letzteres ebenfalls ersetzt wird durch abstrakte Linien und Formen, die dem Antlitz der Mutter unterschoben wurden. Es gelingt auch keine Persönlichkeitssynthese in unserem Sinne, da sich das Kind kein Bild, kein Ebenbild von seiner Mutter machen konnte. Damit scheitert auch die naturgegebene Ich-Synthese auf dem Gebiet der menschlichen Entwicklung, und auch das eigene Bild wird dargestellt durch abstrakte Formeln und Zeichnungen, so wie wir es bei gewissen Schizophrenen beobachten können oder bei modernen Kubisten und Futuristen und vor allen Dingen auch in der Ornamentik der arabischen Kunst. Hier sind wir an dem Punkt angelangt, wo sich das bei uns als pathologisch Betrachtete mit dem bei unserem «Wüstentypus» Normalen kreuzt. Es ist unmöglich für uns, die arabische ganz abstrakte Kunst, das mathematische Denken, das Geometrische der Wellenlinien usw. zu verstehen,

wenn man nicht dazu gekommen ist, das für uns in der Kunst Patholo-
gische mit dem beim Wüstenmenschen Normalen zu vergleichen.
Beim Wüstenmenschen genauso wie bei unseren frustrierten Kranken
kommt es zu keiner wirklichen Synthese des Ebenbildes des Menschen,
weshalb letzteres zerstückelt dargestellt, durch geometrische Steinorna-
mente sozusagen depersonalisiert oder verdaut wiedergegeben wird.

So wirkt sich beim «Wüstentypus» das Gebot von Moses aus:
«Du sollst Dir von Deinem Gott kein Abbild machen», und es ist
kein Zufall, wenn auf dieser Linie beim «Wüstentypus», d. h. das
menschliche Antlitz, das Gottesbild, durch strenge Gebote ersetzt
wird und menschliche Bindung durch strenge Gesetze, welche dem
Affektiven unterschoben sind, und die ihm praktisch oft keine Rech-
nung tragen. Der durch diesen Geist geformte Menschentyp ist normal in der ganzen Bandbreite der Wüste von Afrika bis nach Indien,
und in dieser Bandbreite wird er einwandernde Völker nach kurzer
Zeit ziemlich restlos assimilieren, selbst die romanischen Völker,
deren Kollektiv-Ich sonst eine starke Widerstandskraft entwickelt.
Die Vandalen in Nordafrika dauerten trotz hervorragender militäri-
scher Organisation und Macht nicht länger als 70 Jahre, und auch der
moderne Europäer untersteht dieser zwangsmässigen Assimilation.
Diese Kulturleistung ist den Semiten der Wüste glänzend gelungen.
Wenn wir ihnen auch keine Meisterwerke auf dem Gebiet der bildenden Künste, z. B. der Malerei und der Bildhauerei, verdanken, so
haben sie Grosses geleistet auf dem Gebiet der Mathematik, der
Astrologie, der Alchemie, der Gesetzgebung (ich erinnere an die 10
Gebote) und auch des kritischen und analytischen Geistes. Ich erinnere an die arabischen Zahlen, an die Algebra, d. h. an all jene
Kulturleistungen verrichtet auf dem Gebiet des abstrakten Verstandes,
der glatten Buchführung und Kalkulation, ganz abgesehen von der
oft meisterhaften Organisation dieser Völker auf militärischem Gebiet.

Natürlich wirkt sich dieser Geist entsprechend der oben erwähnten Ich-Struktur und des Charakters durch das Vorherrschen des
Intellektuellen über das Affektive auch ethisch, religiös und sozial aus.

Das dieser Ich-Struktur entsprechende Ideal ist die Allmacht des
einzelnen Menschen in Analogie mit dem Bedürfnis nach Allmacht
des isolierten, frustrierten Kindes, das im Zentrum seiner Welt mit
dem eigenen Kote spielt, allein auf sich gestellt. Dieser Situation entsprechend ist jeder Wüstenmensch allein auf weiter Flur, sein Antlitz
ist verschleiert, vor allen Dingen das der Frauen. Alle reagieren sie
mit demselben Muster nach demselben Modell und sind nach denselben

Mechanismen, denselben Linien und strengen Gesetzen ausgerichtet, innerlich wenn nicht auch äusserlich.

Wie schon gesagt hat auf religiösem Gebiet die Gottheit kein Antlitz und wird wie z. B. in Mekka durch einen Stein, die Kaaba, symbolisiert. Der Gott der Araber, d. h. Allah, ist trotz aller Vertuschungsversuche der Christen, so wie die Araber es betonen, ein einziger Gott, allein auf sich gestellt und keine Dreifaltigkeit im christlichen Sinne, d. h. dreidimensional strukturiert dem occidentalen Bedürfnis entsprechend, was den Christen bei den Arabern den Vorwurf der Vielgötterei einbringt. Und mit dieser abstrakten Gottesfigur, der einzigen, ist der Wüstenmensch mehr verkettet als der Europäer mit dem seinigen. Im wahren Sinne des Wortes stellt dieser unsichtbare Gott ja sein Vaterland dar, denn er hat ausser ihm ja fast nichts an Land sondern nur Sand. Deswegen sind auch die Regierungsformen der Semiten immer mehr oder weniger theokratisch und totalitär im Gegensatz zu Europa, wo wenigstens bis heute noch die Regierungsform nicht totalitär vom Religiösen aus beherrscht wird.

Wie schon gesagt, wird das soziale Leben bei den Wüstenmenschen geregelt durch strenge, unerbittliche Gesetze, die die Abwesenheit affektiver Bindungen und Verpflichtungen ersetzen. Diese Gesetze erscheinen uns oft unmenschlich, denn es ist schwer zu begreifen, dass dieselben die einzige Möglichkeit sind, die Individuen sozial zusammenzuschweissen, und dass sie ohne diese Gesetze wie Sand zerrinnen und verweht werden würden.

Auf sozialem Gebiet wirkt sich dies durch die Gesetzgebung aus, welche gewissenhaft ausgearbeitet automatisch das Benehmen jedes Individuums in jedem Einzelfall genau regeln soll durch Zwang und wenn nötig durch Gewalt.

Deshalb nimmt die Zahl *Eins* bei dieser Geistesrichtung einen besonderen Platz ein, sogar aus Paaren machen die Araber eine Eins und zählen mit Paaren wie mit Einheiten. Die Sprachwurzeln, von denen wir oben schon gesprochen haben, sind isoliert genauso wie die geometrischen Motive der Ornamentik nebeneinandergestellt und nur durch Vokalisierung und nicht durch affektive Assozierung ihren Sinn erhaltend. Die oben erwähnte Arabeske, d. h. die rhythmisch geschwungene Linie, in der Schrift und auch der monotone Gesang stellen sich ebenso wie die «Eins» würdig in Analogie mit dem einzigen Gott und mobilisieren den Sinn für das Ästhetische, für das Heilige, den Sinn für die Heilige Schrift und den Koran, deren Buchstaben Ewigkeitswert beigemessen wird.

Sie entschuldigen, wenn ich so lange auf die Entwicklung dieser Psyche, oder wenn Sie wollen dieser Ich-Struktur eingegangen bin, aber es ist diese Kollektiv-Psyche mit ihren Imperativen, die wir genau kennen müssen, um ihren Einfluss auf die Gestaltung des menschlichen Lebens besonders für unsere nordafrikanischen Leptosomen begreifen zu können. Wir können da nicht mit allgemeinen Begriffen wie dem eines gemeinsamen kollektiven Unbewussten und seiner Archetypen auskommen. Diese Auffassung des Unbewussten scheint uns dem Bedürfnis zu dienen, alles schematisch unter einen Hut bringen zu wollen. Die Begriffe FREUD's vom unbewussten Über-Ich und der unsrige vom kollektiven Über-Ich und vom Kollektiv-Ich, letztere geschaffen durch das Bedingende des Milieus, des Klimas. Sie sind dadurch charakterisiert, dass das eine Über-Ich vom anderen von Grund auf verschieden sein kann, und sie scheinen mir da zum Verständnis der Dinge besser geeignet zu sein. Dieses wie oben beschriebene Über-Ich ist es, das beim «Wüstentypus» zwangsmässig handelt, das durchgreift und das jene Leptosomen formt, von denen SOLÉ-SOGARRA spricht, wie schon am Anfang erwähnt. Und dies Über-Ich hat eine ganz besondere Struktur und absorbiert den weitaus grössten Teil der psychischen Kraft des Individuums, das auf affektivem Gebiet verarmt, und dessen Ich von den Forderungen seines Über-Ichs vollständig beherrscht wird. Deshalb auch erlaubte ich mir, den Spezialfall unserer arabischen Leptosomen zu erwähnen, so wie man sie besonders rein im Hinterland von Agadir findet, um an Hand dieser Beobachtungen darzustellen, wie die Psyche sich auf die Konstitution auswirken kann, d. h. die Gestaltung des Geistes in diesem Einzelfall, gesehen vom analytischen Standpunkt aus.

Vielleicht ist es mir nicht gelungen, die starren Forderungen des oben erwähnten arabischen Über-Ichs stark genug hervorzuheben, damit Sie sich ein Bild über seine Wirkung machen können, aber ich hoffe, Sie können nun verstehen, weshalb AVERRHOES, der berühmte hispano-maurische Philosoph, glaubt: der Intellekt sei ewig und die Seele sterblich. In unserer Sprache ausgedrückt besagt dies: Das intellektuelle Über-Ich des Mauren ist ewig und sein Ich sterblich, d. h. sein Über-Ich ungeheuer stark und sein Ich schwach. Nicht nur ist es dieselbe Tracht, dasselbe Benehmen, die sich seit Jahrtausenden trotz der vielen bei uns in Europa wechselnden Moden und Änderungen bei den Arabern unverändert erhalten haben, sondern auch ähnliche Sitten und Gebräuche, rhythmisch-rituell geregelt, vererbt von Generation auf Generation. Sie sind so stark fixiert, dass auch die sogenannte moderne Kultur im Grunde daran nicht vieles hat ändern können, ausgenommen vielleicht die Fassade. Und mit der Sprache steht es ähnlich. Genauso wie vor Jahrtausenden zu Zeiten Babylons, d.h. Bab-el-Eon, die Pforte der Eonen, schon das Wort Bab die Pforte bezeichnete, genauso bezeichnet das Wort Bab im modernen Arabisch die Pforte, z. B. Bab-el-Mandeb oder Bab-el-Mansur, das erste eine Meerenge, das zweite eine Pforte der Stadtmauer von Meknes. Genauso wie bei den Babyloniern das Leben durch die Gestirne, die Astrologie, nach starren Gesetzen vorherbestimmt war, so auch für den Nordafrikaner durch das Mektoub, d. h. «es steht geschrieben», was besagen will, alles ist voraus bestimmt. So war es auch schon für St. Augustin, der in diesem Punkt von der Kirche als ketzerisch abgelehnt wird.

Die Starrheit, das Stereotype, dieser Psyche hat zur Folge, dass sie aus jedem Individuum denselben Typ herauszuarbeiten versucht, und zwar den des Leptosomen. Betrachten Sie die Leptosomen dieser Gegenden, vor allen Dingen z. B. die Einwohner vom Souss, dem Hinterland von Agadir. Jedes Individuum, wer es auch sei, ist schlank wie eine Arabeske und geht im rituell-rhythmischen Gang seines Weges, so wie es nicht nur durch das Ich sondern durchs Über-Ich zu jeder Führung angeleitet wird. Es sieht nur nach einer Seite, kennt nur eine Richtung, eine Idee, die oft zur fixen Idee wird, alle anderen Ideen blockiert und damit innerlich zur Härte und äusserlich zum Fanatismus Anlass gibt. Wie schon gesagt, ändert die moderne Schulbildung nicht viel an diesem Verhalten, höchstens, dass durch sie der Mensch in grössten Zwiespalt mit seiner ererbten oder seiner traditionellen Über-Ich-Struktur kommen kann und deshalb gehemmt, neurotisch und oft sogar paranoisch wird. Die Hemmungen als Symptom werden oft beobachtet von den Lehrern in technischen Schulen, die überrascht feststellen, was für sie unerklärlich ist, wie der nach europäischem Muster ausgebildete Schüler in seinen Bewegungen diskordanter ist als jener, der die Wohltat dieser Schulen nicht genossen hat. Ein anderes für viele Amerikaner und Europäer paradoxes Phänomen ist die Feststellung, dass die Wohltaten der europäischen Kultur, der Überfluss an Nahrung und Verbrauchsgütern und auch an Geschenken und Wohltaten statt Dank eher Agression und Feindschaft hervorrufen, und dass überhaupt eine Periode des allgemeinen Wohlstandes bei den Arabern oft rasch mit einer der Not und des Verfalls wie zwangsmässig ausgeglichen werden muss. Wer mit den harten Forderungen dieses spezifischen Wüsten-Über-Ichs nicht vertraut ist, kann sich diese unserer Logik und unserer Mentalität widersprechende Haltung nicht erklären, und es erscheint dem nicht Eingeweihten unverständig und verrückt zu sein. Dies umso mehr als oft der durch sein Gedeihen im Zwiespalt mit seinem Über-Ich sich befindende Araber darauf mit Angst und Schuldgefühl reagiert, die sich nicht nur sozial, sondern auch auf psychosomatischem Gebiet äussern. Welches sind nun die hauptsächlichsten Auswirkungen dieser Situation auf die Konstitution dieser Menschen, und wie stellt sich uns in diesem Spezialfall seine Konstitution dar, soweit wir dies überblicken können?

Beginnen wir mit dem zweiten Punkt, d. h. mit der Konstitution. Wir haben es, wie schon gesagt, da mit einem Menschenschlag zu tun im Körperbau leptosom, ein geschmeidiger, gelenkiger Bewegungstypus, extravertiert, aber doch irgendwie verhalten und in seinen affektiven Ausdrucksmöglichkeiten stark beschränkt. Das einzelne Individuum dieses Types schwitzt gewöhnlich wenig trotz des heissen Klimas. Seine Haut ist rauh und gefurcht. Sein Urin ist konzentriert. Die Azidität des Blutes und der Urinsäure ist höher als durchschnittlich, der Mensch neigt sehr früh, vom 7. Lebensjahr ab, zu Nierensteinen, er neigt auch zu Verstopfungen, und der Arzt stellt bei ihm im Gegensatz zu der der Europäer eine *trockene* Diarrhoe fest, wenn dieselbe auftritt, und nicht eine nasse Diarrhoe wie bei den Occidentalen. Die Widerstandsfähigkeit gegen Krankheiten und Infektionen ist sehr hoch, das Niveau für Schmerzgefühl stark herabgesetzt im Vergleich zu unserem. Die Wunden verheilen rasch, und auch Schädelbrüche und sehr schwere Verletzungen werden gut ertragen. Es ist deshalb nicht immer leicht, Verunglückten oder Patienten die nötige Behandlung zukommen zu lassen, da sie sich mit ihren Leiden persönlich nicht in Betracht ziehen können oder wollen und der Tod, das Nichtsein, für sie eine sehr relative Bedeutung hat: der eigene Tod ebenso wie der Tod der anderen, weil das Individuum in seiner Ich-Struktur durch das Über-Ich gehemmt sich nur schwer als Ich-Persönlichkeit existenziell konzipieren kann und deshalb leicht auf jeden persönlichen Besitz bei sich und anderen verzichtet, selbst auf den Besitz des Lebens. An Frustrierung von Jugend auf gewöhnt ist die eigene Existenz etwas sehr Nebensächliches, die Selbstzerstörung, d. h. das Masochistische, ist bei diesem Typ erotisiert und überbetont und ebenso das Sadistische, was zu besonderen Symptomen Anlass gibt, vor allen Dingen zu dem Symptom des Blutrausches. Mit wahrer

Wollust können sich diese Menschen töten lassen oder auch im
Raptus andere töten sowie alles, was ihnen dann in den Weg kommt:
Kinder, deren Schädel an der Wand zerschmettert werden, Weiber,
denen mit dem Messer der Leib geöffnet wird, Hühner, Haustiere,
alles was lebt und bluten kann. Psychoanalytisch ausgedrückt sagen
wir: Das Individuum ist vorzüglich oral in seiner Libidoorganisation,
und diese Tatsache erklärt uns auch, wie SOLÉ-SOGARRA es durch-
blicken lässt, deshalb die Verbrechen bei diesen Typen viel häufiger
sind als bei Athletikern und Pyknikern z. B. Als Gegenbesitzung zu
diesem Zwang braucht natürlich das Individuum strenge Regeln wie
schon oben gesagt, Regeln denen auch die Nahrung sowie das Ge-
schlechtsleben streng untergeordnet sind. Es ist kein Zufall, wenn
das dicke, gemästete Schwein als Nahrung vom kollektiven Über-Ich
dieser Leptosomen und auch vom Koran verboten sind sowie alles,
was, wie Kaninchen, angemästet werden kann. Die Tiere unterliegen
derselben Magersucht wie die Menschen und sind in gewissem Sinne
auch sozusagen leptosom. Auch für sie gilt die Linie – die Arabeske –
als einziger Gott, und auch sie werden der Form geopfert. Weder die
Tiere können üppig gedeihen noch Felder, Wälder und Wiesen.
Komplexuell werden Bäume abgeschnitten, oft in fanatischer Wut,
und es ist deshalb schwer, in diesen Gegenden die Wälder wachsen
zu lassen. Ich nehme an, dass auch die starken Tiere, die im Stier-
kampf geopfert werden, ihr Ende im Grunde diesem Über-Ich verdanken.

Wie hart diese Forderungen des Über-Ichs sich durchsetzen,
ergibt sich aus der Art, wie Frauen und Kinder als zum Stamm ge-
hörende Objekte sichtbar wie Herdentiere abgestempelt werden, d. h.
sie sind gezeichnet. Aber im Grunde genommen sind auch die Männer
gezeichnet diesen Über-Ich-Forderungen gemäss. Sie sind ja beschnitten, und in weiten Gegenden, in Mauritanien z. B., werden die
Frauen der Excision der Clitoris unterzogen. Auch diese rituelle Einstellung, religiös gerechtfertigt, unterliegt viel mehr, als man es gewöhnlich annimmt, einem Zwang, der vom Über-Ich ausgeht und
dem Individuum die strenge Linie des Wachstums vorzeichnet. Der
Zwang eine bestimmte Linie zu kultivieren und stets dieselben Regeln
einzuhalten, von Generation auf Generation dasselbe Verhalten und
durch Jahrhunderte hindurch dieselbe Arbeit, der Zwang zum Fasten
von Jugend auf erduldet – zum rituellen Fasten ebenso wie zum will-
kürlichen und zu dem von der Hungersnot aufgezwungenen –, der
Zwang auch alles, was nicht der einzigen Linie entspricht, rücksichts-

los auszurotten oder abzuköpfen, hat ja zu einer ganz bestimmten Zuchtwahl im Rahmen der Gesellschaftsordnung geführt, wo immer derselbe Typ kultiviert wird, und nur er allein sich fortpflanzen durfte auf Kosten aller anderen. Damit würde sich unserer Meinung nach die ganze typische Konstitution der Leptosomen dieses «Wüstentypus» erklären.

Fügen wir hinzu die Rolle, die, wie schon gesagt, in der grenzenlosen Leere das Auge spielt – die Spezialisierung, der es unterliegt auf Kosten des Gehörsinnes, – dann werden wir uns eine im grossen und ganzen befriedigende Vorstellung machen können über den Einfluss dieser Psyche auf die Konstitution dieser Typen. Der Gehörsinn entwickelt beim Menschen den Sinn für Harmonie, für das Zugehörige, für Hierarchie, Disziplin und Unterordnung nicht durch Zwang, sondern durch Liebe für Akkorde, für das Zugehörige, das Mitschwingende. Beim «Wüstentypus» ist alles eingeteilt und zugeteilt, d. h. zerschnitten und zerstückelt ausgenommen die Zeit, die endlos ist. Wir wissen, wie unsere Schwerhörigen leicht paranoisch werden, und wie sie sich nur mit Mühe einordnen lassen, aber nichts dergleichen bei den Blinden, was psychologisch und auch sonst grosse Folgen hat, wie ich es in einer Arbeit über die Rolle von Gesicht und Gehör bei der Heilung unserer Patienten darzustellen versuchte. In gewissem Sinne sind unsere Wüsten-Leptosomen Schwerhörige.

Sollen wir aus diesen Überlegungen schliessen, dass unter diesen Umständen bei den uns interessierenden Leptosomen durch die Psyche eine hereditäre Situation geschaffen wird? Nach meinen Erfahrungen: nein. Es genügt, dass, wie wir es beobachtet haben, das Kleinkind aus diesem Milieu herausgebracht wird, und man ihm mütterliche Liebe und Schutz in unserem Sinne angedeihen lässt, so wie wir es in gewissen Fällen getan haben, und die Orientierung seiner Affektivität nimmt eine andere Richtung sowie die seiner Körperstruktur, besonders dann wenn nicht Sprache, Religion und Geist dieser Orientierung entgegenwirken. Ich glaube, dass durch eine Änderung der Erziehung, d. h. der mütterlichen Einstellung zum Kind, in drei oder vier Generationen aus unseren beobachteten Leptosomen eine ganze Reihe zu Athletikern und sogar zu Pyknikern werden könnten, falls man sie in eine waldige, gebirgige Gegend bringen würde. Aber diese Änderung der Erziehung bringt eine Desadaption an das ursprüngliche Milieu zustande und lässt sich also nur durch Verpflanzung in andere Gegenden und in ein Milieu mit anderer Mentalität erreichen, was schwer durchführbar ist. Es würde infolge der Fixierung der Charaktere lange Zeit brauchen, bis wir diese Leptosomen von ihren ursprünglichen Bindungen befreien können, um sie einer anderen Mentalität, z. B. der unsrigen, zu integrieren. Für den Augenblick machen wir uns über diese Möglichkeiten nicht zuviele Illusionen, besonders weil mit dem Vorherrschen des Maschinismus bei uns heutzutage eher der Europäer es riskiert, dem harten Wüsten-Über-Ich integriert zu werden als umgekehrt. Das zum Teil durch die Automatismen, die dieser moderne Maschinismus in uns entwickelt. Die Reinkultur des Intellekts auf Kosten des Affektiven schafft auch beim modernen Europäer die Bedingungen, die den Menschen auf einen Nenner bringen, wie wir es in der ganzen Bandbreite der Wüste Afrikas und Asiens beobachten können, und wie es auch schon auf dem Gebiet der Dekoration und der modernen europäischen Architektur zum Ausdruck kommt. Auch bei uns werden schon ohne Rücksicht auf die psychologischen Folgen darauf, automatisch aus sogenannten hygienischen Gründen die Knaben mehr und mehr beschnitten. Ist doch die Hygiene und die Ideologie der Gleichheit der Zwang, dem wir Europäer unterliegen, und wir betrachten dies alles als ein Zeichen der durch den Maschinismus entstandenen Milieuänderung bei uns, die vielleicht in der Folge einen neuen Menschenschlag selbst bei uns schaffen könnte, um uns Ameisen oder Bienen vergleichbar dem strengen Gesetz eines totalitär waltenden kollektiven Über-Ichs unterzuordnen. Das Wissen um diese Dinge verhilft uns zum Verständnis für das Walten des Geistes und der Psyche, die die Konstitutionen jeweils formen, so oder so den Umständen angepasst und an das Milieu gebunden, ob wir es wollen oder nicht.

Ganz besonders lehrreich ist es, den Einfluss der Psyche auf die sexuelle Entwicklung des Individuums zu beobachten. Bei unseren erwähnten Leptosomen spielt die Homosexualität, oder besser gesagt die Homoerotik, eine grosse Rolle. Schon im siebten Lebensjahr werden die Mädchen durch Frauen in die raffinierte Technik der Selbstliebe und der Homosexualität eingeweiht. Die Knaben werden von den Männern zuerst zur passiven Einstellung erzogen und späterhin durch die Männerliebe orientiert. Diese Orientierung der Sexualität hängt natürlich zusammen mit den vom Über-Ich geschaffenen Konflikten. Das Mädchen muss durch sein Werben das mütterliche Über-Ich beschwichtigen und bezaubern, der Knabe das väterliche, das im Grunde genommen ein mütterliches ist, da sich der Mann stark mit der Frau und nicht so sehr mit dem Vater identifiziert.

Beide Geschlechter sind so sexuell aufgepeitscht durch das übermächtige, drohende Über-Ich und reagieren mehr oder weniger paranoisch mit sensitiven Beziehungen. Die Frauen sind glatte, schlangenwüchsige Typen mit maskulinem Einschlag, die Männer lang aufgeschossene Typen mit oft eunuchoiden Proportionen. Schon 1925 stellt MAUZ in einer Studie über «die Bedeutung körperlicher Dysplasien für die Prognose seelischer Störungen» fest, dass «erotischer Beziehungswahn, wahnhafte Eifersucht, sexuell-neurotische Konflikte in ihrer Genese nicht selten in derartigen konstitutionellen schwachen Punkten wurzeln sowie in der mangelnden und unausgeglichenen Ausreifung körperlicher und psychischer Sexual-Struktur». In der erwähnten Arbeit hat MAUZ seinerzeit als Hauptursachen für die Störungen die Keimdrüsen-Funktion sowie die innere Sekretion im Auge, wobei er sich vielleicht noch kein klares Bild darüber machen konnte, wie sehr diese Störungen nicht allein von ererbten Faktoren sondern auch vom Einfluss des Milieus auf die Psyche und von der geistigen Ansteckung durch die Familienneurose abhängig sein können.

Was nun unsere Gruppe von Leptosomen anbetrifft, so sind die dazu gehörigen sexuell aufgepeitschten Kinder frühreif, die Mädchen schon im achten bis zehnten Jahre in der Pubertät, die Knaben mit einer ebenfalls künstlich aufgepeitschten Phantasie einer zwanghaften erotischen Betätigung ausgeliefert und zwar in einer nach unseren Normen mehr perversen als normalen Art. Die Beschneidung, die gewöhnlich erst im dritten Lebensjahr vorgenommen wird und zu starken psychischen Reaktionen Anlass gibt, trägt ebenfalls zu diesem übersteigerten Erotismus und zur unausgeglichenen Sexualität der Knaben bei sowohl auf der Ebene des Auto-, des Homo- oder des Hetero-Erotismus. Natürlich haben diese ganz besonderen psychischen Bedingungen einen grossen Einfluss auf das Konstitutionelle da, wo sie immer dieselben Tendenzen fixieren und zu abnormen sexuellen Betätigungen und Organentwicklungen Anlass geben.

Es ist mir nicht möglich, im Rahmen dieser Arbeit unser Problem erschöpfend zu behandeln. Wir haben, wie schon gesagt, einen Spezialfall gewählt, um an Hand der dabei gesammelten Erfahrungen den Einfluss der Psyche auf das die Konstitution Bedingende besser beobachten zu können. So wie bei unseren erwähnten Leptosomen eine besondere Beziehung besteht zwischen dem Wüstengeist und dem Körperbau und der Konstitution, so vielleicht ebenfalls bei unseren Pyknikern zwischen Waldgeist und Körperbau. Gewiss ist, dass die soziale Struktur, die der Wüste angepasst ist, eine ganz andere Form hat als jene, die sich im Wald-, Berg- und Wiesenland entwickelt hat. Nicht nur das Soziale ist anders sondern auch die Denkvorstellungen mit ihrem kategorischen Imperativ, die Gefühlswelt mit ihrem Leben und Wirken, ja sogar der Begriff der Realität wird dann relativ, da die Realität der einen nicht mehr die der anderen ist, und sich bei den einen das Denken in vorgezeichneten Bahnen abwickelt ohne jede individuelle Freiheit, während sich bei den anderen das Denken und Fühlen symphonisch ordnet, oft mehr durch Akkorde akustisch bedingt, akustisch dem Gemeinsamen eingeordnet und zugehörig und nicht so sehr durch harte, allen sichtbar vorgezeichnete Gesetze. Wir müssen es anderen überlassen, auf dieser eröffneten Bahn unsere Untersuchungen weiter auszubauen, um so zu erlauben durch die analytische Sicht mehr und mehr den Einfluss der Psyche auf die Konstitution im einen und im anderen Milieu kennen zu lernen.

Author's address: DR. R. LAFORGUE, 62, Rue de la Tour, *Paris* (France).

The Concept of "Constitutional" *

J. O. WISDOM, London

I propose mainly to discuss the concept of "constitutional" and say little about the concept of "the constitution". That little may be said straightaway.

There would seem to be two interpretations of "the constitution". Thus BAUER (1) regards the constitution as the contribution

---

* I wish to acknowledge useful discussions with DR. ALAN THOMPSON and MR. R. F. T. WITHERS.

made by genotypical factors. He notes, however, that this is not generally accepted. The opposite view may be found in DRAPER (2), where it is a compound derived from genotypical factors modified by environment, this compound determining the reaction of the individual. Either interpretation can enable us to make sense of "sound constitution", "good constitution", and the like, though the second is more relevant to such ideas as capacity to recover quickly from a disease, seldom succumbing, i.e. good prognosis based on a good health record. Neither interpretation bears on the causes of disease.

The concept of "constitutional" is frequently mentioned, hardly ever explained, and, though one would get the impression that everybody who uses it and hears it knows intuitively what it means, further reflection makes one somewhat sceptical about this. Does it pose as an explanation of or partial explanation of medical phenomena or pathological changes? Or does it play the rôle of what SPINOZA calls the asylum of ignorance? Do we fall back on the use of constitutional factors when we are defeated and cannot explain some feature of a disease? In short, what is the rôle of the concept?

If the concept is seen to be useful in the sense of playing an independent part, it should certainly be different from that of "hereditary" and there should rightly be some relationship between "constitutional" and "hereditary". Our first task therefore is to try to have a clearer understanding of what exactly "hereditary" involves; this may seem a totally unnecessary feature in medical circles were it not for the fact that the concept of "hereditary" is fraught with many difficulties and misunderstandings, the outcome of which is as a rule that whenever something is regarded as hereditary it is *ipso facto* regarded as unchangeable. The very fact that this is a widespread misunderstanding necessitates coming to grips with the concept of "hereditary".

On this matter I propose to take some ideas (3) from WOODGER (4), (though my way of elaborating them cannot be laid at his door). A factor is "genotypical" in one sense if all zygotes that live long enough to develop into a phenotype have the factor in question no matter what the environment may be. Here it will be seen that the rôle of the environment is minimal, there has to be an environment, otherwise the zygotes would not develop into a phenotype; but apart from that, the environment has no modifying influence. It is clear that a genotypical factor in this sense cannot be altered. An example would be the possession of blue eyes which cannot be altered by any change of environment. It should be carefully noted that in this context the focus of interest is on what a person develops as a result of genotypical factors, which are, at least in part, potentialities at the moment of conception, and has nothing to do with what is hereditary in the sense of running in families*.

We are, however, just as often interested in factors that are genotypical in a different sense. We are often concerned with specific capacities, such as the capacity to run very fast or the poor capacity of the blood to clot. One might be called a "hyper-capacity" and the other a "hypo-capacity". One reason why this is important is that the opposition between "hereditary" and "acquired" ceases to have any application. No doubt the effect of a hypo-capacity is hardly susceptible of improvement, at any rate at all easily, though in principle it is not impossible to alter. On the other hand, the effect of a hyper-capacity may at times be altered very easily. The ability to run very fast may be interfered with only too easily; therefore although a capacity may be inherited it may be possible to alter its use, and in an adverse way, and therefore the capacity is inhibited. This only *seems* to conflict with the idea of heredity. Thus if a person has inherited the capacity to run very fast and due to some accident is no longer able to do so, we have a blend of hereditary and acquired capacities and there are no real opposition between the two. In other words, a genotypical capacity may be prevented from manifesting itself. Milk excretion is perhaps an example in which the genotypical capacity may be easily inhibited or may possible be augmented.

It is now simple to distinguish between "hereditary" in the sense of running in families and "genotypical". The hyper-capacity to run fast may or may not have a hereditary factor but the mere capacity to run certainly has not. On the other hand this mere capacity to run is certainly genotypical. It is plain therefore that we are concerned with "hereditary" only if it is equated with "genotypical". To eliminate the irrelevant question of what is inherited, I would use the concept of "genotypical endowment" for the organism at conception.

---

* The clinical importance of finding that a disorder runs in families would seem to be that it facilitates diagnosis and removes (wrongly) the obligation to cope with a gloomy prognosis.

If now we are to link "constitutional" with "hereditary" we shall attempt to do so in terms of genotypical properties on the one hand, and on the other, specific capacities. The importance of bringing out that the operation of a genotypical specific capacity may be subject to alteration is, as we can see, that whatever is built up out of genotypical capacities may be capable of modification. The importance of this conclusion is perhaps a negative one; the rôle that the idea of a constitutional factor is apt to play is that an organism, if limited by constitutional defect, cannot hope to develop beyond it, but we now see that this is not necessarily so. It becomes increasingly questionable therefore, whether the concept of constitutional has any fruitful use.

We have now to turn to a basic question and enquire how far a constitutional factor in such a sense might in principle be likely to govern the subsequent course of disease. It might, however, be maintained that, in the case of a disorder where a genotypical incapacity was a striking feature, the organism was likely to fall ill on account of this lack of capacity. If we take as an example poor visual acuity, which we will suppose has been inherited in the sense described, it might very well play a part in leading to eye-strain and consequential headaches. This situation, of course, would only develop if there was a more or less standardised social pressure requiring the eyes to be used to such and such an extent each day. In this way a genotypical factor can be a significant pathogenic condition bringing about some disorder.

Thus it is quite clear that genotypical factors can and should play their part in the explanation of disease. What, however, is wrong is in the tendency to attribute power to unknown constitutional factors. It is true that there may be unknown constitutional factors and that they may influence the course of a disease; but what is wrong is the tendency to ascribe our ignorance to these things when we might just as well ascribe our ignorance to quite different sources. So far as there is something not understood about a disease, the answer might of course lie in something constitutional, but it might equally well lie in an environmental condition or in a number of other possibilities, some of which may never have been considered at all. All I wish to suggest here is that it is unscientific to put in clauses, supposedly safeguarding, about genotypical factors.

Now the same sort of comment applies to constitutional factors especially if we tend to think of them as built up from genotypical factors in the sense described, but even if we do not and we think of them in some other way, we should still refuse to suppose that the explanation of a disorder lies in part in some unascertained constitutional factor when we might just as well look for explanations in some other domain. If we do really have need to introduce a *caveat* about constitutional factors, we should surely regard it as an obligation to try to say specifically what the factor is and not just refer completely generally to constitutional factors. After all, if one is discussing the explanation of any phenomenon or any disorder one does not refer to physiological factors, environmental factors, completely generally and vaguely; one is giving a serious scientific discussion only if one puts forward these in some specific form and it should be the same with regard to constitutional factors.

Let us lastly turn to the question of the relevance of constitutional factors to psychosomatic disorder. When a point like this is in people's minds, they are presumably suffering mainly from a lack of real knowledge; ignorance about the aetiology or pathogenesis of a psychosomatic disorder is apt to make one think of the possibility that a constitutional factor may play an important rôle. But what exactly is the point of thinking like this? It would appear to be in part to find a reason for one's past ignorance, in part a reason why one may not expect to improve one's knowledge, and in part a reason for being satisfied that little or nothing can be done to improve the lot of those who suffer from such disorders. But it should now be clear that these consequences do not follow and are not justified. The fact that they are unjustified, however, does not mean that constitutional factors may not play a rôle and indeed may not play an interesting rôle; but once the misunderstandings that I have described have been removed and one approaches "hereditary" and "constitutional" not as a refuge for ignorance and as an excuse for remaining ignorant and being unable to offer help, but as just one of the possible places where a contributory cause might be sought, then the subject at once attains the same scientific interest as any other.

Let us consider a possible example. Suppose that a patient on account of genotypical factors has large glands secreting stomach acid and inherits a hyper-capacity for secreting acid and later develops a stomach ulcer. If the hyper-capacity to secrete acid in the stomach is attributed to genotypical factors what exactly does this amount to? From the preceding discussion it will be seen that it means that hyperactivity of the acid secreting glands will occur in an environment which supplies an appropriate opportunity, that is, in simple terms, more acid is secreted than is necessary to digest a certain amount of food. Now it certainly seems possible in principle that a factor like this could determine either a number of instances of some psychosomatic disorder or even in the limit instances of all psychosomatic disorders, but it is difficult to see just why one would pursue a hypothesis of this sort. There is nothing particular to make it a plausible line of research to pursue, and again one is driven to suppose that interest in it is motivated by the present state of ignorance and helplessness. There is nothing in such a hypothesis that makes it more worthy of consideration than other sorts of hypotheses in the field. There is one other feature about it: it is the sort of hypothesis that would be extremely difficult but probably not impossible to test. Presumably it either is in some cases or will in the future be possible to measure such secretions. In a fairly new-born baby or in an infant of a few months old, it may become possible to estimate the acid secretion, for example, and to establish what is the normal secretion, and likewise in other cases. It would, indeed, be highly desirable that such a piece of research should be undertaken if for no other reason than to find out what grain of truth there may be in the possibility of constitutional and genotypical factors governing psychosomatic disorder and if, as is likely, their rôle does not turn out to be particularly significant we shall be freed of a red-herring and able to give our attention more wholeheartedly to more fruitful ideas.

Again consider another example. Consider those suffering from an allergy where histamine is liberated significantly. Such liberation may seem to be genotypical; but it could be constitutional—a reaction developed in reacting to a certain sort of environment. It is enormously difficult to establish the first possibility; yet it is the conclusion we tend to jump to. The second possibility leaves it open that social or psychological pressures lead to the excessive liberation of histamine. Hence, though correct to label this phenomenon as constitutional, to do so may distract the attention from the more significant social and psychological pressures.

Perhaps the most relevant matter to mention in connection with psychosomatics is the cautions appeal to constitutional factors when one is unable to give an explanation. One point is that it is no more reasonable to do this than to appeal to other factors that might be at work—dietary deficiency, sunlight deficiency, social stress, and psychological stress. The other, here more important, point is that when a psychogenetic hypothesis is offered for a psychosomatic disorder, to appeal as well to constitutional factors is either irrelevant or a sign of intellectual confusion. For a psychogenetic account is designed to centre around a person's constitutional reactions; but if, as is likely, the use of constitutional factors in such a context is a covert expression for something physiological, it would be better to say so, and this would at once raise the question of how a constitutional hypocapacity might lead to a psychosomatic disorder. The real point here is that, if by some great advance we gained knowledge of relevant constitutional factors, our problem in psychosomatics would then be not solved but only beginning; for we should then have learned that some constitutional factor had something to do with the matter—the prime nature of which would still be a mystery. And finally if a constitutional factor has been built up not only as a result of genotypical factors but also as a result of their reaction to a certain sort of social or psychological environment, the important point to decide on would not be the constitutional factor but the social or psychological factors contributing to it.

Bibliography

1. BAUER, J.: Constitution and Disease (Heinemann, London 1945).
2. DRAPER, G.: Human Constitution (Saunders, Philadelphia 1924).
3. WISDOM, J.O.: Metabiology. Brit. J. Phil. Sci. *4*: 339–344 (1954).
4. WOODGER, J.H.: Biology and Language (University Press, Cambridge 1952; What Do We Mean by Inborn? Brit. J. Phil. Sci. *3*: 319–326 (1953). I but see HALDANE, J.B.S.: A Logical Basis for Genetics, Op. cit. *6*: 245–248 (1956), and WOODGER: A Reply to PROFESSOR HALDANE. Op. cit. *1*: 149–155 (1956).

Author's address: DR. J.O. WISDOM, School of Economics, Houghton Street, Aldwych, *London W.C.* 2 (England).

The Constitutional Reaction Types as Evidenced by Clinical Experience

G. LANGFELDT, Oslo

The relation between constitution and psychosomatic disorders has been the object of more speculation than research. In fact, in spite of many postulations, little is until now agreed upon as to the existence of a specific correlation between special constitutional types and special psychosomatic diseases.

As the topic; *Constitution and Neurosis* has been put on the program of this congress, I thought it might be of interest to stress what we from clinical experience can state as to the importance of constitution in clinical psychiatry as a whole. The experiences to which I will refer in the following, are predominantly based on the clinical material of the University Psychiatric Clinic of Oslo. This is an open Psychiatric Institute with 96 patients, mostly neurotics and psychopaths, of which I have been the leader for 18 years.

To avoid a misunderstanding, let me start with my definition of *constitution* as the *total psychobiological outfit of a personality* which, because of inherited and external factors has been stabilized to such a degree that it can be changed only by severe psychic or physical influences.

Clinical experience with patients admitted to the University Psychiatric Clinic of Oslo has evidenced that different constitutional types may dispose to quite special reaction types. And these reaction types may be *neurotic, psychopathic* or *psychotic*. If you are familiar with the constitutional types in question, the reactive symptom formations will frequently be comprehensible without any deeper analysis being necessary. In the psychopathic and psychotic reaction types it is as a rule the question of an exaggeration of constitutional character traits—as met with for example in the paranoid psychoses in suspicious psychopaths or in compulsive psychoses in individuals characterized by a compulsive character.

In *neurotic* reactions the symptom formation may also be conditioned in the constitutional disposition proper, for instance the depressive symptoms or the signs of self-reference in sensitive neurotics. However, in most of the neurotic reaction types the symptom formation will be an expression of the intrapsychic dynamic processes taking place.

As all of you will know, many and varied suggestions have appeared, aiming at a differentiation of typical personality types. Most of them are based on direct description of the dominant characteristics, for instance the different psychopathic types described by GRUHLE, KURT SCHNEIDER and E. BLEULER in almost the same terms, such as the depressive, the sensitive, the passive or the aggressive psychopath. Another kind of description is that of the introverted and extroverted personalities of JUNG, or the integrated or disintegrated personalities of JAENSCH. A description according to endocrine types or to fundamental interests has also been suggested. Other systems differentiate *psychodynamic* typologies aiming at a deeper understanding of the *ethical, moral* and *religious* sides of the personality. Also many *structural-analytical* typologies of ADLER, EWALD, FREUD, JUNG and KRETSCHMER should be mentioned. All these typologies have certainly contributed much to a better understanding of the psychodynamic processes in neurotic as well as in psychopathic individuals, but the value of these types in *practical* clinical work is rather disputed. The aim of this paper is therefore to present some clinical experiences regarding abnormal reaction types regularly met with in individuals suffering from quite special constitutional dispositions which are well circumscribed, and which should by that reason also be suited for *international* comparative psychiatry.

Let me in the first place state that experiences from normal characterology, from hereditary investigations and from clinical psychiatry strongly support the assumption of the existence of quite typical abnormal characters, disposing to special pathological reactions. The many characterological studies as well as hereditary studies have evidenced that as to abnormal personalities we most frequently meet with such ones in the field of intellectual, emotional and will-life. In good agreement with these experiences, in the daily practical clinical psychiatry the abnormal constitutional types most frequently met with are characterized by intellectual, emotional or will—and drives disturbances. And these abnormal constitutional types again dispose to quite special abnormal reactions in which the symptom formations to a large degree are characterized by the abnormal constitution traits in question. Most known and generally accepted are probably the reaction types met with in *cycloid* and *schizoid* psychopaths. *Paranoid* psychopaths are disposed to reactions characterized by an exaggeration of the constitutional disposition to suspiciousness, ambition or querulousness. Also the *hysterical* psychopath as well as the *compulsive* charactertype with the disposition to obsessions, phobias and compulsions, should be mentioned.

However, the constitutional type most frequently met with in the daily psychiatric clinic is the *sensitive* constitutional type. In this connection sensitivity means an increased tendency in an individual to react emotionally to different psychic stimuli. Such a disposition to sensitive reactions is to be found in all normal developed children and adults, but there is a great difference as to the sensitivity of mind and the associated feeling of guilt. Clinical experience speaks strongly in the direction that an increased sensibility and a hypersensitive mind are to be found as a general disposition to most of the psycho-neuroses.

In these neuroses the sensitive disposition is the cause of the tendency to *introjection* of the feeling of guilt, which in these individuals is regularly the result of even small hurting stimuli. In addition we also find a hypersensitive mind in *some* types of psychopaths, but due to the fact that these types *project* the feeling of guilt, probably because of another disposition, the symptom formation is quite another one than in psycho-neuroses. While we in these disorders find anxiety, depression and the feeling of guilt, in the sensitive psychopaths we find susceptibility, aggressivity and paranoid traits.

It is not possible for me to describe in 15 minutes the symptom formation in the different constitutional types met with in clinical practice. I only wanted to stress the fact that we by simple observations and descriptive psychiatry have succeeded in differentiating quite special constitutional types which are well characterized and which regularly dispose to quite special neurotic, psychopathic and psychotic reactions. If we have sufficient clinical experience, we will never fail to diagnose the types mentioned and the reactions met with, like the hypomanic, respectively melancholiform reactions in cycloid psychopaths, the selfreference neuroses, respectively psychoses in sensitive neurotics and psychopaths, as well as the paranoid, the paranoic, the hysterical and the compulsive reaction types. All of them are easily recognizable and comprehensible without any deeper analyses.

As to the *therapy* of these abnormal character-types themselves, let me say that a trait common to probably all therapeutic methods is that it will be successful if it results in a desensitization of the basic sensitive disposition. Such a desensitization can, as you will know, in many cases be accomplished by physical as well as by psycho-therapeutic procedures. The reduction of the sensibility, among other things, brings about the ability of the individual to face his personal difficulties in another way than he has been used to. This common attack of all psycho-therapeutic procedures is probably one of the reasons for the fact that the psychotherapeutic theory and technic itself seems to be of little significance as to the final outcome of the therapy.

It is my impression that also many *psychosomatic disorders* are associated with a hypersensitive constitution, so that the clinical experiences derived from the study of the usual psycho-neuroses should be turned to account also in this field.

In this connection I should also like to mention that the most interesting studies of the transmitting substances at the synapses as well as the many studies of the actions of chlorpromazine and other preparations on the physiological actions must be assumed to be of great interest to psychosomatic medizin. Such biological products are acetylcholin, adrenalin, nor-adrenalin and serotonin. It is reasonable to assume that the sensitive disposition in man is conditioned in quite special biochemical relations especially at the synapses. Therefore the modern studies in this field can well be thought to contribute towards a clarification of the psychosomatic relations in the hypersensitive constitutional type forming the pre-disposition to most of the psycho-neuroses. The next step will be to find the chemical preparations which can bring about a normalizing of the *pathological* biochemical conditions at the synapses and thus find the *proper* way to normalize among other things the pathological sensitive reactions. If the scientists working in this field can succeed in this, we may hope that among other things the length of the psycho-therapeutic procedures necessary will be at any rate considerably shortened.

Author's address: Dr. G. Langfeldt, Vinderen, Psykiatriske Klinikk, *Oslo* (Norway).

Body-Build of Male Homosexuals

A. J. Coppen, London

Studies of the body-build of homosexual patients have produced conflicting reports. Weil (1924) in Germany reported that homosexuals had a narrower bi-acromial and a wider intertrochanteric diameter than did a control group. The latter unfortunately was obtained from a different part of the country and measured by a different observer. Wortis (1936) could find no abnormality in the body-build of homosexuals. Sheldon (1949) found there are no distinctive features of homosexual physique recognisable from a somatotyping photograph. He states, however, that the majority of homosexuals are recognisable by what he terms secondary gynandromorphy, that is "the measures of the feminity of the face, hands, skin and skin appendages; manner of movement and co-ordination; voice and facial behaviour; in short the covert gynandromorphy that escapes the photograph". This is in agreement with the common clinical impression that the effeminate appearance that many male homosexuals show is the result of mannerisms of gait and dress affected consciously or unconsciously by the subject rather than due to any abnormality of body-build.

The present investigation was undertaken to determine whether homosexuals have an abnormal discriminant androgyny score—an index of body-build—which as will be shown below, is related to the sexual development of the individual. The discriminant androgyny score (Tanner, 1951, 1955) of a patient is obtained by measuring the bi-acromial and bi-iliac diameters and substituting in the following formula:

$$3 \times \text{bi-acromial} - 1 \times \text{bi-iliac diameters (in cms)}.$$

The term androgyny may be defined as the presence of android features in a woman and gynaecoid features in a man. TANNER obtained a score of 90.1 with a standard deviation of 4.75 for men; the comparable figures for women were 78.9 and 4.57. This sex difference in physique arises at puberty and before this age the androgyny score fails to discriminate between the sexes.

There is evidence that the androgyny score, or its most important component the bi-acromial diameter, is correlated with sexual characteristics and abnormalities. FERRIMAN ET AL. (1957) found that women with hirsuitis had an increased urinary 17-ketosteroids output, a tendency to oligomenorrhea and an increased bi-acromial diameter. RABOCH (1957) found a decreased bi-acromial diameter in hypogonadal men and men with female sex chromatin. LINDEGARD (1955) showed the size of penis was correlated with the androgyny score. Patients suffering from pre-eclamptic toxaemia and frigidity have been found to have abnormally masculine androgyny scores (COPPEN, 1958). Thus there is evidence that subjects who suffer from certain abnormalities related to sexual function will show abnormalities in their androgyny score. The hypothesis tested in the present investigation is that homosexuals have abnormally feminine androgyny scores.

A second androgyny score was used in the present series. This was based on the relative thickness of subcutaneous fat and bone of the calf obtained from a soft tissue X-ray, and will be referred to as the fat-bone index of the calf (REYNOLDS, 1949; TANNER, 1955). This score is obtained by substituting in the following formula.

$1 \times$ bone diameter (m.m.)—$0.4 \times$ fat diameter.

The measurements are made at the maximum diameter of the calf. The index differentiates the sexes better than the discriminant androgyny score and misclassifies only 5% of a normal population of men and women (TANNER, 1955). This sex difference also arises at puberty.

The Investigation

Three groups of subjects were investigated: a group of homosexual patients, a control group and a group of neurotic patients. The homosexual group consisted of 31 patients who had been either exclusively homosexual or predominantly homosexual with only occasional heterosexual activity. The patients had attended the Maudsley Hospital primarily for homosexuality; the majority had been referred from the courts after they had been convicted of homosexual offences. Psychiatric symptoms—mainly depression or anxiety—were present to a varying extent in these patients but in none to a severe degree. However, in view of this another control group of 22 hetero-sexual neurotics was studied, as any differences found in the homo-sexuals may be related to the differences widely reported in psychiatric patients rather than to their specific sexual abnormalities.

All measurements were performed by myself, using a Martin anthropometer; the patients were measured standing, their shoulders relaxed. The X-rays of the calf were performed as described by TANNER (1955).

Results

These are presented in the tables and the figure.

Discriminant androgyny score

Homosexuals differ from the controls in their bi-acromial dia-meter and androgyny score. There is no difference between the groups as far as the bi-iliac diameter, weight, height and age are concerned.

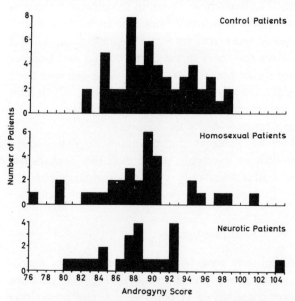

Because of the differences in body-build between subjects in different social classes that have been reported (CLEMENTS AND PICKETT, 1954; Board of Trade 1957) both controls and homosexual patients were divided into five social classes according to the classification of the

Registrar-General (1951). Both the control and the homosexual group have the greatest number of patients in social class III. Table 3 shows that when patients of this social class are compared with controls of the same class the difference between the groups is increased.

The neurotic group has an androgyny score and bi-acromial diameter very similar to the homosexual group, and in addition has a decreased bi-iliac diameter.

Table 1. Body measurements in the control, homosexual and neurotic groups; comparison of homosexual and neurotic groups with the control group

Group	Number	Mean	S. D.	Compared to control group	
				t	p
Control	53				
Androgyny score		90.3	4.1		
Bi-acromial diameter (cms)		39.8	1.7		
Bi-iliac diameter (cms)		29.3	1.3		
Weight (kg)		71.9	7.6		
Height		172.6	6.1		
Age		41.5	10.5		
Fat/bone index	10	35.2	4.4		
Homosexuals	31				
Androgyny score		88.5	5.6	1.68*	.05
Bi-acromial diameter (cms)		39.1	2.0	1.68*	.05
Bi-iliac diameter (cms)		28.8	2.2	0.71	Not significant
Weight (kg)		73.0	10.8	0.54	Not significant
Height		172.5	7.9	0.07	Not significant
Age		40.0	9.7	0.65	Not significant
Fat/bone index	31	34.6	3.1	0.47	Not significant
Neurotic patients	22				
Androgyny score		88.4	4.8	1.74	Not significant
Bi-acromial diameter (cms)		38.9	1.9	2.26	0.05
Bi-iliac diameter (cms)		28.3	1.0	3.17	0.01
Weight (kg)		66.7	9.8	2.50	0.02
Height		173.6	6.7	0.70	Not significant
Age		35.1	11.8	2.37	.05

  * One tailed test.

Correlation coefficient between Androgyny Score and fat/bone index 0.26— not significant.

Fat-bone index

The results in the patients and in the controls are shown in Table I. There is no difference between the homosexuals and the controls. There is no correlation between the fat-bone index and the androgyny score.

Table 2. Distribution of subjects and mean androgyny score according to class

Social Class	I	II	III	IV	V
Controls	(9) 92.6	(0)	(46) 90.1	(0)	(0)
Homosexuals	(0)	(8) 89.3	(15) 87.0	(7) 90.7	(1) 89.7

Number of patients in brackets.

Table 3. Results in Subjects belonging to Social Class III

Controls (46)	Mean	S. D.	Compared to homosexuals	
			t	p
Androgyny score	90.1	3.2	2.78	0.01
Bi-acromial diameter (cms)	39.7	1.8	2.17	0.05
Bi-iliac diameter (cms)	29.5	1.6	1.71	Not significant
Age	43.1	10.7	0.71	Not significant
Height	172.2	5.6	0.36	Not significant
Weight (kg)	71.5	8.6	0.26	Not significant
Homosexuals (15)				
Androgyny score	87.0	3.1		
Bi-acromial diameter (cms)	38.5	2.26		
Bi-iliac diameter (cms)	28.6	2.15		
Age	40.8	11.7		
Height	171.6	5.2		
Weight (kg)	71.5	10.7		

Discussion

The results show that homosexuals have a decreased androgyny score and bi-acromial diameter compared to the control group. This difference however is not specific for homosexuality as the neurotic group in this study also differ from the controls to approximately the same extent both as regards androgyny and bi-acromial width. The androgyny score does not discriminate between homosexuals and controls better than does the bi-acromial diameter although as the figure shows 3 homosexual patients have very low androgyny scores, outside the range of the other two groups. It appears therefore that homosexuals are similar to other psychiatric disorders in having decreased breadth measurements (REES AND EYSENCK, 1945) but that their sexual abnormality is not specifically related to these. Rather it seems the homosexual is influenced by the similar (unknown) factors that produce the abnormalities in body-build found in other psychiatric patients.

The androgyny score is unrelated to the fat-bone index. As both these sexual differences arise at puberty it might have been expected that both would have been dependent on the same factors and hence related. However the androgyny score is dependent on skeletal development alone, whereas the fat-bone index is dependent on soft tissue development as well as bone.

Summary

The discriminant androgyny score, a measure of physique related to sexual development, was obtained on a group of 31 male homosexuals. The scores of the homosexuals were significantly less than that of a control group. A group of heterosexual neurotics, however, showed a similar deviation from the control group. The androgyny score, moreover, did not differentiate the homosexuals from the controls any better than did the bi-acromial diameter which is less in these patients. It was concluded that homosexuals have an abnormality related to that found in other psychiatric disorders and that it could not be specifically related to their sexual abnormality.

I should like to thank Dr. R. D. Hoare and Miss A. Parker for taking the soft tissue x-rays, and Dr. H. S. Friend for arranging the examination of controls at Unilever House.

Bibliography

Board of Trade: Women's measurements and sizes (H.M.S.O., London 1957).
Clements, E. M. B., and Pickett, K. G.: Chest girth of men related to stature, age, body-weight and social status. Brit. J. prev. soc. Med. *8*: 108 (1954).
Coppen, A. J.: Psychosomatic aspects of pre-eclamptic toxamia. J. psychosom. Res. *2*: 241 (1958).

FERRIMAN, P.; THOMAS, P.K., and PURDIE, A.W.: Constitutional virilism. Brit.
    Med. J. 2: 1410 (1957).
LINDEGARD, B.: Body-build, Body-function and Personality (Gleerup, Lund
    1956).
RABOCH, J.: Thirty-one men with female sex chromatin. J. clin. Endrocin. 17:
    1429 (1957).
REES, W.L., and EYSENCK, H.J.: A factorial study of some morphological and
    psychological aspects of human constitution. J. ment. Sci. 91: 8 (1945).
GENERAL REGISTER OFFICE: Classification of Occupations (H.M.S.O., London
    1951).
REYNOLDS, E.L.: The fat-bone index as a sex differentiating character in man.
    Hum. Biol. 21: 199 (1949).
SHELDON, W.H.: The Varieties of Delinquent Youth (Harper, New York 1949).
TANNER, J.M.: Current advances in the study of physique. Lancet 1: 574 (1951).
TANNER, J.M.: Growth at Adolescence (Blackwell Scientific Publications, Oxford
    1955).
WEIL, A.: Sprechen anatomische Grundlagen für das Angeborensein der Homo-
    sexualität. Arch. Fruenk. Eugen. 10: 23 (1924).
WORTIS, J.W.: A note on the body-build of the male homosexual. Amer. J.
    Psychiat. 93: 1121 (1936).

Author's address: DR. A.J. COPPEN, Maudsley Hospital London S.E. 5 (England).

Constitutional Differences Between Two Strains of Rats with Different Behavioural Characteristics

R. H. J. WATSON, London

In studying the effects of drugs on the behaviour of rats it was considered useful to compare strains which had known behavioural differences. For this purpose we used adult male albino rats which had been selectively bred for differences in a behavioural criterion—The Maudsley "Emotional" and "Non-Emotional" Strains (1). Experiments were being conducted into the effects on rats of Methylpentynol (3, 4, 5)—a tranquilliser which reduces some sympathetic responses in human subjects (2). In contrast similar experiments were conducted using Ephedrine.

It was found that these two strains differed in their response to these drugs as determined by a behavioural index, namely, Rearing Behaviour occurring during five minutes exploration of a novel environment (3). Fig. 1 shows the differences in Rearing Behaviour with and without drugs.

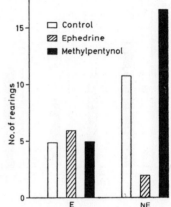

Fig. 1. Effect of Ephedrine and Methyl-pentynol on Rearing Behaviour during exploratory test in "Emotional" and "Non-Emotional" strains of rats.

It is clear that the "Emotional" strain (E) failed to respond to the drugs whereas the "Non-Emotional" strain (NE) showed marked changes in behaviour with the same doses of drugs (Methylpentynol 125 mg/kg, Ephedrine 100 mg/kg given orally 15 minutes before testing).

Since the two strains had been created by selective breeding, it was considered most likely that, in addition to the known behavioural differences, there would also be physiological and biochemical differences which had been genetically determined, and which might account for the above psychopharmacological differences. A number of such possible differences were therefore investigated.

It had been noted that the E strain was heavier than the NE strain, and that their food and water intakes were different. A more detailed metabolic investigation was undertaken by DR. S.E. DICKER, Pharmacology Department, University College, London, and the results are shown in Fig. 2. It will be seen that the E strain has a lower general metabolism than the NE strain. This suggested two possible hypotheses:

(i) *The E strain shows premature ageing when compared to the NE strain.* A comparison of the differences between the strains with changes in metabolism due to age showed that the differences between the strains were very much greater than would be the case on this hypothesis alone.

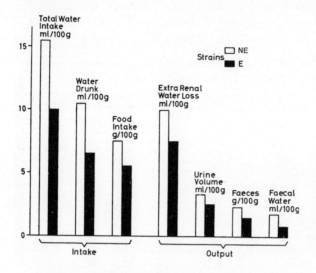

Fig. 2. Food and Water Intake and Water Excretion in "Emotional" and "Non-Emotional" strains of rats.

(ii) *The E strain is relatively hypothyroid when compared to the NE strain.* This hypothesis was supported by further investigations. Body build measurements indicated that the heavier E strain showed no difference in long bone growth when compared to the NE strain, but was more pyknic due to fat deposition. This latter finding was further confirmed by chemical estimation of body fat which showed the E strain (16.4 g/ 100 g) higher than the NE strain (13.1 g/100 g).

Since the strains had been bred in terms of a measure of "Emotionality" it was thought that some differences in adrenal activity might account for the differences. Indirect measures of adrenal activity namely, body temperature, changes in relative white cell count with stress, and adrenal ascorbic acid level (the latter and the body fat estimations were undertaken by DR. A. L. GREENBAUM, Biochemistry Department, University College, London) did not provide evidence to suggest that the E strain was characterised by greater adrenal activity. In fact in the case of the ascorbic acid level the NE strain showed a much lower level (243 mg/100 g) than the E strain (366 mg/ 100 g) which in view of the fact that the animals had just been stressed would suggest that the NE strain were in fact giving a larger adrenal response than the E strain. This paradoxical finding will be discussed later.

The thyroid difference suggested above was now followed up. More detailed investigation of endocrine gland weights was undertaken. Owing to the greater hydration of tissues in the E strain, the glands were dehydrated before weighing. Fig. 3 shows the differences in pituitary, adrenal, and thyroid glands between the two strains. Again the lower adrenal activity of the E strain is supported, and

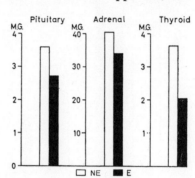

Fig. 3. Endocrine Gland weights (dehydrated) in "Emotional" and "Non-Emotional" strains of rats.

perhaps the most striking of all the differences is that of the thyroid weights in keeping with the thyroid hypothesis above. However, it is well known that mere size of thyroid gland may not be a good guide to the output of thyroxine. Histological preparations were made by DR. DONIACH, Postgraduate Medical School, London. Using cell height as an indirect measure of colloid present in the cells, he was unable to find any significant difference between the strains. In the circumstances, it was considered that the difference in gland size could now be regarded as stronger evidence of differences in thyroxine output.

Further proof of this could be made by experimentally reducing the thyroxine output of the NE strain. Animals from this strain were given methylthiouracil in their drinking water for six days, and then tested with and without drugs. Fig. 4 shows the effect of the reduction of thyroid activity on Rearing Behaviour and compares it to that of normal animals from the E strain. It will be seen that, animals so treated respond much more like the normal E strain animals, although the Ephedrine is still producing some effect. Metabolic studies confirmed that their metabolism had similarly altered so that they were more like the E strain.

It now remains to consider how far the original basis of selection (emotional defaecation) might be considered also attributable to the thyroid differences. It is known that the hypothyroid condition results in a tendency for faeces to be overdehydrated (constipation similarly accompanies human hypothyroidism). This feature of the differences between the strains is confirmed in Fig. 2. Since the E strain will

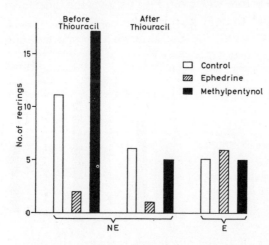

Fig. 4. Effect of Ephedrine and Methylpentynol on Rearing Behaviour in rats of the "Non-Emotional" strain before and after treatment with Methylthiouracil compared to untreated rats of the "Emotional" strain.

therefore retain faeces longer, it follows that under stress more faecal bolusses will be available for voiding. If this index is used solely, it may give rise to such animals being considered as "Emotional" when there is no evidence of autonomic responses of the kind usually associated with "emotionality" being present. In fact our investigations suggest that the animals of the NE strain more closely resemble the physical type that one would associate with "emotionality" in the human sense. In the circumstances such nomenclature may be very misleading to those undertaking psychosomatic research. In spite of this difficulty in the present instance, the investigations reported above indicate that animal experimentation can play a very useful role in psychosomatic research, and in many cases can bring to bear on a problem techniques which are not possible with human subjects, for example, selective breeding and experimental pathology.

Bibliography

1. BROADHURST, P.L.: Studies in psychogenetics: the quantitative inheritance of emotionality in the rat investigated by selective and cross-breeding. Bull. Brit. Psychol. Soc. *34*: 3A (1958).
2. DICKER, S.E., and STEINBERG, H.: The effect of methylpentynol in man. Brit. J. Pharmacol. *12*: 479–483 (1957).

3. DICKER, S.E.; STEINBERG, H., and WATSON, R.H.J.: Effect of methylpentynol on the activity of rats: J. Physiol. *137*: 88–89 (1957).
4. WATSON, R.H.J.: Effect of methylpentynol on learning in rats. J. Physiol. *142*: 30 (1958).
5. WATSON, R.H.J., and STEINBERG, H.: Different effects of drugs on two responses to "stress" in rats. Bull. Brit. Psychol. Soc. *38*: 14A (1959).

Author's address: DR. R.H.J. WATSON, Medical Research Council, Group for the Experimental Investigation of Behaviour, Psychology Department, University College, *London* (England).

III

Training for Psychosomatic Medicine

Training for Psychosomatic Medicine

(Introduction)

A. JORES, Hamburg

All of us who are assembled here know that the number of patients whose complaints have a predominantly psychological background, is considerable. According to estimates it amounts to approximately one half of all patients visiting the doctor. We further know that one can help these patients only in an unsatisfactory manner with pharmacotherapy or even operation. Most of them become chronically ill, their joy of living is clouded, their capacity to work impaired and they become prematurely disabled. We also know, however, that if these patients are treated with psychological methods, this sad fate can be averted at least in a part of them. Here the difficult question arises, however, as to who shall carry out this type of treatment. In European countries the number of trained psychologists is rather small and apart from this it would mean that the practitioner would lose approximately one half of his patients, an impossible situation. Certainly it will not be necessary to carry out psychotherapy in the whole of this 50% of cases in general practice, but every form of psychotherapy, even if only restricted to a few conversations, requires knowledge in the field of deep psychology. Here the question is: how can such knowledge be conveyed to the practicing physician?

One could suggest that knowledge in psychosomatic medicine could be passed on by the well established vehicles of postgraduate courses, lecture and periodicals, through which physicians receive information on the progress in medicine, new medications etc. Unfortunately, however, this is not possible. The decisive point here is not only the accumulation of new knowledge but above all to acquire an entirely new type of viewpoint and method of thinking and, especially, to accomplish something very decisive with regard to ones self: for only the truly mature physician, who has conquered his own bit of neurosis, is in a position to be able to help other psychically ill individuals. There are only two ways of attaining this goal: personal psychoanalysis of the psychotherapist or group analysis. Personal psychoanalysis (Lehranalyse) is an exclusive, long lasting and expensive way.

The way of group analysis of physicians was undertaken by Balint. We are therefore particularly grateful and happy to welcome him in our circle today and we are eager to hear what he has to say concerning a question which is of extremely great importance for the further development of medicine and for the future of the psychically ill.

Author's address: Prof. Dr. A. Jores, II. Medizinische Universitätsklinik, *Hamburg-Eppendorf* (Germany).

Training for Psychosomatic Medicine

M. Balint, London

It may be taken for granted that all of us assembled here for this Conference will agree that psychosomatic medicine sooner or later will establish itself as a special branch of our profession. However, I wish to call your attention to a somewhat amusing but puzzling complication that this innovation will create. It is well known that it is rather difficult to classify the various branches of our profession into a logical system. This difficulty will turn almost into an impossibility by introducing psychosomatic medicine which will upset every classificatory principle used hitherto.

May I just survey the present situation briefly. First we find the great division which cuts across the whole of medicine separating medicine proper from surgery. This division is based, in the first instance, on the therapeutic method used by the specialist; the one handles, and cuts with, a knife: the other does not but writes prescriptions. Recently a new third branch was added: radiology, in which the specialists use neither knives nor prescriptions, but rely on magic lamps. An utterly different classificatory system is based on the age of the patient, we get in this way paediatrics and geriatrics. A third principle is based on the organs or systems with which the doctor is concerned, irrespective of whether he uses a knife or not; in this way we come to ophthalmology, neurology, psychiatry, cardiology, dermatology, urology, gynaecology, endocrinology, otorhino-laryngology, and so on. Then there are specialities which are concerned only with one sort of disease, for instance, acute infectious diseases, tuberculosis, rheumatology, or venerology, etc.

Thus we have at least four classificatory principles—the doctor's customary method of treatment, the patient's age, the organ or system affected, and the disease attacking the organism. Moreover this system is inconsistent; a tuberculous kidney in a woman is not treated by a specialist in tuberculosis, or a gynaecologist but, as a rule, by a urologist, and so on. This chaos could be further increased if we would try to classify the various theoretical and administrative specialities which avoid getting into contact with patients and the various subtle delineations between the neighbouring or overlapping specialities. Instead of pursuing this somewhat philosophical question I would like to ask what is it that differentiates psychosomatic medicine from any of the other branches of our profession? What is it that qualifies a patient or an illness to be considered as psychosomatic? It is certainly not his age or sex, neither the specificity of his illness, nor the organ or system affected. Any age, any illness, any organ or system, might be considered as belonging to the sphere of psychosomatic medicine. To quote a striking example, a broken leg might be due to accident-proneness and thus might qualify as a psychosomatic condition.

Is it then possible to define at all what decides whether a patient or an illness should be our concern or not? I would propose as a classificatory basis the doctor's philosophy that determines his approach to the problems arising out of the patient's illness. According to this definition the decisive factor will be *what the doctor tries to do with his patient.* Of course there always will be extreme cases in which no such decision need or even can be taken, but this is the same in the whole field of medicine. No physician or paediatrician will prescribe medicines for a cleft palate but sooner or later will ask a surgeon to operate on it; in the same way no surgeon will operate on an acute pneumonia or meningitis but will ask one of his colleagues to treat it with suitable antibiotics. Roughly the same will hold true for psychosomatic medicine. On the other hand there are and, almost certainly, always will be patients who may be treated by any of the three great specialities— the two old ones, medicine and surgery, and the new one, psycho- somatic medicine. In a moment I shall quote cases to prove this point.

This leads us to a very awkward problem. What is the specific method of psychosomatic medicine that differentiates it from any other branch of medicine? With this problem we arrive at our main topic because only if we know what techniques should be used in psycho- somatic medicine can we decide what sort of training is necessary to acquire the requisite skills in these methods.

As any other branch of our profession, psychosomatic medicine too has two aspects. One is its philosophy and the other its practice. The one decides what sort of patients and what sort of diseases should be the concern of psychosomatic medicine, these considerations lead then to a pathology, and on the basis of it to diagnostics. The other starts with clinical observations and experiments, out of which in due course therapeutic methods and technical skills will develop. Of course, both philosophy and practice must be checked and rechecked by further clinical observations and experiments.

It is a most interesting historical fact that in our branch philoso- phy—or if you prefer, theory—has far outstripped practice. We have very fine and erudite theories about the nature of psychosomatic conditions, after all the relationship between mind and body has been incessantly discussed at least ever since SOCRATES. In contrast, the practice and technique of psychosomatic medicine are rather primitive, . are still in a largely empirical stage. Moreover, while there is a general agreement, if not about every detail, but certainly about the broad principles, of our theory, I expect that we shall hear sharp arguments in the discussion after my paper.

The discussion of what psychosomatic medicine is and should be, that is what I call its philosophy and pathology, has been dealt with at this Congress by another symposium, consequently I propose to leave it on one side. True, the results of that other symposium will have an important bearing on our topic, the training for psychosomatic medicine, but time prevents me from dealing with it beyond mentioning this fact. So I will concentrate on how to teach the practice of psychosomatic medicine, that is, how to enable students to acquire the technical skills necessary in it.

This, most probably, will prove to be a controversial subject which, as a rule, leads to a disappointingly abstract, or even abstruse discussion. I shall try to prevent this outcome by quoting two concrete clinical examples. The two patients were observed in general practice, a real goldmine for any branch of medicine. However, to avoid misunderstandings I had better introduce myself. I am not a general practitioner but a psychiatrist or, more precisely, a psychoanalyst. My familiarity with general practice stems not from direct knowledge, but from a research that we have been conducting now in the Tavistock Clinic for more than ten years into psychological implications in general medical practice. It started in a very modest form, a handful of general practitioners and a psychiatrist meeting once a week to discuss "problem" cases as they occurred in the practices. The research has developed into a training and we are proud that by now we have ten groups of doctors meeting regularly at our Clinic with a sum total of over 100 participants.

The two cases were reported recently in our advanced group in which at that time we were discussing—what one of our colleagues called jokingly—"30 second psychotherapy".

"Miss S, a plump, pleasant girl, aged 18, has been on our list for a few months only; she came with 'N'. She had severe abdominal pain on a Sunday night, which I thought was acute appendicitis. I sent her into hospital and they sent her out—nothing wrong. Since then I have seen her intermittently during the last few weeks. Never much talk. She said to me the other day 'Of course my step-father does not think I am well enough to go back to work'. 'Step-father' struck a cord. I asked 'What about your father?'. She said 'He committed suicide three years ago'. I said 'Really? What happened?' She said 'He was a homosexual. He was charged by the Police, was going up to Court, and he committed suicide.' I said 'That must have been a blow'. She said 'Not in the least. I can't even say I was sorry. I hated him. I knew all about it'. She added then, she did not want to fall in love and get married; but her boy-friends did, which I can understand as she is rather an attractive girl. I rounded the interview off by saying 'Perhaps the source of your difficulties with boys is that your father preferred boys rather than you, a girl'. She said 'Maybe'. A few days later she charged in, fine and well, and said 'Can I go back to work?'."

A simple case and it is very likely that, provided the doctor can keep up this kind of relationship with the patient, she will not be referred again to a hospital and possibly instead of having abdominal pains she will be able to devise some other methods for coping with her problems. We must add, however, that our colleague needed quite a few weeks till he noticed that he had to treat something else than abdominal pains and on one occasion he referred Miss S. as an emergency case to a surgical hospital—admittedly on a Sunday. It is easy to imagine what could have happened to this girl if her doctor had been, and would have continued to be, less observant. All of us know the many young girls in puberty and adolescence who go on complaining about recurrent abdominal pains till they find an obliging surgeon who takes their appendix out. The appendix then is either not sent for a pathological examination or, if sent, the report is equivocal or, as often as not, negative. On the basis of our experiences we think that this girl will now have a fair chance to keep her appendix and thus avoid starting off on the road which leads to an unending series of abdominal operations. The first station on this road is invariably either an appendicectomy or dilatation and curettage.

Sceptics may say that our result in this case is not much better than that of a surgeon who, having taken out an innocent appendix, discharges his patient after a week or so with perfect results. Of course, only a long follow-up, say about ten to fifteen years, can definitely answer the question, which of these two is the better treatment? So let us turn to our second case where there was some sort of follow-up:

"Mrs. K. aged 55, a very pleasant and jolly woman, came in wanting something against her sweats at night. I said 'It sounds like hot flushes. When did you finish your periods?'. She said 'This January. I wake up 8–10 times every night, and then this awful cough. My husband said I must come to you. I have had this cough for ten years since my father died. His illness was congestion and he had an awful cough when he died. He was a wonderful man. One doctor said I had got his cough'. I said 'What did he mean by that?'. She said 'I'm not sure, just that I picked it up. I am quite well otherwise'. I said 'Perhaps what he was getting at is that you cannot allow your father to die, you hang on to his cough'. She said 'I hadn't thought of that. He was a most wonderful man, very happy and jolly'. Then she added 'Perhaps that is what you meant when years ago you told me I could not relax, I could not let go, as if I would explode if I got angry. True, I never get angry'. Then, after a further pause: 'I never told you about my father and the cough. Perhaps that is why it has not made any difference.' So my clever interpretation a few years ago that she could not get angry and could not relax did not have any effect on her."

Here we tried in the seminar to point out to our colleague that his self-criticism was only partly justified. After all, the patient remembered his "clever interpretation". We thought that he had been on the right track, only he had not gone far enough, and we queried whether he had not repeated the same mistake this time. For instance, did he ask his patient how to her mind her husband compared with her beloved father?

The doctor reassured us that he did ask this question. "She said 'My husband is so good and kind. He never gets angry, only laughs. Last night I was coughing and coughing and wanted to wake him up. I told him this morning and he said 'Why didn't you?' She answered 'It would have been no good if I had, you would only have gone to sleep again'."

There are a great number of points to be discussed in this report Let us start with criticism. In the discussion following the report the doctor was chided for not noticing this broad hint. It is not only the husband who goes to sleep after being woken up, but he, the doctor, did exactly the same. It was only then that he realised, somewhat amused, that the woman who sensed in a way that she needed further help, told him in this roundabout way to get on with his job, instead of falling asleep on his laurels. He was able then to recognise that Mrs. K's "awful cough" was also a reproach against her menfolk—husband and doctor—who are by far not so wonderful as she thinks her father was.

Then there was the ominous sentence in which Mrs. K. described her husband as "kind and good". A description of this kind almost invariably means that the husband is somewhat impotent and tries to compensate for his shortcoming by kindness; on the other hand, it means also that under the appreciative facade of an understanding wife there is considerable bitterness and resentment, if not much more than that. Moreover neither wife nor husband can get angry, apparently both of them must be jolly and laugh. If this does not prove helpful the only thing they can do is to fall asleep—true, to be woken up by the "awful cough".

I wish to emphasise here that all this and some more possibilities for further therapeutic work became available to the doctor only after he realised that in fact he went to sleep too—may we add now, because he too was somewhat frightened, sensing the intensity of emotions behind Mrs. K's jolly and appreciative facade.

Another important point is what may be called a follow-up. Mrs. K. remembered not only that some years ago her present doctor had pointed out to her that she could not relax, could not let herself go, as if she knew that she would explode if she might get angry, but also that even some years earlier her previous doctor had remarked that she picked up her father's cough. Moreover, when her doctor enabled her to understand that bit of her personality somewhat better and deeper, the two other remarks made several years ago fell into their places and made sense to her.

This is a highly important point. Both of the previous remarks were correct and to the point but apparently they did not have sufficient effect. It is anybody's guess whether the present interpretations—of the thirty-second-psychotherapy—namely that she cannot allow her father to die, that she must hang on to his cough, will or will not have a better therapeutic effect. It is possible that in a few days time Mrs. K. will charge in to the doctor's surgery, as Miss S. did, and announce in her jolly manner "you are a marvellous doctor, you took away my cough". However, it is also possible that the doctor has not done enough this time either and some further efforts will be needed to enable Mrs. K. to get in touch with her anger and resentment, which are possibly expressed by her "awful" cough, unpleasant—though to a varying degree— to herself, to her husband, and to her doctor.

Before going any further I have to deal with a likely objection. It might be argued that the two cases have nothing whatsoever to do with psychosomatic medicine, they are simple cases of hysteria and what the doctors did was some sort of primitive psychotherapy. Is this argument valid? Do we know what makes an abdominal pain hysterical or psychosomatic, or what turns an hysterical cough into a psychosomatic condition or even into a chronic bronchitis with atrophies and compensatory emphysema? I certainly do not assume to know the answers, but a cough lasting more than ten years is definitely somewhat suspicious, and we may agree that a few more hysterical attacks of abdominal pain would very likely land Miss S. on the operating table. I wish to emphasise here that—as I have already mentioned—it is largely the doctor's philosophy which will decide whether Miss S's abdominal pains should be treated by sedatives, antispasmodics, tranquillisers, by a surgical operation, or should be considered a psychosomatic condition and then treated by what?

The two cases reported here were considered by the doctors as psychosomatic; though both patients got some medicine, the main treatment they received was psychotherapy. Does it mean that we must take it as proven that the therapeutic technique of psychosomatic medicine is psychotherapy pure and simple? Unhesitatingly I would answer: No, but equally emphatically I would state that *by far the most important therapeutic technique in psychosomatic medicine is psychotherapy.* Even if the doctor prescribes some medicine, examines his patient's body, or massages it, or whatever else he decides to do, he must always be aware of the psychological effects of his physical treatment; and his main concern all the time must be his psychological impact on the patient, no matter whether it has been achieved by physical means or by psychotherapy. Thus we arrive at the question, should every doctor intending to practise psychosomatic medicine be trained as a psychotherapist?

Before answering this question I wish to clear the decks by stating that any training in psychotherapy must be in addition to and parallel with—but certainly not in place of—a thorough medical training. Although throughout the whole of my professional career as a psychoanalyst I have been fighting for equal rights and status of medical and non-medical psycho-analysts in our own profession, this does not mean that the equality could be extended to the field of psychosomatic medicine. The obvious reason is that one cannot properly assess the therapeutic requirements of a case without a reliable physical diagnosis. A statement of this kind is usually interpreted as demanding that any patient whose illness might be considered psychosomatic should first be subjected to an exhaustive physical examination and to a series of medical and possibly surgical treatments before offering him psychotherapy. In many, probably in the majority of, cases this would be a much too expensive procedure for the patient; over and above paying for the various examinations and treatments it would entail a serious loss of time amounting to months or even years. What I am advocating here is, *equal status and equal rights for painstaking physical and psychological diagnostic examinations:* in other words, neither of them should have precedence over the other, both of them should be conducted parallel and with equal emphasis. To be able to do this or, at any rate, to see to it that this should be done, the doctor must be properly trained in medicine but must also know a good deal about psychotherapy and psychodynamics.

This good deal has, of course, a minimal and several higher levels but, as in any other professional knowledge and skill, no maximum. At the minimal level the doctor is required to recognise whether or not his physical findings explain satisfactorily the patient's troubles and how far any physical or pharmacological therapy based on those findings will help, and how much of the troubles might remain unrelieved. At the next higher level the doctor will be expected to form some idea about the probable psychological origins of the patient's troubles, and also about how much these assumed psychological factors have affected the patient's mind, character and human relationships, about what sort of therapeutic intervention will be needed to remedy the whole situation, and, last but not least, to know which specialist should be asked to carry this therapy out. I hope it will be quite clear from my description that at these two levels what is expected from the doctor is considerable theoretical knowledge and some skill in diagnosis—more at the second than at the first level—but no skill in therapy. Training in psychosomatic medicine up to these two levels may be done by the traditional means and methods of the teaching hospitals, that is, by lectures, ward rounds and case demonstrations.

If the doctor aspires to do more than diagnosing his patients and then sending each of them who needs this kind of treatment to specialists, that is, if he wants to try his hand at some therapeutic work, then he must acquire the necessary therapeutic skills, exactly in the same way as in any other branch of medicine, say midwifery or paediatrics. There may be several methods in use to train doctors who are not psychiatrists in this kind of psychotherapy, but I have no first-hand knowledge of them; so may I be allowed to use our own experiences at the Tavistock Clinic. We have found that it is possible to train a selected group of doctors—I wish to stress emphatically that the possession of a medical diploma in itself does not qualify everybody automatically for psychotherapy—to carry out psychotherapy at about the level reported in our two cases. Here too we encounter two different levels; the lower level presupposes that the doctor while doing psychotherapy takes part in an on-going seminar of the kind we have developed, and a higher level when he can do it on his own. The difference between the two levels clearly emerges in the discussion following the second case quoted.

This sounds fairly simple but it means much more than meets the eye. There are quite a number of skills that the doctor has to acquire before he will be able to conduct psychotherapy. The sum total of these new skills amounts to, what I described in the chapter on Training in my book, The Doctor, His Patient and the Illness, as *a limited though considerable change of personality*. This change is the basis of every kind of psychotherapy and this fact is the reason why the present traditional methods of medical training are insufficient and inadequate in our field. To prove this point may I quote some details of our work at the Tavistock Clinic.

The doctor must be able to observe and, still more important, report about his observations to the seminar. It is easy to state that his observations must be conscientious and his report sincere so as to enable the seminar to get a realistic picture of what has happened between doctor and patient. This, however, is not a simple task because every report is followed by a fair criticism of the doctor's methods and, over and above it, by interpretations of why he said or missed something and made the correct interventions or the mistake he made. When it is realised that our skills as well as our mistakes and blind spots are expressions of our character and personality, it will become clear that a frank discussion of them goes far beyond what is required from a student during under- or even postgraduate medical training. Hardly any one of us is so healthy that he could stand un-ruffled a searching criticism of his professional behaviour and the showing up of some of his shortcomings and blind spots, yet this has to be accepted in our seminars; moreover, after listening to all the criticism of his handling of the case the doctor is expected to return to his patient and test out in the subsequent therapeutic work whether the seminar was right or he himself. This is perhaps the most difficult task for most of us like to prove, at any rate to ourselves, that after all it was we who were right and the seminar and its leader were wrong when criticising us. On the other hand, it is almost equally difficult to avoid humbly and penitently accepting that of course one was wrong and all the others, especially the great leader of the seminar, were absolutely right. It is a hard school to learn not to be swayed too

much by either of these powerful emotions and to conduct the subsequent sessions of the psychotherapy so that they might throw some
light on the various problems and show at what point and how much
the doctor was right and how much his colleagues in the seminar or
its leader.

In our scheme a constant watch is kept on the doctor's feelings
and emotions towards his patient as well as towards the seminar,
and on the basis of every case-report we try to demonstrate how these
emotions colour, influence, or even determine his handling of the
patient's problems. A good illustration of this is Mrs. K's case.
Although the doctor made a good start in understanding the etiology
of the "awful cough", at one point he too went to sleep. It was only
the discussion at the seminar that brought to light that he did so
because he sensed his patient's very intense critical and possibly
hostile sentiments and in a way became over-cautious or—one may
say—intimidated.

What we study all the time is the interaction between the patient's
physical and mental problems and the doctor's therapeutic approach
as determined by his own personality and emotions. If the patient's
problems are properly diagnosed and the doctor's individual approach
is adequately assessed, it is not too difficult to predict the probable
course of events during treatment. It is largely under the influence of
these experiences that the doctors acquire sufficient familiarity with
human psychopathology and psychodynamics.

In our experience—provided the doctors were properly selected
at the start—the first level mentioned above can be reached in about
two years or so. Our system is based on weekly case conferences
lasting about two hours each; we meet regularly during University
term time which adds up to approximately 40 weekly sessions in a
year. I wish to emphasise that these are merely approximate figures,
they depend to a great extent on the individual doctor, on the constitution of the group he is attending and, of course, on the ability,
skill and experience of the group leader. All these factors interact
in a most complicated manner so the figures quoted must be taken
only as first orientation. The uncertainty is still greater about how
much work is needed to arrive at the second higher level which enables
the doctor to do psychotherapy unaided. On the whole I would say
that a minimum of another two years is necessary for it, but I wish
it to be understood that this is the minimum, and not the average,
time required.

I do not think it is possible for a doctor—no matter whether he is a general practitioner or a non-psychiatric consultant—to go further and undertake deeper psychotherapy if he wants to remain in his profession. As far as I know everyone who ventured beyond the second level just mentioned and underwent a proper training in psycho-analysis or in any other brand of systematic psychotherapy, eventually gave up his former practice and became a psychotherapist pure and simple. May I quote my own case as a warning example. I started my career as a promising general physician with a strong bent for mathematics, physics and bio-chemistry, to the extent that after taking my M.D. I graduated also as a Ph.D. in chemistry. However, parallel with my studies in bio-chemistry I underwent psycho-analytic training and the result is that I have been a practising psycho-analyst for more than 35 years. I know of several practising doctors who went through a similar change of mind while training in psycho-analysis.

On the other hand, it is with pride that I state that of all the doctors who attended our training seminars at the Tavistock Clinic, numbering by now about 200, we have not lost one to psychiatry or psycho-analysis. All of them remained in their own practices. Rightly you may ask me, why am I so proud of this fact?

True there is a great need in the ranks of the International Psycho-Analytical Association for psycho-analysts with a thorough theoretical and practical training in general medicine, thus each experienced doctor is a most welcome candidate. However great our need is, it is incomparably smaller than the need for both general practitioners and specialists who can understand the patient's physical and emotional problems equally well and, in consequence, can assess their relative pathogenic effect correctly. At present general medicine is based on reliable physical diagnosis and rationally applied pharmacology; consequently he is a good doctor who has adequate skills in these two fields. The future medicine will require, over and above these, adequate skills in psychotherapy. Nowadays the combination of these three skills is called psychosomatic medicine; I have no doubts that in a couple of decades this term will become superfluous and antiquated because the combination will be called simply medicine. The few doctors having trained or training now at our seminars are the first pioneers, each of whom counts such a great deal; that is why I am so proud that not one of them has left our ranks.

Summary

The establishment of psychosomatic medicine as a special branch of our profession will upset the traditional boundaries between the various medical specialities. By far the most important therapeutic technique used in it is undoubtedly psychotherapy, in consequence every doctor intending to practise psychosomatic medicine should be trained as a psychotherapist. As in every other speciality, here too the required therapeutic skill will have a minimum and several higher standards. The training scheme developed at the Tavistock Clinic is described briefly.

Author's address: DR. M. BALINT, Regents Park, 7 Park Square West, *London N.W. 1* (England).

Psychiatric Training Problems in Psychosomatic Medicine

J. BASTIAANS, Amsterdam

In their recent book on teaching and learning of psychotherapy, EKSTEIN AND WALLERSTEIN (1) state, that "the best training system is one which combines stability and a shared viewpoint with room for flexibility, individual difference, and an opportunity for creative and imaginative work on the part of the teachers". I think this statement can be used very well in our discussions on the psychiatric training in psychosomatic medicine.

Firstly the question arises what will be the nucleus of stability and our shared viewpoint in the training process. As an analyst I had the opportunity to train non-psychiatric co-workers as well as psychiatrists of the Amsterdam Psychosomatic Team and of the Amsterdam Psychoanalytic Institute. And although I don't have the same systematic experience as BALINT (2) in the training of groups of general practitioners, I am very glad that I am allowed today to refer to his work and to discuss some differences between his approach and ours, as far as it concerns a more or less specific training in psychosomatic medicine.

The nucleus of stability in our Amsterdam work and a central tool in our training programme is the very detailed life history and analysis of the personality structure of the psychosomatic patient.

In our approach we try to combine the advantages of an intensive phenomenological description of the first contact with the patient with systematic data on childhood, development and conflict situations, which partly determined specific aspects of the patient's character, partly psychosomatic syndromes, which we have usually studied from the point of view of psychosomatic specificity.

I think, that in this respect our approach differs from BALINT's, and, as far as I can see, his case histories are directed especially on the elucidation of those main psychodynamic aspects, which are of immediate value to psychotherapy. The nucleus of stability in his approach is the doctor-patient relationship, especially the counter-transference, and I think, that in a training programme for identical and non-identical psychotherapy—a formulation used by WEYEL (3)—, which can be carried out by general practitioners, BALINT is entirely right. In all fairness it must be said, that the interest in psychosomatic problems coincides to a large extent with the interest in psychotherapy. But from the methodological point of view, we have to differentiate training in psychosomatic methodology quite clearly from training in the different methods of psychotherapy.

Perhaps, we can say that there can be no cure without diagnosis, without structuralization. In my opinion detailed structure analysis of the patient may automatically lead to the development of that psycho-analytic, psychotherapeutic or other therapeutic technique, which is the most appropriate in the individual case and the most adequate for a specific psychosomatic group.

As you know this basic principle "structure leads to therapy" helped GROEN and me (4) in finding and formulating lines of action for the psychotherapy of patients suffering from ulcerative colitis. Later on we learned how our approach resembled partly the analytic approach to psychoneurotics, partly the direct analysis of psychotics. And with our growing insight in the early processes of Ego-development, in individuation and separation, in the intense anxiety of the very immature Ego to loose itself in the symbiosis with the first key-figures, we became aware of the great symbolic value of, for instance, the dietetic measures and of an active and positive maternal approach by all the members of the staff, of doctors, nurses, social workers etc. One may compare the psychotherapeutic experiences as described by VANGGAARD (5) for borderline cases with the different therapeutic measures, which may be useful in the therapy of psychosomatic cases. In both ways there is much the same. The difference, however, is determined by the "normality", by the specific mechanisms of defence of the psychosomatic patient, who always tries to his utmost to appear normal and mentally healthy (6). The meaning of this barrier of defence, specific in psychosomatic adaptation to stress, has recently been rendered into objective terms by BARENDREGT (7), who found that psychosomatic patients are significantly more sociable than psychoneurotics, as we see them in the psychotherapeutic and psychoanalytic institutes.

These findings imply, that our psychosomatic patients may be very young babies, children of four to five and adults at the same time. In training psychiatrists and non-psychiatric co-workers in a psychosomatic team we must equally pay attention to the patterns of normal as well as of abnormal behaviour and to the physiology of feeling states as met with in the different phases of individual development. Unfortunately the interest of our trainees in description of normal processes usually is far less pronounced than the interest in abnormal processes. Our students mostly are keen on the analysis of "deeper" structures. They want to see behind a veil, past which they could not see before and they constantly fail in describing the veil itself. Here the students have to go the same way as psycho-analysis itself, i.e. from Id to Ego, from the description of one dynamic aspect to that of the integration of many aspects of personality.

I may illustrate how phenomenological vagueness and inaccuracy may give rise to misunderstanding in many discussions on the essence of behaviour and feeling.

A year ago, during an interesting discussion on an excellent paper of HAMBLING (8) read before the British Psychosomatic Society, everybody seemed to agree with the concept that inhibition of aggression gives rise to elevation of the blood pressure. Nevertheless, there was no agreement with VAN DER VALK (9), who accentuates the significance of anxiety as well as of aggression in the psychogenesis of hypertensive disease and of the ratio anxiety-aggression for the discrepancy in the separate elevation of systolic and diastolic pressure. I wondered how there could be so much difference of conclusion between two such investigators in this field. I think the solution of this problem may be found in a more detailed clinical description, in a better phenomenology of aggression and in a more exact definition of what we mean by stating that the patient is aggressive or anxious. There is a difference between suppressed and repressed aggression, and there is also a difference between destructive, sadistic and creative aggression, or between a feeling state, in which conscious aggression is experienced or in which anxiety indicates that feelings of aggression are more operative on a lower level of consciousness. To a certain extent, our phenomenological difficulties can be compared with those which mostly are inhaerent to the description of the manifest and the latent dream-content.

What we have therefore to teach the student in psychosomatic medicine is to verbalize which criteria he consciously or sub-consciously uses, while stating that the patient is aggressive. In this way the student may get interested in the psychosomatic aspects of normal behaviour, of normal mimicry and other aspects of psychomotoric expression.

The problem of clinical accuracy was mentioned by WISDOM (10) in his interesting paper on the problem of hysteria, in which he accentuated the fragmentariness and the incompleteness in the use of criteria and definitions concerning the hysterical syndrome. Much controversy or divergence in opinion could have been avoided, if the hysteric behaviour and the hysterical feeling states would have been described more carefully. Of course, we constantly have to make abstractions out of the wealth of human behaviour and human feelings, but I think that, for the development of psychosomatic medicine, the initial descriptions cannot be good enough.

As a matter of fact it seems superfluous to state that detailed description is fundamental in every good clinical work. Yet it remains difficult to fulfil this condition. In our own work we noticed how much improvement could be found in the case histories we make nowadays, compared with those of 1947, when we started the Amsterdam Psychosomatic Team. In one of the first case histories, a woman suffering from obesity was described as "a rather fat hysteric with oral traits". Thus we typified the first contact. This may be compared with the first impressions of one of my co-workers concerning a 40 year old lawyer, who came to us complaining of difficulties in his private life. The psychiatrist, who worked with the psychosomatic team during some years, wrote:

The at a rough estimation 35 year old patient gives in the first
contact the impression of being a jolly good fellow, loving wine,
women and song.

He looks quite well and suntanned; wears gay sporting dresses,
blue linen jacket, brown suède shoes, jaunty ties. His habit is that of
a pycnic. He has a chubby head, getting slightly bald, dark brown
hairs, and large and lively velvet brown eyes.

Psychomotorally he behaves supple and lively in a Latin way;
his mimicry is quite nuanced; he has a warm baritone that is richly
modulated to which the accent of the dialect of the southern part of
Holland gives a nice colour.

In his contacts he is intrusively personal, charming to the utmost
with a strong tendency to flirt.

His mood is constantly changing: now he is radiant with bon-
homie, then he is dysphoric, sometimes manic, sometimes down,
inhibited, and then again he looks quite defensive and paranoid. His
affects are not quite adequate. As to his complaints and his personal
difficulties, he tends to bagatellize and sometimes he behaves in a
rather childish and naive way.

His main mechanism of reaction to questions is what could be
called the Pilatus-manœuvre: "Truth—what's truth?", and with the
help of this mechanism of defense he bites his feelings to pieces. His
complaints make the impression of being genuine, but one feels that
his sense of illness remains rather intellectual and that he avoids the
essence of his emotional difficulties to come to consciousness.

His intelligence seems rather good; by clinical estimation his
I.Q. is 120. His way of thinking is rather orderly and rectilinear,
although he tends to jump. The level of consciousness is clear. There
is a marked preoccupation with his problems. It makes the impression
that he comes "spontaneously", but he feels ambivalent towards a
psychotherapeutic treatment.

Phenomenological descriptions like this one, which are the starting point for further exploration, make high demands on the trainee.
He must have the disposal of a certain capacity to express and to
verbalize everything that usually in the contact with the patient is
experienced as self-evident. To a great extent flexibility is required as
well as a nuanced sense of accuracy. A valuable help at the psychiatric
examination, too, is a photo, an instantaneous photograph. And often
the assistent, who drudged on a complete structure analysis for many

hours, hears from his supervisor: well, just show me his photo now. This indicates how difficult it may be to be clear and complete at the same time.

I don't want to discuss in detail the elaborated schemes of life history and summary as we use them in Amsterdam. Especially our summary-scheme puzzled us during many years and now we seem to have found one in which phenomenological, psycho-analytical, psychological and other data are collected and integrated more or less harmoniously.

But there is a special aspect of our examination technique, important to training, that I want to discuss with you. In the supervision of the case histories of our co-workers, we can soon notice which categories of the case history are described better and which categories apparently activate emotional problems in the examinator, which may give rise to distortion of the picture. Only a few trainees are able to complete a life history evenly. One student describes first impressions much easier than the first associative material related to, for instance, the parents, the other one avoids puberty problems or over-accentuates actual problems in comparison with traumatic experiences of the patient's past. It is our experience that a clear analysis of actual conflict situations which give rise to psychosomatic syndromes, is mostly neglected by those students who have actual problems themselves. Much discrepancy in opinion in our groups seemed to be determined by this personal aspect of the investigator. And the answer to many questions of psychosomatic specificity appeared to be difficult as a consequence of contrasting descriptions by different investigators of the actual conflict situation of the patient.

Another difficulty is found in the number of associations we need in the answers to the questions of the scheme. The purely scientifically thinking investigator, who prefers the mechanism of regulation and defence of "isolation" in his intellectual activity, usually needs more associative material, in order to construct valuable hypotheses, than one who works more intuitively and who tends more to be wrapped up in the whole situation. The latter mostly is more therapy minded, whereas the "isolator" mostly is more research minded.

To nearly every investigator, who has to make detailed psychosomatic case histories, it is difficult to find the right balance between closeness and distance in the contact with the patient, a balance so basic in all our therapeutical work.

Another difficulty in training a staff of psychiatric and non-

psychiatric co-workers in a psychosomatic group is, that group interactions hamper the construction of a standardized case history
mentioned above. Some members of the group are able to use the
model after some training without much trouble and mistake. Other
members experience their task as something they have to do for the
leader of the group and they react to him in accordance with their own
neurosis. Then we see the mechanisms of protest, anxiety, competition
and other well known dynamisms, reflected in the inability of the
trainee to complete his task. An important point is, whether we have
to interpret these disturbing factors in the group. It is my experience
that, if the scientific work is really threatened by too much personal
group interaction and by its own nucleus of stability, group discussions
can be useful. However, it has to be done very carefully, especially
when some members of the group undergo their training analysis at
the same time. It would be interesting to hear BALINT's opinion on
this subject.

I think this the right moment to say something about the second
part of EKSTEIN AND WALLERSTEIN's formulation concerning stability
and flexibility in training.

In using the standarized examination technique as mentioned
above, one has to be flexible. For instance, the trainee may not ask
all the questions in the same order. If the patient needs to speak
without restriction during the first interviews, one has to postpone
questions related to objective data till a later session. It is a technical
fault if the patient experiences the interviews as if he has to answer
a questionnaire. Therefore, it may be useful if the leader of the group
shows how he talks with the patient, especially how he analyses precipitating conflict situations, the analysis of which may be so difficult
in the beginning. Doing the examination together with a trainee may
stimulate his insight, that in spite of the need for systematization
every case history leaves enough room for creative and imaginative
work. Not seldom we can see that the case history is a baby who has
to be born. The process of this delivery is subjected to as many
inhibitions and resistances as birth itself in women and men. Thus we
have found that we have to pay equal attention to every case history
made by members of the team. One has to help the students especially
making the summary, which is often incomplete at the moment that
the case history is discussed in the staff conference. In this summary
the student has to formulate his opinion on the influence of early
traumatic experiences and neglect on later behaviour, mood, feeling

state, characteranomalies. And it is remarkable how many problems arise, if the student has to answer systematically how Ego-functions as perception, memory, regulation, reality-testing, integration etc. have been impaired by acute or chronic traumata. Likewise it is worth while to try to formulate the details of transference reactions as found during the examination and how far these reactions may have been determined by the early relations with key figures. Other aspects of the summary, which give rise to many discussions, that often have great training value, are those concerning the criteria which consciously or pre-consciously are used when stating, that the patient needs a special form of therapy.

Our examination technique has especially been criticized by those psychiatrists, who are used to make short case histories, who don't have much research experience, especially not in correlating psychic events with somatic data. If one is used to working with neurotics and psychotics, one is mostly not aware of the advantage of psychosomatic complaints and psychosomatic syndromes, which function as a hold for much correlative work in the psychosomatic team. It is my experience, that the possibility to compare one's own data with those of the physiologist, the psychologist, the internist, the sociologist and the other members of the team, is of great importance for the psychosomatic psychiatrist, who mostly has not had much systematic training in this field, while working in a department of neuro-psychiatry.

Do we have to use the detailed biographical technique always? It depends on the aim as well of our research as of the training. Daily psychosomatic practice necessitates us to use abbreviated examination techniques. In the team of QUERIDO in Amsterdam WEYEL (3, 11) developed a psychosocial history scheme, which enables us to collect many relevant and important data in one interview. This technique is especially useful for psychiatrists working in a general hospital, where they have to see many patients, and it has to be decided in the first place whether social or psychic problems and conflicts, found in patients suffering from organic diseases, are of psychogenetic importance or only functioning as parallel syndromes, which are independent of the organic syndrome.

The next step in the development of reliable examination techniques is to find out which categories of the case history scheme are the most valuable in relation to prediction. In the Psychoanalytic Institute in Amsterdam we'll try to comprise our present examination scheme to one, that only consists of question categories, the answers of which, as collected by the average trainee, are the most reliable in prognosis and indication. We presume, that the answers of our patients as given in the first interviews are to a certain extent independent of the investigator and of the doctor-patient relationship, the same as in relation to prediction with respect tu future behaviour, mood the Rorschach technique and other projective tests. In a well organized team it usually is not difficult to eliminate too much individual variations determined by the investigator. This process of elimination may have training value itself.

The use of abbreviated techniques—and once again I want to mention the study of WEYEL—may be especially useful when having to convince others of the importance of psychogenetic and sociogenic factors in the genesis of certain organic diseases. With such a technique QUERIDO ET AL. (11) made a follow-up investigation of 1630 patients admitted to a general hospital. It was attempted to assess how far they were suffering from social and/or psychic stresses to the extent of impeding their wellbeing. This assessment (the integrated evaluation made by a team consisting of a general physician, a social worker and a psychiatrist) as well as the clinical prognosis of the cases was compared with that of the actual condition of the patients about half a year after discharge from hospital; the last one was made by other members of QUERIDO's team independently of the first assessment. It was found that 871 patients of 1630 lived under stressful conditions at the moment of admission. Unambiguously it appeared to be necessary to give—help—after-care, social work, case-work, psychotherapy etc.—to nearly all those patients who were in distress at the moment of admission.

A significant difference in the chance of recovery was found to exist between patients who had to cope with problems apart from their physical illness and those who did not. A favourable clinical prognosis was made in 1128 of 1630 cases. This means that medical science offers a possibility of recovery to over 69 per cent of the sample of the patients from a general hospital. But the follow-up study showed that only 660 (60 per cent) of the 1128 favourable clinical prognoses were realized. This accentuates the inaccuracy of clinical prognosis in general. It was proven that the forecast of recovery as based on the integrated assessment was accurate in 75 per cent.

The results of this study underline the importance of a systematic socio-psychosomatic or integrative approach as to the problem of illness and its treatment in general. Besides the need of a systematic training programme in this field is stressed unmistakably.

Lastly I would like to tell you something about my experiences with courses and group therapy. For many years I had to give introductory courses for non-psychiatrists in the Psychoanalytic Institute. Psychosomatic problems appeared to be of great teaching value. I noticed that there was little interest in theoretical discussions on problems of drive energy, instincts and other aspects of drive theory, unless they could be illuminated with the help of ethology. There was more interest in problems of Ego-regulation, mechanisms of defence and Super-ego details as far as important to pathology. But there was a sudden increase of interest when we compared a case history of a psychosomatic patient with that of a patient suffering from a disease which only slightly differed from the former. An example may be found in the comparison of patients suffering from dyspepsia or gastritis with those suffering from peptic ulcer. This approach enables the members of the group to compare first associations to the questions of the scheme as given by different patients.

The importance of associative processes can also be illustrated by the discussion of exact records of group sessions of psychosomatic patients. Groups merely consisting of asthmatics or ulcer patients demonstrate the specificity of the mechanisms of defence much better than the records of an individual case therapy. Besides the group study of group records confronts the investigators quite naturally with problems of transference and countertransference, and sometimes correction of faults in the doctor-patient relationship is easier in a group than in an individual teacher-pupil relationship.

You will understand that I as an analyst prefer psychoanalytic training for psychiatrists working in a psychosomatic team. But at the same time I must say how much I have been impressed by what could be done in group therapy and individual therapy by psychiatrists and non-psychiatrists, members of a psychosomatic team, who did not have psycho-analytic training. The condition that had to be fulfilled was that they had worked in the team during many months or perhaps years and that they had assimilated the essence of this kind of group work, especially the essence of our psychosomatic sthetoscope, the detailed case history discussion, which remains our nucleus of stability.

Bibliography

1. EKSTEIN, R., and WALLERSTEIN, R.: The teaching and learning of psychotherapy (New York 1958).
2. BALINT, M.: The doctor, his patient and the illness (London 1957).

3. WEYEL, J.A.: Psychiatry in general practice. Thesis (Amsterdam 1958).
4. GROEN, J., and BASTIAANS, J.: Studies on ulcerative colitis: personality structure, emotional conflict situations and effects of psychotherapy. In: Modern trends in psychosomatic medicine (London 1955).
— Psychotherapy of ulcerative colitis. Gastroenterology *17*: 344 (1951).
5. VANGGAARD, TH.: Schizophreniform pseudoneurosis. Paper read before the Dutch Society for Psychoanalysis (Amsterdam 1958).
6. BASTIAANS, J., and GROEN, J.: Psychotherapy of internal disease. In: The affective contact (Amsterdam 1952).
— Some problems of the transference in the treatment of psychosomatic patients. Acta psychother. psychosom. orthopaed. suppl. *3*: 292 (1955).
7. BARENDREGT, J.T.: Lijders aan psychosomatische kwalen als sociaal aangepaste neurotici. N.T. Geneesk. *42*: 2044 (1958).
8. The Nature of Stress Disorder. Conference of the Society for Psychosomatic Research. May 1958, London. Hutchinson Medical Publications, London 1959. p. 37.
9. VALK, J.M. v. d.: in: BASTIAANS, J., Psychosomatische gevolgen van onderdrukking en verzet, p. 382 (Amsterdam 1957).
10. WISDOM, J.O.: A methodological approach to the problem of hysteria. Paper read before the Dutch Society for Psychoanalysis (Amsterdam 1957).
11. QUERIDO, A.: Inleiding tot een integrale geneeskunde (Leiden 1955).
Forecast and follow-up. Paper to be published in J. Prev. Soc. Med.

Author's address: DR. J. BASTIAANS, Memlingstraat 11, *Amsterdam* (Holland).

One Year's Experience in Psychosomatic Group Training of General Practitioners

H. BAERWOLFF, Hamburg

Training in analytical psychotherapy has long ceased to be a problem of method. Accumulated experience has had its effect upon the conditions of training prescribed in the corresponding institutions.

Practitioners so trained are generally occupied exclusively in psychotherapy. They are specialists mostly working in isolation. In their daily practice they are so often confronted with the psychological errors, omissions and blunders in medical practice, and the almost always serious consequences of their implications for doctor and patient, that they are faced with the choice of either falling into resignation, or exerting themselves to communicate psychological knowledge to their colleagues.

Factual criticism of efforts of that kind (discussions, letters to doctors, lectures, courses) shows unfortunately that they are almost invariably unsuccessful, if one accepts as a criterion that the doctor not only recognises psychological circumstances, but also introduces psychology into his therapeutic treatment. Furthermore, partial knowledge is always more dangerous than utter ignorance—particularly for the patient.

But against such scepticism are the facts of medical practice. The figures for the proportion of psychogenic illness among patients of general practitioners and physicians vary between 20 and 50 per cent. In the catamnestic examination of patients in our earlier psychosomatic clinic we found as an average length of illness with psychogenic symptoms 12 ½ years.

Furthermore an increasing number of doctors demand a training adequate to equip them to carry out well-founded diagnoses of psychogenic disturbances. Further, they confront the fact that they are either unable or unwilling to refer all cases of psychogenic illness to psychotherapists. Thus recurs constantly the concept of training in "minor" psychotherapy.

This the majority of serious psychotherapists, upon the grounds of the experience described, are disinclined to accept. Psychotherapy can be learned only in an extremely thorough training; just the desired "minor" therapy is the most difficult. And no psychotherapist will expect a physician to assume the burden of a full training for this purpose. Thus disappointment upon both sides is accompanied also by contradictions in facts.

Our own long years of discouraging experience had led us to resignation. Then about a year ago BALINT's book appeared and stimulated us, through a seminar, to resume our efforts to communicate our experience to our colleagues in the manner he describes. At that time upon the occasion of an intern congress, PROF. JORES instituted a round-table conference attended by 200 to 300 members. BALINT's recommendation was discussed. The demand for the further training indicated by him was welcomed and supported.

PROF. JORES gave notice of our intention to begin such a seminar in the Hamburg medical paper. Upon the appointed day eight doctors appeared.

The resulting disillusion was increased as the group gradually reduced itself to four members.

If we do not wish to evade examination of the realities of this disappointment, it must be recognised that we were disappointed because our expectations and our demands resulting from an insight into the subject were not shared by others.

It is, however, natural that not everyone is prepared to sacrifice time and money for something with which he is unfamiliar, or which he consciously or unconsciously opposes. And just that effort—made upon false promises and expectations upon both sides—the effort to communicate psychological facts, brings with it the described disillusions. It is a reality that, under our present conditions of living—one needs to think only of the features of German health-insurance—the number of medical men and women who come to us will remain small.

And this is the prime requirement: willingness. Only he who comes to psychotherapy of his own will be able to assimilate and make critical use of it.

Now let us turn to our Seminar:

In a preliminary discussion we had explained our procedure. For at least twelve months we wanted to meet for a weekly two-hour period. We wished neither to follow a training programme nor to give any kind of theoretical or practical advice in therapeutic technique. Free discussions were to be held about patients upon whom the members should report, in order communally to establish the psychical problem that might lie behind the illness itself. Simultaneously we wished to attempt to make conscious our own attitude in the approach to the patient.

What we did not tell the members at that time was our firm conception that our intention necessitated the creation of such a group atmosphere, in which the intimate details of daily procedure and one's own experience could be revealed. Besides, we had the more or less secret principle so to confront the members with themselves that, where necessary, they would correct themselves in their attitudes, expectations, approach and criteria.

In other words, we saw our task as that of forming a special kind of group-therapy whose detailed characteristics were not yet known to us.

The development of our seminar to this point permits division into two phases. We might call the first the emotional; the second the analytic attitude.

We were very quickly faced with the fact that the problem of the "doctor as a drug" is an emotive one, and not a question of knowledge, learning, or of technique.

Consciously object and manner of working had been willingly accepted by all members.

Although the desired free discussion was lively from the beginning, what followed the first reports on patients was nevertheless the discussion of a psychological problem. In content, long discussions of differential diagnosis occupied first place. Further considerations of how to deal with any rare "Case of", considerations of the therapy by drugs their efficacy, constitutional and other hypotheses, considerations later characterised as scientific paths of escape, occupied a considerable space. Several members soon protested against this, remarking that they wished to discuss psychological questions. The atmosphere remained relaxed and friendly, but soon achieved its dynamic form through the fundamentally different personalities.

In some there appeared a strong tendency to use the group to exchange experience of normal medical procedure. "Psychology" was then the attitude: one must be able to get on with people, they are actually quite simple. This was coupled with very active advice in regard to general measures on even somatic therapy as well. Generally a proven "recipe" for getting on with people would be offered.

In the discussions following therefrom it became evident—although only to a degree just for those members actually concerned—that hopes of immediate success, of recognition and thankfulness played an essential part, as also the attitude that patients uncritically accepted advice as to their approach to life. Authority of position, knowledge, education and confidence through mastery of medical routine were not only a therapeutic medium, but also a very personal affair of these members of the profession.

In some cases psychotherapy would be considered as useless, the patient being too old, too long ill, or because general experience shows one that nothing can be done for such people.

Such observations were accepted with ever increasing contradiction. But the discussion remained friendly in tone, even although tending to become increasingly more personal.

The shaping of the group-form was closely connected with the with-drawal of four members. One member moved, and would have had a journey of several hours to and from the meeting.

Another doctor, in an official post with a small private practice, explained that he found it all very right and interesting, but, as in his practice he found no immediate necessity to master psychotherapy, he wished to give it up again. This attitude, that one must really acutely have felt a need inclining one to psychotherapy, was confirmed as a motive by the other members. Another member we lost, had always referred to possible organic illnesses and therapy through drugs and was obviously unsure not only of psychological enquiry, but of himself.

We lost a further member on account of lumbago. Through a colleague he informed us of it beforehand, with the remark that he always suffered from it when anything placed him under a strain.

He was the one who always reverted to proven recipes for handling people, and was evidently disquietened by the progressively more analytical discussion of one's own behaviour.

We see that the will to try psychology for one's therapeutic treatment is not enough. This penetrates the sphere of the personality, where a final decision for or against will be made.

After three months this state was reached. The composition of the group remained the same. One late-comer to the group stayed away after the group had made clear to him, certainly over emphatically, the necessity of the decision for the psychotherapeutic approach as alternative to a practice within the health-insurance scheme.

Meanwhile the group had worked out certain guiding aspects for the understanding of a case. The relation between the patient's history and the origin and or course of the illness was established; that is to say, situations of conflict were sought. Together with this went the effort to secure a picture of the patient's personality. In this would be noted the ways of behaviour which affect the ability to make contact the emotional inclination and sexuality; and in addition many conflicts resulting from inadequate modes of behaviour in self-assertion and realisation were rendered understandable. Also problems relating to behaviour in relation to give and take were to be observed always and again.

Besides the not systematically presented case-histories, the question of the reporter's own behaviour recently came especially to thefore.

This is connected with the fact that now, after a long period of considerable success, reactions and failures appeared to increase. The discussion has been able to explain this either as insufficient comprehension of the problem, or, more often, as the result of the doctor's attitude, which concorded more with his own mode of behaviour and disposition at the time, than with insight into the needs of his patient.

At the present stage every member has achieved an evident certainty in seeking and locating the patient's problem. A directed listening and questioning is at the disposal of each. For therapeutic treatment there is an occasionally formulated premise which seems to us in principle important: One may only proceed psychotherapeutically in so far as one realises the patient's situation. In this the clarifiying of the patient's own problem to him is of lesser importance, rather is he to be advised as to the possibilities leading to insight and treatment. The principal concern is to stimulate the patient in accord with the possibilities present in him.

To make this clear in its efficacy, the comprehensive presentation of a case dialogue and its discussion would be necessary. We can, however, summarise our own experience and state in the first place that this work shows controlled results whose difficult assessment is due to their arising not out of the familiar analytical situation, but rather out of a field of work completely foreign to analytical psychotherapy, namely in the situation of the medical practitioner.

Here we see BALINT's merit in making clear the fact that this sphere of work has its own structure which renders possible a most skilful, effective, and peculiarly formed type of psychotherapy. The thorough training is also necessary here, but is certainly cannot go the way which leads to the comprehensive analytical training. It has to give the practitioner the facts in psychosomatic medicin and the knowledge of himself.

We have to discover and experience this therapeutic situation just as FREUD has done for the effectiveness of the analytical situation.

Author's address: DR. H. BAERWOLFF, II. Medizinische Universitätsklinik, *Hamburg-Eppendorf* (Germany).

Problems and Difficulties in Psychosomatic Training

W. Grodzicki, Hamburg

In psychosomatic training one must distinguish two facts: first, the theoretical training; and secondly the training in psychoanalytic practice. Theoretically we must present to our students today's understanding and knowledge and hypothesis of psychoanalytic psychology. In this area the teacher communicates his knowledge in the usual way of the lecture which is addressing the student. In the training directed toward educating a practicing therapist considerable difficulty arises which is connected with the very complicated special problem which became more differentiated in the course of ongoing psychoanalytic research. Because of the limited time I can only outline shortly the problem referred to.

I am talking about the relationship between patient and analyst during the analytical treatment. From a certain point of view analysis can be described as a continuous working around the relationship between patient and doctor. This relationship is under focus in regard to its momentary structure—with respect to both subject-matter and form—and in regard to its genesis. Since the patient is unable to develop any different pattern in relating except in his every-day life we are able to understand the relationship which establishes itself during the analysis as a model. Within this functional model our work is to show the patient meaning, function and genesis of his specific way of relating.

We know that every human being develops a more or less stable pattern of behaviour in the course of his development. Within this pattern he tries to deal with all the relationship which concerns him. The more plastic and flexible this pattern the better the ability of the person to adjust to reality. All our patients suffer due to their more or less rigid and unflexible pattern from maladjustment. This holds true also for patients suffering from socalled psychosomatic disease. All those patterns of behaviour bring about a typical scheme of relationship. This scheme shows the character of compromise since it tries to justify the striving for pleasureable satisfaction as well as the need for security and the defense against anxiety.

Within the situation of analytical treatment we can observe how the patient tries to establish the relationship with the analyst in the pattern which is specific for him alone. It depends on what kinds of needs of the patient are the most urgent. Accordingly we will see that the patient tries to achieve the satisfaction of all his wishes from the analyst or how he in another case tries to defend and protect himself against the analyst in order to keep the relationship free from anxiety. In this way the analyst finds himself pushed into a certain role by the patient. This role satisfies the needs and anxieties of the patient. It does not correspond, however, with the reality of the analyst. In this area lies the crucial point of the analytical work. It should not accept the striving for pleasureable satisfaction of the patient but it also has to be careful not to reinforce his anxiety. In this way the patient has to realize step by step that his wishes and anxieties are distortions of the reality situation. This knowledge alone will enable him to grow out of his rigid pattern into a more flexible form of behaviour. Due to the fact that the analyst has a certain pattern of behaviour of himself which may even have some rigid trends, the possibility exists that he distorts his relationship to the patient disregarding the reality situation of the treatment. The therapist may for instance misuse the analytical situation in order to satisfy his own narcissistic needs. He also may react with anxiety to a certain behaviour of the patient against which he has to defend himself immediately. In such a case the working of the behaviour of the patient becomes impossible.

The analyst is during the treatment not only confronted with the task of being aware of the pattern of behaviour of his patients but he is, beyond this, obligated to check himself in regard to his feelings, wishes, and fears about the patient. Only in this way a favourable treatment can be achieved. The facts I tried to outline here briefly are usually referred to by the terms of transference and counter-transference.

Since we learned about the dynamics of relationship it becomes obvious that the therapist's personality pattern should be free of neurotic, rigid trends in order to garantee a favourable treatment.

For this reason it is imperative that each analyst has to undergo an analysis himself in order to deal with his own personality problems and in order to work through them as far as possible. Only in this way one can be reasonably sure that the therapeutic action of the analyst does not serve his own uncontrolled unconscious needs, and consequently hinder or make impossible the clarification and working through the problems of the patient.

As long as we deal in a training programme with candidates who undergo training analysis the problems and difficulties of psycho-analytical training are fairly well under control. The real difficulties arise if the trained wants to get acquainted with the basic facts and the theoretical knowledge of psychoanalysis without wanting to become an analyst, and especially then if he cannot undergo personal-analysis. This is especially true for those who want to use the scientific knowledge of psychoanalytical psychology in a practical way; in other words for all doctors who are dealing with patients with psycho-somatic disease without being analysts.

In the course of my lectures given to students of different faculties I made several observations which caused me to consider the question of theoretical lectures. At first I will report in outline form what I observed.

1. During academic examinations I noticed that quite a few well gifted and also well oriented students presented certain parts from the lectures about psychoanalysis in a completely distorted way. When I compared their statements with the notes they had taken during the lecture I found out that the notes were written correctly according to my statements during the lecture. The student had also learned from his notes but he had distorted certain facts. Those were facts which could be recognized as being related to the problems of the individual student. The distortion usually was related to an unconscious defensive tendency.

2. With another group of students the lecture was reported correctly. Frequently the facts of the lecture were elaborated by further studies of the literature and very intensive involvement in the subjects. A few of those students did missionary work, in other words they recommended to many different people to undergo analysis. Very frequently I found that the brilliant mastery of theoretical knowledge hid among other neurotic problems a deep ambivalence. I feel that those also belonged to this group who interpret their own peculiarities or even their neurotic symptom in a theoretically

brilliant way. They argue with themselves and with others that they know themselves perfectly and maintain they are completely able to control their peculiarities since they can explain them. An experienced observer will recognize the defense mechanism of rationalization immediately.

3. The members of still another group became vicious opponents of analysis while the lectures were going on ardent and fanatically. They did a lot of acting out, tried to influence fellow students, got hold of malicious critiques about psychoanalysis from the years of 1900 until 1920 and argued in discussions along the well known misunderstandings. Some of them stayed away from the lectures risking in their exasperation failure in examination. However, I have seen only a few students of this behaviour.

4. Finally there is another group whose members also act out. Unfortunately their acting out is worse than that of Group 3. The acting out takes the form of their trying to do analytic therapy. We call this, "analysis of home sweet home", since the victims were usually relatives or friends. Naturally in those cases their own problems and conflicts were usually acted out in this pseudo treatment.

Those are the observations which I made with my university students. I presented them to you not because I feel they are especially alarming but because I think we should consider them and reflect upon them. The presentation of facts of psychoanalytical psychology can apparently not be equated with the presentation about the location and function of muscles or the pathophysiology of inflammation. Whenever we present facts of psychoanalytical psychology and illustrate those with case histories we will by necessity touch upon problems, difficulties, anxieties and feelings of guilt which are present in each of our students. They are present in our students in a different way than a muscle the anatomist talks about. They are present in a sense that need, anxiety, pleasure and guilt, is reactivated by the presented material and that those will be relived by identification and participation.

In this way it even can be possible that a person who was just carrying on a delicate balance psychologically may lose his adjustment. All presentations of depth psychology mean: tua res agitur.

From our analytical technique we know that we can tell the patient only in limited ways about himself. We have to consider his ego structure and to estimate what he can tolerate. We should be careful not interpret too deeply. In a similar way we should go about in lectures, but these in their traditional form have no possibility for such an approach. For this reason the following modification for lecturing seems to me a better one. The teacher should not lecture about depth psychology to a large number of anonymous pupils. One only should talk to small groups, who are actively engaged in their own training. I have in mind that each student should be asked to present a fictional detailed biography of a person. Then the student has to pick out sex and age of his fictional patient himself. He has to describe the appearance of his fictional character as well as his environment. It seems quite obvious that plenty of the personal data of the student would appear in such a fictional biography. Within the group each biography of each groupmember should be discussed thoroughly. In those discussions one could not only present and communicate facts about psychoanalytic psychology but one could also work around personal problems of the individual student. This method naturally could be expanded in various ways. I would also like to point out that in my opinion the advantage of this method seems to be that the analyst gets to know his students and is able to deal with unbalanced people in a special way. On the other hand one can discuss problems in such a way that they do not provoke the feelings of any special student. If I may say it dramatically: The danger of the anonymous audience lies in the fact that frequently young people experience an actualization of their conflicts, and afterwards have no way of dealing with them. Frequently they have to find a way out what is not helpful to themselves nor to their study.

The presentation of the theoretical material within the group makes it possible for the single student to deal with the material in a way which is more appropriate to his personality structure. He may experience that his own attitudes and patterns of behaviour determine decisively in which way and to what extent he can deal and handle the presented material.

What I said until now was valid for lectures to students who do not want to use their psychoanalytic knowledge for therapy. Let us now turn to the training of medical doctors in regard to psychosomatic problems. Those doctors have the advantage that they are usually more mature people. For once they are older and are confronted with a lot of problems in their patients which have to be dealt with. For this reason there is a sincere interest in getting some training. On the other hand there exists quite a difficult problem. The medical doctor is not helped with his training in psychoanalytical diagnosis. He wants to learn something about the technique of treatment. It is my opinion that this is a problem which practically cannot be solved. In order to cure a psychosomatic disease one needs the full training of an analyst. However, this is practically impossible. A general practitioner or an internal specialist could for external reasons never carry on such a time consuming treatment. What can be done about that? Doesn't every attempt for training necessarily lead to disaster under those circumstances? As much as I admire the work of DR. BALINT I cannot regard it as an actual training but as the attempt for a compromise. The doctors within this groups also become confronted with their own problems but it seems that those are exclusively problems which are quite ego related. Real severe problems as for example neurotic character trend by which the behavioural pattern of the single individual is decisively determined are not touched in this training. In order to deal with them analysis is imperative. In other words marked neurotic personality trends cannot be corrected in this way. Consequently the possibility to treat severely ill patients is not given. To deal with transference and countertransference is impossible on this basis.

However, just this is especially important in psychosomatic disease. While their structure frequently seems relatively easy to understand their defense is mostly very difficult to approach.

I am aware that there is a definite need to create the possibility for training treatment of psychosomatic disease since there are so many of them. I don't know how one could improve or even only change the approach of DR. BALINT. In big hospitals there should be psychoanalytic wards under the direction of analysts where training and treatment of practicing doctors could be carried out. The danger which I see in this kind of postgraduate training is the fact that the doctor may learn how to deal with less difficult cases but that he also tries sooner or later to treat severely ill patients. Since he does not have the equipment, failure seems unavoidable. There is the consolation that the intentions were the best, only the patient cannot be consoled since it is his life which goes on a "messed up way".

Author's address: DR. W. GRODZICKI, *Hamburg 19*, Am Weiher 13 (Germany).

Problems and Difficulties in Teaching Psychosomatic Medicine to Medical Students in Germany

J. CREMERIUS, München

If one wants to teach psychosomatic medicine in Germany one encounters the difficulty that the students have, in general, no knowledge of this area, or even of the basic principles of psychology. The University curriculum does not provide any training in this field. The required one-semester course in psychiatry is hardly enough to give the student a clear picture of the major psychiatric syndromes, let alone medical psychology, psychopathology, or anthropology. We are also not in the fortunate situation of America, in that we cannot count on our students having a general knowledge of this field. The average academician in Germany has, as a rule, only a vague idea of psychology. This situation is not likely to change in the foreseeable future, despite strong efforts from many sides.

What can be done? Three possibilities present themselves: The first would consist of giving the student the basic principles of psychology in a concise form before beginning with the specialized psychosomatic area. The second would be to begin immediately with this specialized field, and the third would be to forego the basic theoretical knowledge and to emphasize the treatment of psychosomatic illnesses. That would mean to teach the student the use of pragmatic treatments such as hypnosis, suggestion and other practical procedures. This last way, however, which threatens to become "fashionable" everywhere, we consider to be a wrong track which could lead to complications and confusion and could endanger the doctor as well as the patient. The requirement that the students learn the theoretical principles and criteria of therapeutic treatment, must be maintained by all means. There remains then only one choice between the first and second possibility. We have decided to devote all the available time to psychosomatics and to forego instruction in the other branches of psychology. Not because we consider the latter unimportant, but for the following reasons: the main goal of instruction in psychosomatic medicine we consider to consist in showing the student, by description of the various syndroms, how as psychological understanding works, how the doctor proceeds to recognize the dynamic forces which are instrumental in the development of such an illness, that is, we lead him directly to the problem: what conflicts and difficulties are present in the patient, suffering from a psychosomatic illness, and what are the relationships between these and his illness. We teach, therefore, motivation psychology. In order to enable the student to comprehend the picture of the above, however, we must introduce him to the basic concepts of psychoanalytical thought, which is the best model today of motivation psychology. With this procedure, we must give up, as a matter of course, the idea of including the main body of students, since the manner of instruction demands a strong interest and individual study, which cannot be expected from the average student, whose schedule is already overloaded. We believe we are thus doing justice to the realities of the present educational system, since this is our only possibility at the present time, when we give most of our attention to those students who are exceptionally interested and talented. We know that we are limiting ourselves but hope, at the same time, in this way, to prevent an accumulation of superficial information and the acquisition of a knowledge which is simply absorbed. Our renunciation of a kind of preparatory course, an introduction to general psychology, which would correspond roughly to physics, chemistry and botany in the pre-medical semesters, indicates a basic departure from the usual medical curriculum, which organizes and arranges the courses according to more didactic viewpoints, so that they can be learned by the ordinary student. We represent, therefore, a form of university teaching which requires individual work, research and independent thought from the student. We show him, by a few examples, the basic principles of the scientific way of thinking; we familiarize him with the theoretical concepts and the method and then leave the working-out of the more detailed material up to his "curiosity" and his critical abilities.

We have been using this procedure for years. Right from the announcement of a course—a course which can be elected by anyone and which is never subject to examinations—only a small number of pupils appear, some of whom discontinue coming as soon as they notice that they are not getting any practical and immediately profitable knowledge. The rest, however, show a genuine interest and are cooperative. Most of them remain through the three semesters of lectures and supplement their knowledge by individual study. Several discover an interest for this field and pursue it further.

But now a new difficulty turns up: the material of our lectures has to do with human beings, human beings whose very existence is imposed on him in a very problematic way as something to be fulfilled rather than simply given to him as the instinct mechanism for example.

The student is also such a human being. The lecture material forces him to come to terms with himself. He will thereby discover problems in himself and reflection is the inevitable result. Above all, contact with the unconscious exposes him to a heavy burden. He is forced out of the role of a mere student, out of the loge of a natural scientific observer and suddenly finds himself in the midst of the play, on the stage of his own life. On hearing the psychosomatic case histories he becomes a fellow-man to his patient. The case shows him "tua res agitur".

The sterile lecture-room becomes a highly infectious place. Above all, in his unconscious forces are mobilized: infantile wishes awaken, repressed I-impulses come out, Super-Ego positions become stronger or weaker and the Ego is forced to orient itself anew. The result of this process is that disturbances, anxieties, and even psychoneurotic and psychosomatic symptoms arise. The latter especially by those students, who chose the courses because they suffer from strong neurotic disturbances.

It is important for the instructor to know this process since often the mobilization of unconscious forces results in the student's having to strenghthen his defenses and activate additional defense mechanisms. One of the most common is that the defense against his own impulses is projected as hostility towards the instructor or towards the field itself. Above all, the lecturer must realize that he enters into a dynamic relationship with his student. Always, when the lecture deals with dynamic psychology, an emotionally-laden area between the lecturer and the student results, an area which is given its very character by the rules of transference. Thus the student often identifies the professor, for example, with what he is lecturing on and from this ensue unconscious feelings of love or hate. Furthermore, wishes arise in the student to confide, like the patient described in the lecture, to the professor, who is at the same time a therapist, and to seek help and love from him. Or else old father—relationships become re-activated and directed at the lecturer. It can be expecially disturbing for the progress of the course if the student's own defense is so weakened by what he has heard that he tries to support it by a fight with the professor or with the field itself. This can lead to endless discussions, and to biased and pointless disputes. Often the student involved argues with views and judgement about our field, which are advocated by University authorities of the place, and tries in this way to conceal his emotion behind the judgements of those. The question arises, then, whether despite these difficulties one is justified in giving a psychoanalytically oriented course in psychosomatics to medical students in the present situation in Germany. To answer in the negative means that untill the creation of a more favorable situation, the field cannot be taught at all. This, in turn, means that the only place where the student can be informed, disappears, and further, that we give up a position, which, in medicine, has an important function: the representation of the Science of Man.

Despite the dangers, however, we should not overlook the positive points of our method. Through contact with our field the student is called upon to indulge in individual thought, self-control and reflection, to become an individual. He leaves the role of a mere pupil and can become a genuine partner of the instructor in trying to gain a deeper understanding of human beings. That he must understand and question himself is actually nothing new in academic education. The professor in philosophy, for example, who, fulfils his task as a successor to the old "know thyself" has always viewed his student not as a mere pupil but as one whose inner development he is personnally concerned about. We are conscious of the fact that we require more from our students than to merely "know thyself", and that the contact with the unconscious renders this knowledge more difficult. We are of the opinion, though, that we can rely on the bold and resolute spirit of discovery of youth, a spirit which has always been ready to strike out for something new.

In conclusion, just a few remarks about how we have tried to minimize these difficulties. To make a greater understanding of general psychology possible for the medical student, and to give him an opportunity to discuss scientific problems from another angle than that of natural science causality for example, we invited the students of the Institute for Psychology and Psychotherapy to this seminar. The result was what we had hoped for. Discussion groups, which afforded much help for the further development of the students, were formed. During the discussion which followed the seminar, there were expecially valuable discussions from the two opposing sides. From the psychologists the medical student also learned what possibilities exist for further study, which rendered the increase of his psychological knowledge easier. The talks had, above all, the effect of showing the students how many of their views which they considered to be scientific theses, were basically only generalized ideologies, "Weltanschauungen".

We took care of the emotional difficulties coming up in the course of our pupils through long talks which we held with them outside the classroom. Many students took good advantage of these discussions. By some, a few conversations sufficed to overcome any approaching difficulties, and by others we had to recommend psychoanalytical treatment.

To sum up: as long as the education of medical students in psychology in Germany is not sufficiently taken into consideration in the curriculum, psychosomatic instruction should use all the available time for the presentation of those dynamic factors involved in the formation of the specific illnesses and should not dwell on general introductory courses. The teaching of essential matters will attract essential men, who will be willing to take on the required additionel research work. The danger to which we expose the student by instructing him in psychoanalytical principles, obliges us to be prepared to aid him as a person and help him in his crises. I should like to emphasize that such a procedure is only justifiable in those places where a sufficient number of psychotherapists are available to take over any necessary analytical treatment of the student. The enlargement of the class by psychology students has proved to be a great help.

Author's address: Dr. J. Cremerius, Medizinische Universitäts-Poliklinik, *München* (Germany).

IV
Free Papers

The Way of Working with "Model" Psychoses

L. van der Horst, Amsterdam

Experimental psychiatry plays nowadays an important role in the investigation of the study of psychoses and neuroses. There exists a close co-operation with psycho-pharmacology. We know that we can produce artificial psychoses with illusions, hyperactivity and even delusions. And in this way we examine whether psychotropic drugs may cure these so-called model psychoses. The same holds for the psychoneurotic and the so-called vegetative syndromes.

To gain insight into the relation between personality and the specific forms of behaviour, we studied the possibility of evoking model psychoses by administering LSD. But the general knowledge we obtained in this way is not an adequate basis to differentiate the specificity of psychosomatics.

In our anthropological work we should attempt to discover specific and verifiable rules. The first question is, whether specific forms of behaviour tend to fall in certain general categories according to their anthropological type.

A survey of the possibilities shows that one of the most important data is the grading of neuroticism and psychoticism, that is the possibility of obtaining psychotic reaction. Here we may find a way for verifiable findings.

And so we started to examine the changes of activity during LSD psychosis, ascertained by PAVLOVIAN methods and we created a test-battery to these questions: the two-factor personality inventory test, the picture recognition, and the worries test to render the grading of neuroticism in order susceptible to discussion and we researched the expressive movement, the tapping, the autokinetic effect and the level aspiration (BOURDON), the conditioning, to get discussible factors of anthropological types under anthropometric aspects.

Secondly we examined whether the experimentally evoked model psychosis is to be regarded as an entity or as a reactive syndrome in accordance with the morphological constitutional type.

Up till now we know that there is a great difference in psychotic behaviour and nervous activity following LSD impact. All our examined persons became disequalibrated or disturbed. But there were qualitative varieties in feelings and emotions, differences in agressive expressions and frustration tolerance. If we try to bring these differences in psychometrical data, we get into difficulties.

In the same way the psychosomatic needs exact data; basing itself on somatological phenomena and distinctions—as they are used in the anthropometries—we in our work seek to detect correlated psychological phenomena and distinctions.

Although these investigations are in full swing, I should like to accentuate that we do not expect much from distinctions derived from characterology, psychiatry and psycho-analysis.

The whole team is organised by DR. VAN REE and we work with a group of 8 men. One of the main topics of our teamwork is the concept of constitution, the questions of constitution and neurosis and also of constitution and psychosomatics. One of us had worked many years ago on constitution and mental illness. Another of our group (DR. VAN REE) noticed that different persons showed different forms of psychosis after taking lysergic acid. This was a rough experience, but it opened the possibility of gaining insight into the relations between personality and the specific forms of behaviour by administering LSD 25. However, the general knowledge, obtained in this way, is not an adequate basis to differentiate the specificity in psychosomatics. So we needed a more comprehensive framework.

We know that the functional disturbances in the psychosomatic field depend not only on the specificity of the administered chemical substance, but also on constitutional factors. Laymen and general practitioners know that there is a close correlation between the bodily structure and the behaviour in illness and health. Well known investigators accentuate the necessity of studying the physical anthropometrical data in connection with the possibility and the way in which the same impact may produce different somatic and psychical symptoms.

Then the question arises whether the model psychosis is to be regarded as an entity—and if so—which psychosis it might be. But as the main topic we put as the central question, whether it would be possible to produce the form of reaction by testing the person before giving him LSD 25.

In the same way as anthropometry furnishes the material, sorted according to sex, race, age and constitutional type, in our team we studied grading of neuroticism, introversion-extroversion, the degree and nature of symptoms under LSD 25, which correlate with the evaluation of psychotic reactions.

We used objective tests *before*, *during* and *after* the LSD impact. The research concerns also physical attributes. E.E.G., handwriting pressure, body swing are used as well as the above mentioned two-factor personality inventory test, the worries test e.o. Moreover we used projective tests in order to find a hypothesis that could give us a lead.

In literature we can read many data built upon unverified hypothesis. In the work of our team there is also more unsolved than positive results. No wonder when you realise with how many side-problems we were overwhelmed.

Not only what is the influence of LSD on performance and behaviour, but also what are the individual differences in the change of performance under LSD?

Furthermore in which way is there a co-ordination between neurophysiological results and psychical data?

Further if there is a possibility of predicting individual differences.

Does it depend from social situation, specific constellation of constitution whether the tested person will suffer from a model psychosis or mere neurovegetative disturbances?

Can we predict, whether he will become psychotic or not?

Is there a schizophrenia-like illness under the model psychosis?

Is it possible to cure the artificial psychoneurosis with drugs as tranquillizers?

And last but not least are we allowed to make experiments like this?

You will agree that the necessity for teamwork was felt more then ever. Only a part of what we are doing can be brought, but additions can be made to the discussion at the end of the morning. I hope that the discussion will bring us further into this interesting subject.

Author's address: PROF. DR. L. VAN DER HORST, Universiteit van Amsterdam, Psychiatrische en Neurologische kliniek Wilhelmina-Gasthuis, *Amsterdam* (Netherlands).

Prediction of Syndromes under LSD-25

F. VAN REE, Amsterdam

LSD is lysergic acid diaethylamide. This substance is since 1943 known as a drug able to induce psychoses. Notwithstanding the fact that there are many clinical arguments which indicate there are many individual differences in reaction patterns after the intake of LSD, only very few studies are known which make this fact their subject. Our investigations are especially directed to these individual differences. During some experiments we did in 1957, we came to the supposition that the form of psychoses someone gets, depends for a great deal on the dimensions introversion-extroversion in the sense of JUNG, and operationally defined by EYSENCK. To investigate this we applied an extensive testbattery, which we used two weeks before and during the experimental psychoses. We gave the male subjects 150γ and the female subjects 100γ by mouth. The ages of our subjects varied between 25 and 50 years. With only a few exceptions our volunteers were professional people. There were three women and 18 men. There were two main problems on which we directed our attention.

In the first place the individual differences in the degree of disturbance, and in the second place the individual differences in the form of reaction. All our 21 subjects showed disturbances but only 12 of them became really psychotic. If the subjects during the whole experiment remained able to realise that their disturbances were artificial and caused by the intake of LSD we named their disturbance instrumental, and spoke of mild reactions, if this was doubted we spoke of border cases or moderate reactions, and if they surely didn't we said they were psychotic and severely disturbed. In order to make a further graduation in the intensity of the disturbances, we reasoned that instrumental disturbances consisting mainly of vegetative symptoms were less severe than those which showed psychological phenomena.

Diagram I. Degree of disturbance

type of reaction	duration	number of subjects
I. D. veg.	1	
	2	
	3	
	4	1
I. D. psych.	1	
	2	1
	3	3
	4	1
B. C.	1	
	2	
	3	3
	4	
Ps.	1	
	2	1
	3	3
	4	2
Ps. HD	1	
	2	
	3	3
	4	1
Ps. X.	1	
	2	
	3	1
	4	1

In the psychotic group we made a further differentiation based upon the following criteria. Occurence of hallucinations and/or delusions in clear consciousness named as factors H and D we regarded as serious symptoms and the most malignant sign seemed the fact that sometimes it was necessary to terminate the experiment before time was over because the behaviour of the subject became dangerous for himself or his surrounding or because the subject suffered so much that it seemed morally not justified to go on with the experiment. This factor we classified with the symbol X. Finally for each group so formed, we used the time during which the disturbance existed as a further graduating factor. We divided based on this criterium in four groups as follows: less than ten minutes duration as group one, 10 to 30 minutes as group two, 30 minutes to 6 hours as group three and 6 hours and more as group four. These facts are shown in diagram I.

Concerning the form of reaction. All our subjects showed certain symptoms in common, namely vegetative symptoms, concentration difficulties, visual disturbances, changes in time perception, and derealisationphenomena. These common symptoms we named *the basic LSD syndrome*. Apart from this syndrome there appeared symptoms distributed over the different subjects, which we called *the specific or individual symptoms*. We based our clinical diagnoses on these specific phenomena. In this way we made four different groups:

1. *Schizophreniform psychoses:* which were characterised by strong autism, together with more or less of the symptoms well known in real schizophrenic patients.

2. *Degenerative psychoses as described by* Prof. van der Horst: with moderate or severe autism, cosmic or degenerative thoughts and accompanied by a variation of other phenomena, but mostly more or less schizophreniform.

3. *Hysteriform psychoses*, mainly characterised by reactive emotional instability or changes in mood, and reactualisation of conflictual situations and frustrations, and a tendency to regressive infantile behaviour.

4. *Maniform psychoses:* with maniac mood, flight of ideas, increased motor activity and hyperirritability.

In our group we found only one case in which the existing psychoses could not clearly be classified in this scheme.

After we made our diagnoses, Dr. Barendregt gave us the pretest scores on the introversion-extroversion scale, measured by the *Maudsley-Medical-Questionnaire*, which questionnaire is well-known in European psychological literature. As a matter of fact we also applied some other introversion-extroversion tests. We found them correlated with the MMQ scores for extroversion. Untill further research is done to increase the number of subjects we based our correlation on the MMQ only.

The scorings on the MMQ scale vary from 0 to 36 in which 0 is the most introvert result and 36 the most extrovert. For each clinical defined psychotic group, we computed the average extroversion score. The results are shown in diagram II.

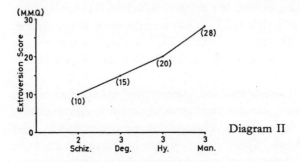

Diagram II

Of course the number of cases is rather small and this correlation has to be crossvalidated in the experiments which are continuing now, but the results seem very promising.

Author's address: DR. F. VAN REE, Wilhelmina-Gasthuis, *Amsterdam* (Netherlands).

The Influence of LSD on the Handwriting Pressure Curve

J. PH. THURING, Amsterdam

Referring to DR. VAN REE's paper about the clinical aspects of LSD psychosis, I would kindly ask your attention for one of the objective tests used in our LSD Experiment, a psychomotor test known as: Handwriting Pressure Curve (HPC).

In this test a subject writes repeatedly the same testword in his own manner and with his own speed, on a surface which is sensitive to pressure and pressure-variations in the depth dimension. These pressure variations are transformed into electric variations by means of an electronic apparatus. The electric variations are recorded in just about the same way as is done in the ECG. The curve so produced is two dimensional. The pressure variations are recorded in function of time.

Extensive work has been done to distinguish relevant criteria in this curve and to correlate them with psychological and psycho-pathological phenomena. Among others by STEINWACHS and co-workers.

The HPC was introduced in the clinic of PROF. VAN DER HORST by DR. VAN HINTEN. From his work as well as from literature this test appeared to be a most useful and promising one. Therefore we used this test in our LSD research. In order to become familiar with this test we tried to evaluate objectively the significance of this test in relation to LSD psychosis, because one of the chief problems in our research was to find objective criteria which correlate with the clinical diagnosis of LSD psychosis.

We asked ourselves the following questions:

If LSD causes alterations in the HPC, is the degree of these alterations correlated with:

1. the degree of the clinical disturbances, evaluated by DR. VAN REE;

2. the degree of the alterations, established by DR. BARENDREGT, in two of EYSENCK's psychoticism tests: the Figure Reconstruction Test (FRT) and the Tapping.

To answer these questions we had to find first of all objective criteria in the HPC.

STEINWACHS and coworkers described about 40 criteria, some of these qualitative, some quantitative.

In the selection of criteria we restricted ourselves in two ways:

1. Concerning the nature of criteria: we chose only those which were objectively to define and easily to quantify;

2. Concerning the number of criteria, we chose only those which constitute together the basic pattern of the HPC.

The result was that we could reduce the aforementioned 40 criteria to 5 criteria.

This is illustrated in the first slide.

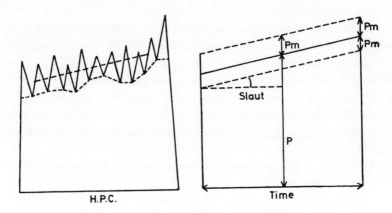

H. P. C. = Handwriting Pressure Curve
P   = Average Pressure
Pm   = Average Modulation Pressure

Underneath the two diagrams is written the testword we used. This testword was introduced in 1930 by ENKE.

The diagram to the left is an example of a H.P.C.

The diagram to the right is the reduced basic pattern with which we worked.

We chose in the time dimension two criteria:

1. the mean of time for a certain set of written words

2. the relative variability of time

In the pressure dimension we chose three criteria:

1. the average Pressure (P)

2. the average Modulation Pressure (Pm), expressed as % from the average Pressure

3. the average slant of the curve, also expressed as % from the average pressure.

The relative variability of the pressure criteria has not been calculated. For the calculation of the pressure criteria we chose two out of 24 curves, one in the first half and one in the second. The criterium for this choice was the mean of time.

Time, average pressure, modulation pressure and the slant of the curve constitute together the basic pattern of the HPC.

For additional information we chose from the handwriting itself two objective criteria:

1. the mean of length for a certain set of written words
2. the relative variability of length.

This enables us to compare in the future two different sets of objective criteria, produced in the same time, in the same act of writing.

The intercorrelation of these 7 criteria is very low. So we may conclude that they are independent factors.

For each of the 7 criteria we calculated the difference between the test under LSD and the pretest, and we expressed this difference as % from the pretest values.

For the calculation of correlations we used SPEARMAN's Ranking correlation coefficient.

The probability of exceedance for the whole group of 7 criteria was calculated by DR. D. VAN DER GON, with the aid of Student's T-test and the Chi-square tables.

The results we got are listed in the following table:

	clinical Rank	F. R. T.	Tapping
I Diff Time	0.39	0.37	0.39
II Diff Var Time	0.56	0.58	0.32
III Diff Aver Press	0.28	0.05	0.00
IV Diff Mod Press %	0.00	0.32	0.04
V Diff Slant %	0.24	0.29	0.28
VI Diff Length	0.36	0.63	0.07
VII Diff Var Length	0.54	0.43	0.27
Number of Subjects	17	15	16
Probability of Exceedance	1 ½ %	1 %	35 %

In the first column our 7 criteria are listed. In the second, third and fourth column are listed the ranking correlation coefficients between the degree of the alterations in our 7 criteria and respectively the dregee of the clinical evaluated disturbances, the degree of the alterations in the FRT, and the same for the Tapping test.

The outlined ranking correlation coefficients are significant below the 5 % level.

From this table we may draw the following conclusions:

1. The very low probability of exceedance in the second and third column indicates that there is a significant correlation between

the degree of the alterations in our whole set of 7 criteria, and the degree of the clinical evaluated disturbances and the degree of the alterations in the FRT on the other hand, but not with the degree of the alterations in the Tapping test.

2. It seems probable, but it has not been proved, that the difference in the relative variability in time and length, and to a lesser extent also the difference in length itself, give the highest correlations. This has to be cross-validated in our second group of experiments.

To illustrate this possibility, we divided with the aid of DR. VAN REE's clinical ranking, the 17 subjects in three groups:

1. the severely disturbed group;
2. the moderately disturbed group;
3. the mildly disturbed group.

We calculated the means of the 7 criteria for each of the three groups.

	severe	moderate	mild
I Diff Time	18.3%	7.3%	— 1.8%
II Diff Var Time	145 %	75 %	— 5.8%
III Diff Aver Press	21.7%	13.1%	5.3%
IV Diff Mod Press %	4.2%	— 5.4%	—15.5%
V Diff Slant %	12.8%	—13.8%	0.36%
VI Diff Length	40.7%	4.2%	1.5%
VII Diff Var Length	89 %	15.6%	11.1%

The greatest alterations are found in the relative variability in time and length and to a lesser extent also in the mean of length itself.

The relative variability in length and length itself are only strongly altered in the severely disturbed group.

If our second group of experiments gives the same result we may conclude that it is not the basic pattern of the HPC that is altered in first instance, but the relative variability in time and length with which one writes.

Author's address: DR. J. PH. THURING, Wilhelmina-Gasthuis, *Amsterdam* (Netherlands).

Performance on Some Objective Tests under LSD-25

J. T. BARENDREGT, Amsterdam

The chief goal we have in mind with our experiment is: the prediction of individual differences in, firstly, the degree and, secondly, the nature of symptoms under L.S.D.-25.

In his paper DR. VAN REE dealt with the clinical assessment of both degree and nature of symptoms. If we want to predict these symptoms we need a more reliable criterion than is obtainable by clinical assessment. For that reason we applied objective tests. Until now our experiment did not proceed so far that we could assess the nature of symptoms objectively. Therefore I shall confine myself to the degree.

L.S.D. is known as luxating psychotic symptoms. EYSENCK AND BRENGELMANN described objective tests discriminating normals and psychotics. Therefore it seemed reasonable to apply some of these tests. EYSENCK also described some tests discriminating normals and neurotics. We also applied some of them. Not so much to test EYSENCK's theory on the relative independency of neuroticism and psychoticism, but also to study the generality of the influence of L.S.D. on behaviour in the abnormal direction.

18 male subjects have been given 150 y L.S.D.-25 and 3 female subjects 100 y. Age range 25–50 years. All subjects were volunteers of high educational level. In table 1 we see the tests applied in pre- as well as during L.S.D. testing.

Static ataxia is known in medical literature as the ROMBERG-test. EYSENCK AND INGHAM described it as discriminating normals and neurotics.

Worries is a pencil and paper test described by EYSENCK as discriminating normals and neurotics.

Picture recognition test is described by BRENGELMANN as discriminating normals from neurotics and psychotics. Subjects have to recognize pictures shown for a very short time.

Tapping is a performance test described by EYSENCK as discriminating normals and psychotics.

Figure reconstruction test is described by BRENGELMANN as discriminating normals and psychotics. Subjects are shown a pattern of geometrical figures for 5 seconds. After these 5 seconds they have to reconstruct the design. There are 12 trials for one design. We applied BRENGELMANN's rotation error score.

In table 1 is given under + the number of subjects with better (more normal) performance under L.S.D. than in their normal state; under — is given the number of subjects with a worse (more abnormal) performance under L.S.D. than in their normal state.

Table 1

	+	—	Correlation with symptoms
Static Ataxia	10	8	+ .09
Worries	11	5	— .12
Pict. Recogn. T.	11	8	+ .12
Tapping	6	11	+ .34
Fig. Reconstr. T.	1	15	+ .72

The results suggest some support for the hypothesis of the independence of neuroticism and psychoticism. The influence of L.S.D. on the performance on neuroticism tests is small as compared with the influence on psychoticism tests. More important for our goal is the decrease in performance of nearly all subjects on the F.R.T.

When we found the performance on the F.R.T. to be very sensitive to the intake of L.S.D., our next step was to relate the individual differences in performance on the F.R.T. with the marked individual differences in the clinical symptoms, which the subjects demonstrated. In the last column in table 1 this relation is expressed in the SPEARMAN rank correlation co-efficient. We correlated the difference of the performances in pre- and during-testing with the order of degree of symptoms under L.S.D. as is described by DR. VAN REE. Here again the F.R.T. gives the most promising results.

When we found an objective criterion for the degree of symptoms under L.S.D., we tried to predict the individual differences. We used the scores of 10 objective tests, administered during pre-testing, as predictors. 3 of them were neuroticism-, 2 psychoticism-, 2 intro-version-extraversion-, 2 intelligence-tests and 1 level of aspiration test. Our objective criterion, the performance on the F.R.T. during L.S.D., was by none of the 10 tests predicted beyond chance ex-pectation. Contrary to the *nature* of symptoms we could not predict the *degree* of symptoms by means of objective tests.

Author's address: Dr. J.T. Barendregt, Psychologisch Laboratorium der Universiteit van *Amsterdam* (Netherlands).

Performance on Some Projective Tests under LSD-25

J. E. van Lennep, Amsterdam

The tests used in Mr. van Ree's LSD-experiment, included several projective tests: these were the Zulliger, which is an abreviated Rorschach-test; further: drawing-tests, that is to say the Three Tree Test, the Drawing of the Human Figure and the Drawing of a House, and finally the Four Picture Test.

The subjects were tested in their normal state and about a fortnight later, after taking the LSD.

Among the many things we have investigated, we tried to discover criteria for the classification of our subjects on the intro-version-extraversion continuum.

The results achieved have not been very satisfactory yet, in my view because the criteria were not sufficiently sharply defined and consequently left too much room for subjective interpretation by the evaluator.

But, as Mr. van Ree has already told you, the classification in introverts and extraverts and consequently the prediction of the *kind* of disturbance the subjects were likely to acquire, was achieved by other means, notably by objective tests.

For predicting the *degree* of disturbance, the objective tests were of *no* avail, as Dr. Barendregt has pointed out. Consequently I intend to talk to you about the contribution that projective methods have made in this respect, especially the Three Tree Test and the Four Picture Test.

The Three Tree Test is an elaboration of Koch's Tree Test. Instead of having to draw one tree, the subjects are asked to draw first a tree, e.g. a fruit tree, after which they have to draw a fantasy tree and finally a dreamtree.

In the FPT, as you may know, the subject is asked to combine four different pictures, which lend themselves to various interpretations, into one story.

In our clinical experience with the Three Tree Test, we have found several pathological signs in the treedrawings of psychiatric patients. I have treated some of these in my book on the pathological aspects of the Three Tree Test, published last year.

We take the following signs to be pathological; Trees without roots, loosely constructed trees, marked leaning of the trunk to left or right, especially when it occurs more than once, unusual position on the paper, e.g. the upper left corner; an impulsive, rash way of drawing, indefinite shape of the tree and poor elaboration, bizar shape, abnormally large or small trees; and insufficient regard for the instructions given. Of course, if several of these signs occur together, it points to a more serious condition.

As these signs are a mean of distinguishing between normal persons and psychiatric patients, we cannot expect to find them in the same gross form and quantity in the drawings made by the LSD-subjects in their normal state. However, the symptoms mentioned might occur in a minor form and this could be interpreted as an indication that these subjects are less stable and more vulnerable than others who do not show these signs in their drawings and consequently they may be more liable to become disturbed under the influence of LSD.

Investigation of the treedrawings of our 21 subjects in their normal state, proved that several drawings showed one or more of the signs mentioned above, whereas the others did not. We have submitted these drawings to an evaluator asking him to award a point whenever one of the indications mentioned above, occurred in the drawings. This might enable us to arrive at a grading, that would tally with the psychiatrists clinical evaluation.

It appeared that of the 12 subjects who according to the clinical diagnosis were severely disturbed, 8 subjects scored three or more points and that of one subject it was dubious whether 2 or 3 points should have been scored. Of the remaining 9 subjects who according to the psychiatrist were only slightly disturbed or were borderline cases, 7 were awarded only one or no points.

Although these were rather promising results our criteria did not, however, enable us to arrive at a distinction between the mildly disturbed and the borderline cases, let alone any subtler distinctions. Other criteria may perhaps be found for this.

In reading and interpreting the FPT-stories of our subjects, in their normal condition, I was struck by the different ways in which the chief characters in the stories solved their problems. The one gets the better of his difficulties in some way or other, the other, on the contrary, does not know how to tackle them, is defeated or runs away from them altogether.

A striking contrast was afforded, for example, by two stories, on the same theme: namely a row with the boss. In the one story the boss, whom the subject despises, falsely accuses him. But instead of his being upset, a plan fostered for some time, suddenly matures. "Now he knows for certain. He will quit and start on his own, even if this is a somewhat risky undertaking. Therefore, even in the heat of the argument, while the boss is covering him with abuses, he feels a liberated man." The subject who wrote this story was only moderately affected by the LSD.

In the other subject's story, the chief character abused the boss and was dismissed on the spot. What was he to do? His wife on hearing the bad news, left him of course. Fleeing from his deserted and chilly home, he roams the streets aimlessly and gets drenched in the rain. Soon this will be the end of him.

The subject who wrote this story was severely affected by the drug.

Taking these and a few other stories as guides, I arrived at the following hypothesis:

People who in their FPT-stories show a certain amount of character, which enables them to tackle life's problems and adversities, or have sublimated their problems, are less liable to become severely disturbed under the influence of LSD .These form group *A*.

Those who in their stories run away from their problems, put too great a distance between themselves and their problems, or are too much involved and consequently harassed by them, being unable to find a sensible solution, are liable to get severely disturbed under the influence of LSD. These form group *B*.

An evaluator was asked to sort the stories into these two groups.

Of the 12 subjects who according to the psychiatrist were severely disturbed, the evaluator placed 9 in group *B*. He placed none of those who were only slightly affected, according to the psychiatrist evaluation, in group *B*. As with the tree drawings the evaluator, however, did not succeed in distinguishing between the subjects who were moderately affected by the drug and those who were mildly disturbed.

All the same the results were significant, at least as far as the investigation has gone. For my hypothesis was an "ad hoc" hypothesis, which will require crossvalidation. This we are hoping to achieve with our next twenty subjects for the Four Picture Test and for the Three Tree Test as well.

Author's address: Dr. J. E. van Lennep, Wilhelmina-Gasthuis, *Amsterdam* (Netherlands).

A Case of Probable Psychogenic Hypertricosis

F. Antonelli, Rome and E. Rottini, Perugia

A 24 years old woman, confined in a State Prison at Perugia after conviction of first degree murder in the person of her mother, exhibits a conspicuous hypertricosis which cannot be explained through organic influences and became evident just after the dramatic event. Therefore the case is apt to be discussed according to the psychogenic theories.

A few words about the well known hormonic causes in this matter: adrenocortical influences are usually accepted as the most important, even in cases where other causes, such as toxic and infectious diseases or metabolic disorders or gonadic dysharmony, seem to play a concomitant role. In our case no clinical sign of adreno-cortical syndrome or gonadic disturbances were found.

The first research about the possible relationship between hyper-tricosis and psychic factors date to 1921 and the constant conclusion was in the direction of psycho-endocrine correlation. This view never excluded a suprarenal interference as a necessary causal link.

Hypertricosis in psychiatric in-patients of State Hospitals, affected with schizophrenia, oligophrenia, dystimia, etc., is frequently met, but our patient is not affected with these diseases. Relationship between emotions and hair-growth have always been considered in connection with alopecia and psychogenic bleaching, and never with hypertricosis. However a few cases of reputedly psychogenic hyper-tricosis, with or without evident pathologic suprarenal involvement, are reported in literature, but they have never been studied with psychodiagnostic techniques and according to psychosomatic and dynamic trends.

MARIA C., 24, was born in a little village of Southern Italy. The environment was constantly tinted with absolute indigence. She is liliterate. She never knew her father. No hereditary taint. Her physical growth was normal and no remarkable illness afflicted her youth. She menstruated at 17, and menstruation has always been regular.

At 18 she was seduced by the man with whom, afterwards, she became engaged. This man was accepted in her own house where he divided the bedroom with the girl, her mother and her younger brother. When she became aware of intimate relations between the fiancee and her mother, home life resulted very disturbed and she was compelled by her fiancee—whose imposingness she always bore very passively—to leave home and to establish herself in a nearby peasant house where the man occasionally joined her. After a while, because of financial reasons, the man requested her return home but he met the obstinate objection of her mother, who was leading a rather free life. In order to reach his goal he convinced the girl to face her mother and to force her to accept them home again. Actually he put a knife into her hands suggesting her to use it at least as a threatening measure. During the dramatic altercation he was backing her and actually pushed her toward hitting her mother. The girl followed the instigation without a clear notion of what she was doing and stabbed her mother, repeatedly.

After the deed she ran away leaving her mother on the ground, without being aware of her death. She knew about this only the day after, when she was arrested. According to the patient, she remained in a semi-conscious state until she was questioned at the police station. She maintains that the first time the related emotional shock occurred to her was only after a certain time, during the confront with her fiancee on the place of the crime. It was just in this circumstance that the patient felt a sudden change in her personality: she finally felt free from the imposingness of her partner and she felt surprised of being able to accuse him vehemently and resolutely. The jury condamned her to a 20 year imprisonment while her partner was given a 26 year sentence.

After 5 months of confinement she noticed the first appearance of hair on her face. This hair growth progressively acquired the shape and the thickness of a masculine beard.

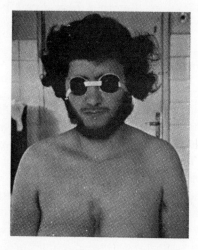

All the possible tests which the patient underwent resulted absolutely normal.

Psychodiagnostic tests and repeated interviews gave the following results: severe affective disorder, global immaturity of character with unresolved dynamic problems, maladjustment with special referment to family problems, low mental level without clear-cut oligophrenic picture, extreme aggressiveness, evident asocial trains, depressive mood, affective obtuseness, complete disappearance of sexual desire.

On summarizing it is possible to conclude for a definite deviation of the personality toward aggressive traits and toward masculine behavior. Since the case did not undergo a real analysis, it can only be described from a phenomenologic point of view. Accordingly, the psychogenic interpretation of the case remains on a pure hypothetical basis which can be formulated in the following way: this hypertricosis represents a parallel somatic expression, eventually with the contribution of adrenocortical influences, of a profound deviation of the entire personality, including psychosexual life, consequent to obscure pathogenetic mechanisms.

However, we are not facing a real personality derangement: an aggressive trait must have been a previous constituent of her character, as it is indicated by the very criminous deed, although the latter was performed in a hypnotic-like state. The latent aggressiveness acquired a new adaptation during the course of events which followed the crime, i.e. during the police investigation, judicial confronts, etc. Aggressiveness became an outward component of her adaptive behavior, after she perceived—apparently under a new light—that the lover was attempting to impose over her again, during the confront, while he tried to convince her that she was the only responsable of the murder. Whether the new situation of the patient—that is being a center of interest for the police investigation—represented a push which radically changed her relationship with the world, and in particular with the previously main object, her partner, or simply represented a feeling of being finally backed by something coherently consistent—although punitive and expiatory—which substituted her lack of ego strength, is a matter of speculation.

At any rate, aggressiveness has become a dominant trait of her personality. Contemporaneously a repulse of her femininity takes place, under a circumstance which actually is preventing her from any sexual acting out for the next 20 years, while sexuality had been previously felt—although obscurely and primitively—as the main drive of the tragedy.

Since the psychic change antedate any manifestation of hypertricosis, obviously the latter cannot be the cause of the former.

The eventual adrenocortical disfunction must be very unconspicuous if it is not revealed by the appropiate tests, as it is the case in our patient. Besides, all treatments—including Roentgentherapy—directed to neutralize an eventual suprarenal hyperfunction, proved useless.

Therefore we are inclined to consider this case under a psychogenic causal determinism, through a psychodynamic mechanism, and with a psychosomatic result.

The very central theory of Psychosomatics is based on the concept of the symptom formation—the somatic one—as a symbolization of a specific affective (emotional) drive. It is definitely accepted that in somatic disturbances of "organic neurosis" the only property which distinguishes their clinical entity is represented by their symbolic and finalistic meaning. A certain disturbance is never the result of pure accident but it is always precisely chosen to fulfill a specific need or to materialize a sort of unconscious compromise.

As far as hypertricosis is concerned, it is not difficult to attribute a symbolic meaning to this phenomenon, since it is well known the psychologic significance of hairiness both as a womanly—attraction, etc.—and as a manly prerogative—strength, virility.

The symbolic aspect of the psychosomatic mechanism pursues the realization of an unconscious need or helps in the solution of a conflict which is felt and experienced as vitally important. In order to fulfill this task the unconscious drive employs the neuro-endocrine-vegetative system, because it cannot reckon upon the cooperation of the ego; the latter, in fact, is completely unawere of those ideative contents which are removed because morally unacceptable. The vegetative system—according to Cannon, Alexander, etc.—exhibits a dysharmony which neither anticipates nor follows the relative psychodynamic mechanisms, but parallels them as one of their means of expression. According to Freud every psychosomatic syndrome requires both a somatic and a psychic contribution, and it cannot materialize without a certain somatic complaisance, which is represented by a normal or pathologic process of that organic district.

In our case, after the dramatic and real experience whose emotional weight is well understandable even in a primitive personality, it is manifest a deviation of personality in the sense of aggressiveness and independence. This attitude detaches from the feminine pattern, which used to be even exaggerate as far as passiveness was concerned, and leans toward the opposite one, i.e. nearer to the masculine behavior.

It seems that hypertricosis favours this deviation, from its somatic ground, and contributes to maintain this new attitude. One can hypothesize that this hypertricosis represents the somatic expression of an analogous phenomenon—a psychic one without somatic component—which is the transvestitism.

The eventuality of a future identification of organic causes in this problem—which at present is not yet evidenced by any diagnostic test—does not seem to be able to counteract our psychosomatic inter-pretation about this case. In fact, psychosomatics consider the organic participation as absolutely indispensable, otherwise it would be simple Psychiatry and not Psychosomatic Medicine. In this case adreno-cortical influences must play a determinant role, even if not proved through functional tests, but they are necessarily moved by psychic motives.

Authors' addresses: DR. F. ANTONELLI, Via Selci in Sabina 14, *Roma* (Italy).
DR. E. ROTTINI, Istit. di Semeiotica Medica Univ., *Perugia* (Italy).

The Problems of Perception

S. CANEVA, Vicenza

The discovery of the eidetic image, i.e. of a phenomenon which appears to isolate a stage intermediate between perception and representation has thrown new light upon the problem of the rela-tionships of sensation, image and hallucination.

The eidetic image can be defined as a physiological perceptive image which is formed during the waking state and the content of which is determined by a genuine perception at some past time.

The study of the eidetic image has greatly facilitated the psycho-logical problem of perception, since it reveals the dissociation of the phase of the perceptive process which normally is less open to positive investigation. It is a known fact that the retinal image is a physical reality, and the image in the proper sense of the word is a psychic reality, and therefore immaterial and without dimensions, and the whole secret of perception lies precisely in the passage from the one to the other. Now, the eidetic image makes it possible for us to approach this secret more closely than the mental image, since from the subjective point of view it possesses the same type of localization as the direct or consecutive sensation.

Recognition is due to the JAENSCH brothers of the Marburg psychological school for repeating the investigations of URBANT-SCHITSCH on a much larger scale and for having made eidology into an exact science. GRESSOT has carried out a profound investigation of the experimental eidetic images in 258 school children of Lausanne, aged between 9 and 13 years: 45 of these children (17.4%), presented definitely verifiable eidetic images.

The "eidetic disposition" which is frequently seen in persons of prepuberal age, is encountered in adults only exceptionally.

The intensity of the sensory contents of the eidetic images varies from a confused reproduction to great clarity and abundance of detail.

The eidetic images are subdivided into two categories, characterized by rigid automatism of appearance (comparable to that of the consecutive images) or by complete dependence upon the affective life (as with mental images): these categories correspond to different neurovegetative and characterological constitutions. A distinction is also made between experimental and spontaneous eidetic images: the latter are projected, unconnected with any systematic investigation, upon some natural screen (a wall or book page), or occur upon closure of the eyes.

As regards the "neuro-physiological mechanism", on which the eidetic process is based, it is to be recalled that, after SCHILDER's experimental demonstration of the relationship of certain visual hallucinations with the labyrinth, BIVRING-LEHNER has found the same relations between the labyrinth and the eidetic image, a finding which explains some of their manifestations, such as the attacks of spontaneous nystagmus.

An image by definition, a sensory, aesthesic or perceptive image, still the eidetic image must always be distinguished from perception, from the mental image, from psychotic hallucinations and from the various pseudo-hallucinatory phenomena of fantastic or oneiric nature.

Using this clearly distinct group, the eidetic images, as a starting point, we have attempted to define the fairly controversial distinctions between sensations and perceptions, between mental images and perceptions, and between hallucinatory images and perceptions, and we present the study of the perceptive mechanism as one particular aspect of the complex problem of the psychosomatic correlations.

Sensations and perceptions

Most theories on perception attempt to explain away some of its inherent contradictions so as to render the phenomenon of perception open to scientific reasoning.

The phenomenological school has shown that it is not necessary to start from a previously elaborated logical representation of perception, but rather to return to the concrete, effective perception, superimposed on the personality as a whole, as to a type of original experience lived through. Analytical psychology cherishes the illusion that through global perception elementary sensations are attained, with subsequent suprasensorial synthesis. From the primitive sensations thus conceived as learning of pure qualities, there are lacking the intuitions of objectivity, exteriority and spatiality which constitute part of perception. It is, however, impossible to link the problem of perception to this artificial representation, because the pure impression is imperceptible (MERLAU PONTY) and not to be found within human experience.

We must no longer fail to recognize that the sensation is determined by the modification of a sensory organ and that its contents depend strictly upon material causes. But although sensation depends on these causes, it cannot be reduced simply to its organic conditions: it is strictly a psychological phenomenon, and therefore immaterial and accessible to one person only, because it represents an awareness of the subject.

The physiologist may know no more than its lower aspect, whereas its formal aspect for experimental science represents a factor that cannot be known in its essence, an irrational phenomenon in front of which positive investigation has to stop.

Sensation does not have to present perfect photographic copies of the visible objects: the existence of the objects registers more rapidly and more accurately than its structure. Its truth or untruth is something to decide for the immediately following judgment which confirms or denies its relation with an object or its similarity with it.

We regard perception as the act of a subject which takes in an object and attaches a significance to it: perception supplies a knowledge which consists in penetrating that which it knows (PRADINES). We use the term "sensible intuition" for this immediate and concrete knowledge: by this we mean that the knowledge directly reaches the singular reality of an object to the degree to which the quality of the latter affects the sensory organ. On the other hand, however acute the perception, the sensible object retains some virtually unassessable aspects and often the perceptive data do not correspond to the data obtained, for example, after accurate measurement.

The perceptive act possesses an internal unity because it is an awareness and perception cannot be separated from the consciousness of reaching the object itself: this consciousness is a component of perception. We therefore use the term perception, in its strictest sense, only for sensation rendered conscious.

The part attributed in classical psychology to attention in the perception process is known. The appearance of the object perceived varies to a greater or lesser degree as the result of the fact that a certain number of elements taken in escape the subjects whose attention decreases: consciousness cannot bring back these elements which have not immediately been integrated in the perception, except by a further effort. Actually, every perception implies a selection from the number of elements observed with the senses, which themselves represent a sort of pre-perception or latent perception, which SHERRINGTON called the subliminal fringe. In this phase of presence, which precedes the appearance of the form, there develops a process of economy and coordination, the useless components being kept back at the threshold of consciousness and ignored. According to FREUD and DELACROIX this function of logical accomodation manifests itself both in the perception and in the secondary elaboration of the oneiric contents.

Other, strictly unconscious effective sensations, such as the colours that change hallucinations or consecutive images and the tactile, auditory and proprioceptive sensations which give rise to certain dreams, remain unable to compel apperception.

The analysis of perception leads us to define the distinction of sensation and perception, no longer establishing a distinct separation between the physiological and the psychological, but within psychism, between the conscious and the unconscious. And to the eidetic image has fallen the role of explaining the problem of perception: it has, as a matter of fact, more than one trait in common with the period of consciousness in which perception takes place. The eidetic attributes to his intuitive images properties which are usually reserved for perception: they seem to be localized externally and appear to have a certain quality of intensity. Their occurrence follows phases which schematically correspond to those of the perceptive process and causes them to imitate objects whose visual preciseness increases as they are regarded more closely: phases of presence, of development of the sensible forms, of completeness.

Mental images

The notion of image has often served to establish a transition stage between the sensation and the conception. However, many of the general theories on psychic life agree only with a "logical equivalent" (SARTRE) of the mental or representative image. We do not regard it as justifiable, for instance, to reduce the image to its physiological concomitant or to assimilate it with the impression of a previous perception, regarded as a material reality.

It is obviously difficult to imagine a mode of existence radically different from the physical existence and the nature of a phenomenon which fits no mechanical or spatial model. Still, although it is subjective, i.e. inexpressible and unexpressed, an image is an irrefutable fact, an "antipredicative evidence" (SARTRE).

The image does not exist outside its relationship with the object it makes known: the particular modality of this relationship makes possible the easy distinction between the image and the perception. Still, the image is not the literal rebirth of a perception. Once the effects of a stimulation end, a sensation disappears without leaving any truly sensory trace. There exist, on the other hand, conscious or unconscious visual records which accidentally contribute to the changing of the sensory impressions, records which are the psychic tracks made by perceptions or images or which derive from such tracks.

An element common to all categories of images and which reveals the functional difference which separates them from perceptions is the fact that the image encloses only a limited number of determinations and frees them all; perception, on the other hand, possesses a virtually unlimited number of determinations and only partly gives them up for investigation. The image, is integral the perception partial.

We see, therefore, that subjectivity is a fundamental characteristic of the image, the intuition of an active genesis, of a production, that is, of retrospective nature.

The world of images cannot be separated from the world of objects and every object, to the extent to which it has evoked a perception, can be authenticated by one or more images.

There exist no images which are not images of something, and both with the image and with the perception, it is the object which we perceive directly and primarily. But whereas the sensation is a psychic fact and its contents depend strictly upon material causes, the contents of the image are in themselves immaterial and cannot be observed with the senses, although representing material and sensible qualities.

SARTRE analyses the conscious nature of the image as follows: "It is impossible for me to form an image without knowing at the same time that I form an image, because the mode of being of an image is precisely its appearing". And further: "The object in the image is never anything more than the consciousness one has of it".

The content of sensible consciousness which constitutes the image is a primary, indivisible fact. As a definition of our attitude in connection with the content of the image, SARTRE uses the word "almost-observation", which refers to the almost-sensible qualities represented.

The material of the image, which forms the object for consciousness, SARTRE calls "analogon mentale": the analogous content of consciousness. It is the nature of this analogon which differs in the eidetic image and in the mental image. The intuition of concrete, stable sensoriness which constitutes the eidetic image is sharply opposed to the fleeting imprecision of the mental image. The images therefore appear as spontaneous acts of the functions of consciousness developed in view of the integration of the sensations. Because of their nature of apparatus of consciousness these functions tend to lead to the external object.

SARTRE's studies have definitely established that the images are original structures of consciousness, manifestations of a distinct, major psychic function. The eidetic and mental images, even if not different for their intensity, but for the nature and frequency, are characteristic of the vigilant consciousness. Other classes of images appear with modifications of the state of consciousness: hypnagogic and oneiric images.

Hallucinatory images

The eidetic image implies a hallucinatory sensoriality: in contradistinction to hallucinatory phenomena, it is not associated with mental or neurological disturbances. Introspective study of the eidetic phenomenon makes it possible to analyse the subjective nature, the structure and the content of the hallucinatory process.

In the eidetic as well as in the hallucinating subject, there is a direct conflict between the effectively active genesis of the visual image and the feeling of passive genesis with which this same image imitates perception. Whether hallucinatory or simply representative, the image is undoubtedly an act; and the hallucinatory image is dependent upon the whole of the psychic life, it is a dramatic segment of the mental life of the individual (POLITZER).

A hallucination, according to ESQUIROL's classical definition, is a perception without object. This definition presupposes a perfect identity of the hallucinatory with the perceptive process and moreover the patient's conviction that the external object actually exists. In pseudo-hallucinations, on the other hand, the psycho-sensorial phenomena are not regarded by the subject as directly deriving from the world outside him, but as the effect of an action transmitted from afar by others. And the voices, which are the most representative aspect in these cases, are heard in a particular way which distinguishes them from genuine perception, and which the patient interprets as the effect of transmission from a distance: their localization in space never corresponds to that of a normal perception.

The intuitive image which constitutes the basis of the pseudo-hallucinatory disturbance is a fairly modest phenomenon which essentially does not differ greatly from an image which in normal conditions may arise spontaneously.

Another element which characterizes the pseudo-hallucinations as distinct from representations is that they interrupt the course of thought suddenly, unrequired by the apperceptive process and without immediately apparent logical linkage with what the subject is thinking at the moment of their appearance.

As regards the relationships between hallucinations and delirium, our School, headed by BERLUCCHI, interprets the hallucination as a fact secondary to delirium; the latter is thought to be a primary fact of the intelligence, not attributable to either hallucination or disturbance of affectivity. Our leader, however, emphasizes the psychogenic origin of the pseudo-hallucinatory phenomena and insists that the intuitive image has very little significance in this respect.

Concerning the structural analysis of the hypnagogic pseudo-hallucinations and of the pseudo-aesthesic material of dreams, we may say that the oneiric thought develops through concrete images, mostly of visual nature, which are often the result of combination of several images or ideas (coalescence of images). In the dream there is a predominance of visual temporo-spatial intuitions, i.e. the succession of images assumes the visual form of a change of the pattern (as in a film).

There is nowadays a tendency to recognize in the oneiric states not only the prototype but also the origin of hallucinations: the latter are thought to be only the result of interpolation of oneiric activities or fragments of such activities into the psychic life during waking (JANET).

The incomplete character of the reality of the images and the lack of belief in them are characteristic of oneiric states, of which the peduncular form is typical: the images which appear to patients with lesions limited to the mesodiencephalon possess sensoriality and spatiality, appear in an incoherent manner, on the occasion of visuo-tactile associations, and occur preferably during twilight time or at the moment of nocturnal rest.

For some of its aspects, analysis of the eidetic process cannot go far beyond the general problem of hallucinations, and there exists a too strict correlation between hallucinoses and the eidetic images for the neuro-dynamic state which conditions the appearance of the hallucinatory images not to be largely common to them.

Thus, the eidetic image appears to be destined to bring the problem of hallucinatory aesthesia into the field of normal psycho-biology.

But however exciting the problem of the physiological concomitants of the hallucinatory image, we must emphasize that each of its aspects leads us to two classes of phenomena, of which some characterize the integration of the phenomenon in the entirety of psychic life and the others contribute to the genesis of the image itself.

As regards the ultimately physical nature of the hallucinatory process (modifications of the neuronal chronaxias according to PIÉRON), the hope that it would be open to precise exploration by electro-encephalography has unfortunately proved vain. In our hospital practice, we have carried out systematic EEG examination of hallucinating patients: in the majority of the cases the curves remained completely as before. This finding would appear to confirm that hallucinations are in general not due to cortical irritations but to dissociation phenomena.

Thus, the transformation of the stimulus into immaterial sensation, the rise of imagining consciousness above the physiological plane, the rush of thought beyond the sensible data, the appearance of hallucinatory images, all remain phenomena of such complexity, that all positive investigation up to now has had to stop on the threshold: and this must inspire us to tackle with ever increasing zeal the difficult problems of neuro-physiology and psycho-biology.

Author's address: DR. S. CANEVA, Ospedale Psichiatrico S. Felice, *Vicenza* (Italy).

From the Psychosomatic Research Unit, Wilhelmina Gasthuis, Amsterdam (Director: Dr. J. M. v. d. VALK) and the University Department for Pulmonary Diseases, Groningen (Director: Prof. Dr. N. G. M. ORIE).

Allergy and Neurosis in Asthma *

E. DEKKER, J.T. BARENDREGT AND K. DE VRIES

Several attempts have been made in the literature to classify asthma patients according to the predominant etiological factor. Thus some authors distinguish patients with allergic asthma from patients with psychogenic asthma. This distinction only makes sense if it can be proved that in some asthma patients the importance of the allergological factor predominates over the psychological factor whereas in other patients it is the psychological factor which is of greater importance than the allergological factor; in other words this distinction only has any meaning if there is a negative correlation between allergological and psychological factors. So far comparatively little actual research has been carried out on this topic and such research as has been done had led to contradictory results. MCDERMOTT AND COBB (1939) and HARRIS AND COWORKERS (1959) were unable to find such a negative correlation between allergological and psychological factors, whereas the work of MITCHELL (1947) AND COWORKERS

---

* These researches were in part supported by the Organization for Health Research T.N.O.

and that of REES (1956, 1956a) implicated the actual existance of such a negative correlation.

But so far the methods of assessing the relative importances of the causative factors have been greatly influenced by the subjective judgement of the investigator as far as the psychological factors are concerned. The significance of positive skintests in asthma patients is still open to discussion and the interpretation of allergological history, results of skintesting and/or the results of desensitizing treatment—which have been applied as methods to obtain an answer to this question—also introduce an important subjective element.

The proof however, that there actually exists a negative correlation between allergological and psychological factors in asthma patients, should not be obtained by subjective methods. It should not be obtained as a result of a compromise between workers in different fields discussing their findings in a number of patients, but it should be obtained by objective methods measuring psychological and allergological factors.

We tried to provide such evidence for the hypothesis that there actually exists such a negative correlation between allergological and psychological factors.

Method: The allergological classification was done with the aid of inhalation tests. A number of extracts of inhalation allergens i.e. grasspollen, treepollen, haydust, housedust, fungi, feathers and animalhair were inhaled by the patients in a nebulized form. The vital capacity was measured at regular intervals.

The patients were divided into an "allergic" and a "non-allergic" group defined by the following criteria:

The "allergic" group was composed of patients who responded with an actual attack of asthma to the inhalation of a nebulized allergen, causing a decrease of the vital capacity of at least 10%.

The "non-allergic" group was composed of patients who either had no single positive skin test or in whom no single positive inhalation test could be obtained after testing every positive skin-reaction which was obtained.

We also chose an objective criterion for the assessment of the psychological factors at play. In the literature asthma patients are described as neurotics. We therefore chose a Dutch version of the two part personality inventory of HERON (1955) as a criterion. This test consists of a simple questionaire which must be answered by the patients with yes or no. It asks a 110 questions of which 42 are related to neuroticism. Each of these 42 questions has been shown to distinguish statistically highly significant between groups of healthy individuals and patients suffering from neurosis. The neuroticism-score of a person is defined as the number of questions which he answers in the "neurotic" direction. So the minimum possible score is 0, the maximum score is 42.

BARENDREGT (1958) did a validation study with his Dutch version of this test in a group of normal individuals and a group of neurotic patients. It was shown that it distinguishes very well between these two groups. A further advantage is that the test result is hardly influenced by age, intelligence and sex of the subjects.

With these methods two groups of asthma patients were examined. All were females between 21 and 55 years of age. The first group was examined in Amsterdam, it was composed of 39 patients. And then to minimize the influence of selection factors a similar investigation was done in 40 patients at the allergological outpatient department of the University of Groningen where antiallergical treatment is emphasized.

Using these methods we came to the following definition of our problem: Is the neuroticism-score in our "allergic" group lower than in the "non-allergic" group?

Results: these are summarized in table 1.

Table 1. Neurotiscism scores in "allergic" and "non-allergic" asthma patients

	Total number of patients	manifest allergy number	scores	SD	p values	no manifest allergy number	scores	SD
1st investigation	39	18	18.7	5.5	0.78	21	20.8	6.6
2nd investigation	40	16	18.2	6.2	0.70	24	16.4	7.9
combined results	79	34	18.5	5.9	0.85	45	18.5	7.5

It is evident from these figures that there is no significant difference between the neuroticism scores of the "allergic" and the "non-allergic" asthma patients.

Fig. 1 shows the frequency distribution of the neurotiscism scores in the "allergic" and the "non-allergic" groups.

Discussion: Our investigations do not support the hypothesis that there is a negative correlation between allergological and psychological factors in asthma patients. Although these results cannot be considered as definite proof that such a negative correlation is non-existent, they stress the need for convincing objective evidence supporting

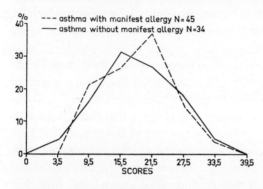

Fig. 1. Frequency distribution of neuroticism scores in "allergic" and "non-allergic" asthma patients.

the view that asthma patients can be classified in an allergologic versus a psychogenic group.

But from our figures a more positive conclusion can also be

Table 2

	neurotiscism-scores	
79 female asthma patients	M = 18.5	SD = 6.8
100 female psychoneurotic patients	M = 19.1	SD = 6.6
30 normal females	M = 7.3	SD = 5.3

drawn. This becomes obvious if the neuroticism-scores of our asthma patients are compared with the scores of a group of 100 psycho-

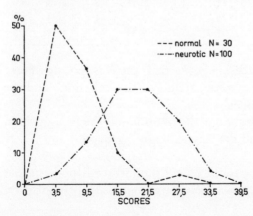

Fig. 2. Frequency distribution of neuroticism scores in "normal" individuals and in a group of psychoneurotic patients.

neurotic female patients and with the scores of a group of 30 normal females (Table 2).

Fig. 2 gives the frequency distribution of the scores in the normal individuals, the asthma patients and the psychoneurotic patients.

There is a statistical difference between the normal individuals and the asthma patients (p < 0,01) and also between the normal individuals and the psychoneurotic patients (p < 0,01), but there is no statistically significant difference between the asthma patients and the neurotics. Thus accidentally we did find support for the hypothesis that asthma patients are neurotic.

Summary

1. Several attempts have been made in the literature to group asthma patients according to the predominant etiological factor. A classification of asthma patients into an "allergic" and a "psychic" group can only be justified if a negative correlation between allergological and psychological factors can be demonstrated.

2. Seeking support for this classification 79 adult female asthma patients were divided into two groups. Those patients in whom attacks of asthma could be provoked by the inhalation of nebulized allergens, were considered to be "allergic" (34 patients). The "non-allergic" group was composed of patients who either showed no positive skin reactions or in whom all positive skin reactions were followed by a negative inhalation test (45 patients). In all patients the neuroticism was quantitatively and objectively determined by an independent observer by means of the "Two Part Personality Inventory", described by HERON.

3. No significant difference was found between the neurotism scores of the "allergic" and the "non-allergic" groups.

4. It was concluded that there is no convincing evidence available to support the classification of asthma patients into an "allergic" and a "psychic" group.

5. There was no significant difference between the neuroticism scores of these asthma·patients (18.5 ± 6.8) and those of a group of 100 female psychoneurotic patients (19.1 ± 6.6).

6. The asthma patients had a considerably higher neuroticism score than a control group of 30 normal female subjects of the same age group (7.3 ± 5.3).

Bibliography

Barendregt, J.T.: Lijders aan psychosomatische kwalen als sociaal aangepaste neurotici. Ned. T. Geneesk. *102*: 2044 (1958).

Harris, I.D.; Rapoport, L.; Rynerson, M.A., and Samter, M.: Observations on asthmatic children. Amer. J. Orthopsychiat. *20*: 490 (1950).

Heron, A.: Personality and occupational adjustment: a cross-validation study. Canad. J. Physiol. *9*: 15 (1955).

McDermott, N.T., and Cobb, S.: A psychiatric survey of fifty cases of bronchial asthma. Psychosom. Med. *1*: 203 (1939).

Mitchell, J.H.; Curran, C.A., and Myers, R.N.: Some psychosomatic aspects of allergic diseases. Psychosom. Med. *9*: 184 (1947).

Rees, L.: Physical and emotional factors in bronchial asthma. J. Psychosom. Res. *1*: 98 (1956).

Rees, L.: Psychosomatic aspects of asthma in elderly patients. J. Psychosom. Res. *1*: 212 (1956).

Authors' addresses: Dr. E. Dekker, and Dr. J. T. Barendregt, Second Medical Service, Wilhelmina Gasthuis, *Amsterdam* (Holland);
Dr. K. de Vries, Department for Pulmonary Diseases, Provinciaal-, Stads- en Academisch Ziekenhuis, *Groningen* (Holland)

From the Second Medical Service, Wilhelmina Gasthuis, Amsterdam (Director: Prof. Dr. D. Durrer) and the Institute of Medical Physics T. N. O., Utrecht (Director: Dr. D. H. Beddering).

Further Experiments on the Origin of Asthmatic Wheezing

E. Dekker, E. van Vollenhoven and J. During

Current thought about the pathophysiology of asthma is divided between those who believe asthma to be an allergic disease in which infection often plays an important rôle and those who think asthma is predominantly a psychosomatic disorder. The allergists localize the main pathophysiological processes in the tissues of the smaller

* This investigation was supported by the Organization for Health Research T. N. O.

airways, especially the bronchioli. Psychosomatic investigators on the other hand have been so deeply involved in problems of personality structure and psychosomatic specificity that the question of the pathophysiological pathways from the brain to the lungs has hardly been considered, and it has certainly not been solved.

Some authors however seem to take it for granted that the autonomous nervous system, especially the vagi, or humoral factors play the intermediary role. During the 3rd European Conference on Psychosomatic Research evidence was presented in support of another possibility first described by TALMA in 1898 and later by STRÜBING (1906) and SAENGER (1917) that asthma patients might be able to narrow their airways by means of their voluntary respiratory muscles. Within the scope of this paper only a brief summary of our findings can be given (DEKKER and GROEN, 1957; DEKKER, DEFARES and HEEMSTRA, 1958; DEKKER, 1958).

1. Asthma patients as well as normal individuals can easily learn to wheeze voluntarily.

2. During this wheezing expiration a considerable narrowing of the trachea and larger intrapulmonary airways can be observed by means of X-rays.

3. During voluntary wheezing expiration a high intrathoracic pressure of about 80 to 100 mm Hg can be measured in the esophagus.

4. Such a positive intrathoracic pressure could easily compress the human airways during experiments with post-mortal human lungs in vitro.

5. We introduced a catheter in the lungs of human subjects. This enabled us to obtain direct measurements of intrabronchial pressure during voluntary wheezing respiration which proved that the main air flow resistance during this type of forced expiration was located in the larger cartilage supported intrapulmonary airways.

These observations made us consider the possibility that emotional influences might affect the diameter of the airways by altering the breathing pattern of the patient in such a way that the voluntary respiratory musculature raised the intrathoracic pressure which in turn compressed the trachea and bronchi, thus producing the increased expiratory air flow resistance which is characteristic of the attack of asthma.

To day I would like to present a progress report of our work along these lines which centers around the question: what causes the asthmatic wheezing?

To the ear there is a great similarity between the wheezing which can be heard from a distance in a patient in status asthmaticus and in a normal individual who is practising voluntary wheezing expiration. Now the question arises whether there is also a similarity between the physical properties of these sounds in the patient and in the normal individual.

Methods

To answer this question a method for the registration and frequency-analysis of breath sounds was developed (KUIPER, DEKKER AND DURING, 1958).

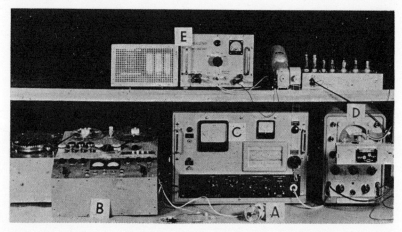

Fig. 1. Apparatus for spectral analysis of respiratory sounds (Description in text).

Fig. 1 shows the apparatus. The breath sounds are picked up from the body of the patient with a microphone (A), they are recorded on a tape recorder (B). Sound analysis is done at a later date in the laboratory. The sound of a single respiration is played back a great number of times by a play back head mounted in the rim of a circular disc revolving in a loop of the tape (Fig. 1, far left). This signal is transmitted to a wave analyser (C) which only transmits signals of a certain frequency band and at the same time measures the intensity of this band. The intensity is made to modify the intensity of the light spot which writes a horizontal line on the screen of the oscilloscope (D). Recording is done photographically with a camera. An example may serve to illustrate this method. Let us assume the wave analyser is set at a frequency of 200 cycles per second. The play back head turning inside the loop of the tape picks up the whole recorded signal during one respiration. The wave analyser picks out the components of 200 cycles per second which are contained in this sound and the. oscilloscope writes a horizontal line. Whenever there occurs a sound of 200 cycles per second, the spot becomes bright and it writes a dark line on the photographic record.

Now the play back head comes to its next revolution inside the tape. The tuning frequency of the wave analyser has in the mean while been automatically changed by an electromotor to 240 cycles per second and the light spot at the same time is vertically deflected so that it now writes a second horizontal line, closely parallel to the first one representing the intensity of the 240 cycles per second frequency, contained in the respiration, and so on.

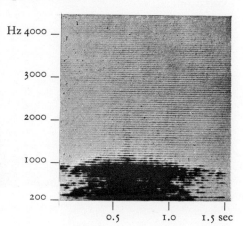

Fig. 2. Spectrogram of normal expiration. Vertical axis: frequency. Horizontal axis: time. Intensity of each frequency indicated by blackning of the record.

Fig. 2 represents such a photographic record of the breath sounds, registered from the trachea of a normal individual during expiration.

On the vertical axis the different frequencies are represented from 200 cycles per second to 4000 cycles per second. The horizontal axis is the time axis. The intensity of each frequency is represented by the intensity of blackening of the record. It can be clearly seen that normal respiration has the character of a murmer; up to a certain frequency all frequencies are represented.

Fig. 3 shows an expiration of a patient during an episode of asthma. The harmonic contents of the asthmatic wheezing can be clearly recognised as black lines.

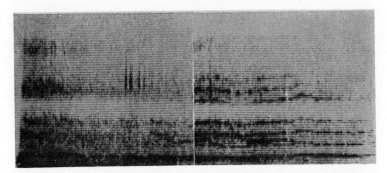

Fig. 3. Spectrogram from an expiration of a patient during an episode of asthma.

Fig. 4 shows a record from an asthmatic who produces voluntary wheezing expiration. It shows similar lines indicating wheezing expiration.

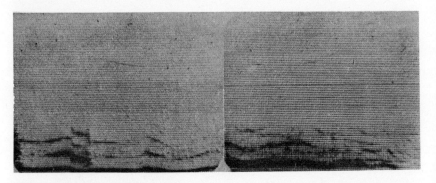

Fig. 4. "Voluntary wheezing expiration" from an asthma patient.

Fig. 5 shows that a similar pattern can also be produced by a normal individual who wheezes voluntarily. From these records we have not as yet * been able to detect any characteristic difference between the sounds of voluntary wheezing expiration of normal individuals and the sounds heard over the trachea in a severe attack of asthma.

So we may conclude that there is also a great similarity between the physical properties of the sounds which occur in an attack of asthma and those which normal individuals can produce with the aid of their voluntary respiratory muscles.

* Of course the possibility cannot be excluded, that such a difference will be found in future.

What is the mechanism producing these sounds? We developed the following theory: If a stream of air is led through a tube and this tube is at the same time externally compressed by an increasing outside

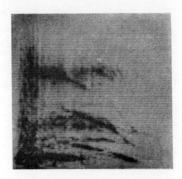

Fig. 5. "Voluntary wheezing expiration" from a normal individual.

pressure its walls will come close to one another and air speed increases which decreases the static pressure on the walls according to the law of BERNOULLI (the principle of the watersuctionpump). The walls are thus sucked inward and they will momentarily very strongly narrow the lumen. Then the inside pressure builds up behind this occlusion and the walls are forced apart. This cycle repeats itself, bringing the walls into a vibration which produces sound.

Model experiments were done with thin rubber tubes through which a stream of air was blown while the walls were at the same time compressed by an outside pressure. In stroboscope light the walls could be clearly seen to vibrate. A loud sound was produced consisting of a basal frequency and several overtones. Fig. 6 shows the spectrogram.

Similar experiments were done in vitro with isolated human airways obtained post mortem through which a stream of air was blown during narrowing by an outside pressure. We did not always succeed in producing sound from each preparation. But some specimens of the postmortem human trachea produced asthmatoid wheezing during external compression.

Fig. 7 shows the sound analysis of a trachea, which is wheezing post mortem. This picture is very similar to that obtained from asthma patients during an attack (Fig. 3). Fig. 7 proves that it is possible to obtain asthmatoid wheezing from the human airways post mortem. It does not prove of course that wheezing in the asthmatic attack originates in the trachea. We have reasons to believe that it is

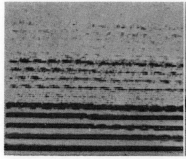 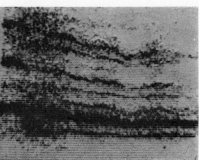

Fig. 6. Sound spectrogram from the "wheezing" produced by blowing through a thin rubber tube which was externally compressed.

Fig. 7. Sound spectrogram from the "wheezing" produced in vitro by blowing through an isolated human trachea which was externally compressed.

rather the cartilage supported intrapulmonary airways which give rise to the wheezing sounds of asthma. Further research is needed to solve this problem.

Summary

1. Results from our previous investigations indicated that psychogenic factors might influence the pulmonary function in asthma by means of an altered breathing mechanism in which the voluntary respiratory musculature raises the intrathoracic pressure thereby compressing the airways. This compression may narrow the lumen and increase the air flow resistance of the bronchi.

2. This hypothesis is supported by the observation that normal individuals as well as asthma patients can be taught to wheeze at will.

3. In this paper the physical properties of breathsounds from asthma patients in an attack of asthma, were compared with the wheezing sounds produced voluntarily by asthma patients and by normal individuals. This was done by a method of sound analysis. No significant physical differences between these different sorts of wheezing sounds have as yet been detected.

4. Model experiments were done with rubber tubes through which a stream of air is led under simultaneous outside compression. This produces a wheezing sound by vibration of the walls, probably as a result of the BERNOULLI-effect.

5. Human airways—if treated in the same way—can produce a

wheezing sound, which may show a great physical similarity to the wheezing sounds of asthma patients.

6. These observations support our hypothesis that the voluntary respiratory musculature may act on the airways of asthma patients creating a positive intrathoracic pressure which compresses the airways. These observations support the hypothesis that such an external compression of the larger intrapulmonary airways might also be responsible for the production of the wheezing sounds which so characteristically belong to asthma. Emotional factors in asthma might act through these mechanisms.

Bibliography

DEKKER, E., and GROEN, J.: Asthmatic Wheezing. Compression of the trachea and major bronchi as a cause. Lancet *I*: 1064 (1957).

DEKKER, E.; DEFARES, J.G., and HEEMSTRA, H.: Direct measurement of intra-bronchial pressure. Its application to the location of the check-valve mechanism. J. appl. Physiol. *13*: 35 (1958).

DEKKER, E.: The influence of intrathoracic pressure on the diameter and flow resistance of the airways in normal individuals and in patients with asthma and emphysema. Doctor's thesis (Groningen 1958).

KUIPER, J.; DEKKER, E., en DURING, J.: Een methode voor de frequentie-analyse van ademhalingsgeluiden en de toepassing hiervan bij asthmapatiënten. Ned. T. Geneesk. *102*: 274 (1958).

SAENGER, M.: Über Asthma und seine Behandlung (S. Karger, Berlin 1917).

STRÜBING, P.: Über Asthma bronchiale. Dtsch. med. Wschr. *32*: 1252 (1906).

TALMA, S.: Über «Asthma bronchiale». Berlin. klin. Wschr. *35*: 1141 (1898).

Authors' addresses: DR. E. DEKKER, Second Medical Service, Wilhelmina Gasthuis, *Amsterdam* (Holland);
    DRS. E. VAN VOLLENHOVEN and MR. J. DURING, Institute of Medical Physics, T. N. O.,
    Da Costakade 45, *Utrecht* (Holland)

Emotional Aspects of Hysterectomy.
A Follow-up Study of Fifty Patients under the Age of 40

B. ACKNER, London

The view has long been held that the operation of hysterectomy, associated as it is with the removal of woman's symbol of femininity, carries with it special psychological risks. KRAFFT-EBING (1890) claimed that operations on the female genitalia caused psychoses more frequently than those on any other organ. More recently LINDEMANN (1941) has shown that post-operative psychiatric reactions were more common after pelvic than after upper abdominal surgery. However, STENGEL, ZEITLYN AND RAYNER (1958) demonstrated that the higher frequency of psychosis following gynaecological operations was related to the large number of such operations performed. Furthermore, they showed that the incidence of all post-operative psychoses increased with age and that while there was a greater liability of hysterectomies than other gynaecological operations to be followed by psychoses this could be accounted for by age differences. The average age of the hysterectomies in their series was 48 but was only 35 for other gynaecological operations.

Despite all that has been written on the subject, the literature contains remarkably few examples of well designed follow-up enquiries into the psychological ill-effects of hysterectomy.

KROGER AND FREEDS (1951) textbook of Psychosomatic Gynaecology only refers to the follow-up study of WENGRAF (1946). However, this paper is merely anecdotal and WENGRAF's (1953) later monograph entitled Psychosomatic approach to Gynaecology and Obstetrics still provides no follow-up figures.

Many studies have failed to separate those cases in their series in which a simple hysterectomy was performed from those which were complicated by the additional removal of both ovaries. LEWIS AND JACKSON (1940) attempted to investigate the importance of endocrine changes in causing psychological symptoms after hysterectomy. They studied the psychiatric state four to five years after operation in a group of women who had undergone simple hysterectomy compared with another group who, in addition, had had both ovaries removed. However, the findings were not conclusive, for the ages of the two groups were not comparable and many of those whose ovaries remained intact were found to have manifested menopausal symptoms in the follow-up period.

MENZER ET AL. (1957) carried out a detailed pre- and post-operative psychological study of a series of hysterectomised women. However, an unspecified number of women who had been subjected in addition to bilateral oophorectomy were included, and no mention was made of the age distribution of the subjects.

DRELLICH AND BIEBER (1958) reported the results of a pre- and post-operative psychological investigation of a series of women all of whom were described as premenopausal, though no actual age distribution was reported. They found a very high incidence of pre-operative fears and post-operative psychological ill effects. It seems likely, however, that their findings were partly related to the fact that both ovaries were removed in every case, many cases were suffering from malignant disease and all were nursed in a ward where other women were undergoing extensive pelvic surgery, often associated with colostomy and suprapubic drainage.

The present study reports the results of a follow-up investigation of women whose hysterectomy had not involved the removal of both ovaries. The patients were all under the age of forty and except for the exclusion of cases of cancer they were an unselected group of fifty consecutive cases all of whom had undergone operation in the gynaecological department of a large general hospital. The indication for operation was commonly severe menorrhagia or pain, and in addition a large number of the patients were found to have complained for some time prior to operation of depression, irritability and fatigue. To avoid prejudicing the follow-up findings, a psychiatric interview was not undertaken before the operation. Shortly after the operation each patient was seen briefly on the ward by the psychiatric social worker who explained the purpose of the investigation, and six weeks later she interviewed the patient at length in order to obtain a social history. Six months following the operation the patient was seen for full psychiatric assessment. Subsequently various features of the personal history of the patients were assessed and rated independently of the findings of their state at the six months follow-up period.

The average age of the group was 36.5 years and only one patient had not been married. The findings at operation revealed significant organic pathology in 66.5% of the cases and in the remainder the symptoms were considered to be functional in nature.

Psychiatric examination six months after operation indicated that the majority of patients had improved markedly in mood, energy and physical health. Many reported that they had not felt so well for years and wished that the operation had been carried out earlier. In many, sexual adjustment had improved and some expressed relief at the loss of their fears of pregnancy. However, in about 30% of the cases the results were considered to be unsatisfactory on account of symptoms which included marked deterioration in mood, complaints of lack of energy, presence of additional psychiatric and physical complaints, sexual maladjustment and feelings of regret for loss of childbearing capacity. No post-operative psychosis occurred, but admission for treatment of a depressive illness during the six months following operation was necessary for one patient.

When compared with the findings in the total group, poor outcome was found to have no correlation with the age of the patient or husband, divorce, religion, intelligence, childhood attitude to parents, childhood stress, duration of marriage, marital harmony, sexual adjustment and fears concerning operation. It is to be noted that LINDEMANN (1941) also failed to correlate the presence of pre-operative anxiety, sexual maladjustments and environmental factors with the occurence of post-operative psychiatric symptoms.

The patients with a poor outcome manifested, however, the following significant features. They had fewer children, their average number being 1.6 compared with 2.4 in the total group. Of the five patients with no children four had many post-operative psychological complaints. Illegitimate children were more common (22%: total group 14%). Desires for more children were more frequently expressed (46%: total group 28.5%).

85% of those with a poor outcome were considered to have shown evidence of emotional instability in their previous personality as compared with 55% in the total group. However, there was no significant difference in the presence of psychiatric symptoms prior to operation (38%) and fewer patients with a poor outcome had had breakdowns prior to operation (7.5%: total group 14%). Furthermore, whilst 33% of the total group were considered to be suffering from some form of environment stress immediately before operation, this was only present in 15.5% of those with a poor outcome. Those with a poor outcome less frequently gained weight after operation (23%: total group 47.5%) and more commonly lost weight (38.5%: total group 14%). They also more commonly expressed feelings of regret for loss of childbearing capacity (38.5%: total group 21.5%).

It might have been anticipated that poor outcome should be more commonly associated with functional uterine disturbance and yet a reverse tendency was found. 85% of those with a poor outcome were discovered to have organic pathology at operation compared with 66.5% in the total group.

Poor outcome was not related to the presence of post-operative flushes which occurred to some extent in about 50% of all cases during convalescence and were still present in about 20% of cases at six months following operation. It is commonly believed that even though the ovaries remain intact the presence of post-operative flushes indicates the onset of the menopause. This view was not, however, supported by a study of the vaginal cytology which was successfully carried out post-operatively in twenty-four cases. Eighteen cases were found to manifest a continuing cyclical ovarian activity, yet post-operative flushes were just as common in this group as in the six cases who showed no persisting cyclical ovarian function.

The findings of this investigation are being analysed in more detail and a follow-up of the patients will continue for a longer period. A few cases have already occurred in which psychological symptoms have emerged subsequent to the first six months following operation and it can be accepted that the frequency of unsatisfactory sequelae now reported, represents a minimum. However, at this stage one can suggest with confidence that in women about to undergo hysterectomy the presence of an unstable personality, childlessness, illegitimate births and a strong desire for more children represent indications for psychiatric supervision.

Bibliography

DRELLICH, M.C., and BIEBER, I.: The psychological importance of the uterus and its functions. J. nerv. ment. Dis *126*: 322 (1958).

KRAFFT-EBING, R.V.: Lehrbuch der Psychiatrie (Enke Leipzig, 1890).

KROGER, W.S.,and FREED, S.C.: Psychosomatic Gynaecology (Saunders, London 1951).

LEWIS, A. J., and JACKSON, J.: Psychiatric comparisons of artificial menopause and the effects of hysterectomy. J. Neurol. Psychiat. *3*: 101 (1940).

LINDEMANN, E.: Observations on psychiatric sequelae to surgical operations in women. Amer. J. Psychiat. *98*: 132 (1941).

MENZER, D.; MORRIS, T.; GATES, P.; SABBATH, J.; ROBEY, H.; PLANT, T., and STURGIS, S. H.: Patterns of emotional recovery from hysterectomy. Psychosom. Med. *19*: 379 (1957).

STENGEL, E.; ZEITLYN, B. B., and RAYNER, E. H.: Post-operative psychoses. J. ment. Sci. *104*: 389 (1958).

WENGRAF, F.: Psychoneurotic symptoms following hysterectomy. Amer. J. Obstet. Gynec. *52*: 645 (1946).

WENGRAF, F.: Psychosomatic approach to gynaecology and obstetrics (Thomas, Springfield 1953).

Author's address: DR. BRIAN ACKNER, Maudsley Hospital *London S.E. 5* and Postgraduate Medical School of London England).

Psychic Factors in Obstetrics *

R. HELLMANN, Hamburg

From remotest antiquity, the very beginnings of mankind, technology has continuously changed our way of life. Besides all progress we must not ignore certain obscure or even negative partial vistas during the recent period of stormy development. Technology touches our lives on every side, even in reproduction—let us only think of the possibilities of artificial insemination—and especially in the sphere of obstetrics.

Development of obstetric technique spans from the invention of the obstetric forceps by the brothers CHAMBERLEN via the first use of chloroform during delivery, applied by J. SNOW in 1853, which was to bring about even farther-reaching effects, up to the modern Cae-

---

* Dedicated to PROF. DR. H. H. SCHMID of the Rostock University on occasion of his 75th birthday.

sarian which under optimum conditions delivers the child to day in barely two minutes. Two centuries ago, J. SMELLIE laid the foundations to a conservative doctrine of childbirth by research into the anatomy of the pelvis and the mechanics of parturition. It is interesting that since the invention of anesthesia both the British and still more extensively the Americans—who are generally taken to be individualists and mainly starting from "ratio" when alleviating pains—have subjected childbirth to an exaggerated mechanization and pharmacologization. Whilst more than nine tenth of all births should and could be spontaneous as a natural event and almost physiologically normal, there are "lying in wards" which show a higher percentage figure of operative deliveries compared with normal parturitions. If possible, all deliveries are performed by general or partial anesthesia. In our medical jargon one might call this "perfect routine anesthesia".

There is no doubt that an obstetrician who is intent on humanitarian ideas will have to avail himself of all possibilities of up-to-date medical technique in order to carry out a delivery, in pathological cases, with a minimum of danger to mother and child. But when the thesis of a gynecologist is still haunting our present time, "without artificial obstetrics the civilized human races would have disappeared on earth in three generations" this appears to be rather a hypothetical supposition. We obstetricians need not to try to prove with fervour our right to obstetric existence in this direction. Without recourse to the rather hackneyed talk about medical ethics one should give dispassionate consideration to the issue in future, whether deliveries should be "handled", in the main, artificially or to a large extent naturally. In the former case it seems to be an "abionomous" procedure in the terms of J.H. SCHULTZ. On the contrary it might be more sensible to streamline obstetrics according to the laws of bionomy to which man is subjected.

Psychology has gained an ever increasing importance in the whole of the medical science. Medical psychology, psychodiagnostics, and psychotherapy assume an ever increasing and wider space and have not left untouched "Ars obstetrica" in recent years. To a larger and larger degree they form a countercurrent for the technical-minded and hitherto only permissible "positivistic-mechanistic" attitude which is prevailing in the whole sphere of modern medical science (J. MEINERTZ). Though the well-known psychotherapist G.R. HEYER recently wrote with a view to gynecology that unfortunately he was not of the opinion that the knowledge of psychotherapy has sufficiently permeated a wide range of the medical world, there appear to be more favourable prospects for our endeavours within the field of Ars obstetrica.

On principle, the gestation processes, with due regard to psychic aspects, should be given greater importance and consideration in our concept of the world. The sublimity of creation which renews again and again in each individual event of parturition, is often ignored or undervalued. War, mass catastrophes and traffic accidents are often given priority, though, strictly speaking, they ought to reduce the Promethean pride in achievements of our technical-minded era and should lead us to attach greater value to the essence of the innermost human emotional sphere. The general feeling of insecurity in our present world frequently finds its expression in an overvaluation of the belief in "exactitude" and the seemingly comprehensible.

The legend of traditional labour pains is still dominating the imaginations of experts and laymen. The essential reason for this is said to be the *erect posture of man* which allegedly makes parturition more difficult with man than with quadrupedes. This assertion admits at least—which some opponents of "natural childbirth" contend—that animals generally give birth more easily than Homo sapiens, especially Homo faber. But does nature actually cut such capers? Can the erect posture of man be traded in for the unilateral commitment to impose on the female partner the "indispensable", depressing labour pains? With the male partner, neither the functional desire is impaired nor is he even punished by "physiological pains" within the cycle of reproduction. Might it not be possible that with these mechanistic explanations, quite instinctively reminiscences of magic-mystical spheres and ancient guilt complexes based on the old Testament play a part like the Fall of Man and, according to MARTIN LUTHER the curse in Genesis related to painful childbirth: "In sorrow thou shalt bring forth children"? Apart from this, there are modern and more correct translations by H. GUNKEL and M. BUBER. In line with steadily growing scientific knowledge we obtain better insight into the inter-relations thus enabling us to understand the reasons which have led to such phraseology. By this we would be able to depart from the Dogma of Sin and the consequent penalty of suffering labour pains. Even when fully appreciating the peculiarities of a change towards an erect posture we ought to judge positively upon the effects resulting therefrom.

A highly experienced obstetrician such as TH. v. JASCHKE gives due consideration to this problem when saying that "with primitive peoples living under natural conditions painfulness of parturition seems to be far less" and "that doubtlessly it has increased in line with progressing civilization". This supposition would be almost a match to G. DICK-READ's concept of painful "cultural labour". Furthermore, this scheme which accentuates pains, gives no room to Partus insensibilis, and possibly many a precipitate delivery, and to the statement by P. A. NIKOLAJEW according to which in the U.S.S.R. about 7 per cent of all women deliver painlessly without any pain relief—so to speak natural talents.

In addition to this there is my own continuous experience with Partus naturalis since 1949, which comes up to the observations made all over the world. During my gynecological practice in South China from 1934 to 1937, I have experienced how easily and with but little trouble Chinese women gave birth to their children, with emotional stability, fully composed. Psychic moments were decisive for this. In the past six months I have been able to perform fifty deliveries in my own Hamburg clinic—among them a sizable number of eldery primipara—who gave "natural birth" to their children in an almost ideal way. It goes without saying that we were fortunate and had not to resort to Caesarian and forceps, but again and again the pre-eminent importance of psychic factors in obstetrics was confirmed. These factors are at least as important as the mechanics of parturition. In the course of recent years we have also abandoned to a large degree the general concept that with normal conditions during delivery labour of the second stage is said to result in "extreme painfulness" by the intensive squeezing and stretching of the muscular pelvic floor, as the relatively large head of the child forces its way through. On the one hand the reason is the psychological preparation and supervision of the parturition, and on the other hand our expectant mothers have an emotion of relief when they help "bearing down" and by their own conscious efforts and achievements can promote the continuance of parturition. At the beginning, when drawing up the Cervix and later on when dilating the pelvic floor, their knowledge, their antenatal training in relaxation and respiration are of greatest importance. Local or general anesthesia mostly proves unnecessary— also with possible episiotomy of the stretched perineum and even when sewing it up, which operation, however, should be done as early as possible.

In 1933, G. DICK-READ started from the idea that labour pains are due to social and cultural influences which cannot be justified by any Law of Nature. Psychological obstetrics does no longer acknowledge physiological pains and prefers psychoprophylaxis of pains right from the outset rather than combatting such pains at a later stage. Consequently, also here prophylaxis is given priority to therapy. The psychotherapist in cooperation with the obstetrician is offered a wide field for his activities. The personality and psychic attitude of the child-bearing woman are of no lesser importance than that of the obstetrician. Co-ordination, or better still, mutual influence as a means towards correlation, might penetrate into deeper psychic spheres.

From the wish to convince the patient by "good words", persuasion and suggestion up to hypnotic influence—though generally unnecessary—there is such a wide scope according to training and therapeutic ability of the obstetrician, ranging from the work of a plain and simple medical "artisan" up to the art of an outstanding medical personality.

When considering the "*Fear-Tension-Pain-Syndrome*" many mal-adjustments of a "woman in distress" which in the main result from fear and anxiety, can be avoided or removed. Gestation neuroses of more or less superficial structure are mainly in the domain of "minor psychotherapy" (J.H. SCHULTZ) and offer favourable possibilities for treatment. G. DICK-READ prefers tranquilizing information, gymnastics, respiration and relaxation training. The "pedagogic" success achieved with this antenatal training can be reproduced by any obstetrician after he has acquainted himself with the basic concept of this. Many factors must contribute towards the objective that the deep-rooted pre-conceived idea "birth equals pains" will disappear.

Among the various shortcomings of the man-dominated world ranks the fact that also in obstetrics certain *knowledge* determined by male ratio has been given priority to female *experience*. In this field the function determined by the female emotional sphere, the core of the female psyche, must again increase in importance. Isn't it odd that in the "progressive" western world many a woman should like to be delivered of her child at home for fear of an "institution"? In.contrast to this, many male managers of clinics stressing the risks involved in domiciliary midwifery (which are probably of minor significance as compared to those of a road-user in motorized traffic) propagate the sterile-sober, perfectionist-technicized delivery in a large hospital. This means, the emotional and sympathetic private atmosphere is contrasted with the more or less spiritually anonymous environment of a mass of people. Does this not show in the subconscious mind a sort of "masculine attitude of protest" (A. ADLER) against the female psyche? Maladjustments in conjunction with the environment during delivery have only been partially uncovered—e.g. in the room for parturient patients. In addition to this, women persistently hold the opinion that childbirth and disease cannot be brought to a common denominator.

Often woman, in the man-dominated order, is forced into situations which are inadequate to her being and way of life (A. MAYER, GRAF WITTGENSTEIN, R. HELLMANN). If the ambivalency of woman is reduced, disharmonies and dysfunctions can be avoided more easily. Antenatal training is to free the expectant mother, to a large extent, from wrong concepts of male intellectual attitude. We try to achieve by an elevated position of the upper part of the body during the expulsion stage an undisturbed relaxation and "bearing down"— abandoning the male "bearing up". Are we at the end of a decaying epoch of paternity and again on the very threshold of matriachate, a revival of the "eternal feminine"? Or is an order in the offing, with increasing equality of both sexes, which WITTGENSTEIN calls "Paar-rechtlich", mutual co-operation of couples? Will then the typical female function of delivery be less painful again?

More essential than alleviation of pains is stressing the *importance of the experience of parturition and how to influence it*. The mother's emotional happiness in childbirth in terms of the ideal of "maximum functional riches in life" as expressed by M. EBERHARDT must be maintained and promoted. Favourable effects on forthcoming births and generations will be in the offing but can only be intimated. Let us follow E. SPEER who considers psychotherapy, and in his full right, from the fact of working up experiences. The obstetrician would do well to apply this knowledge in his sphere, as it has been obtained during a long way of rich experience. It is with good reason that the female psychologist H. DEUTSCH has described childbirth as "the greatest and happiest experience of a woman, perhaps of man in itself altogether".

Within the frame of our small private clinic we have endeavoured to approach the often unexpressed wishes of female psyche. One can largely do away with the "institutional character" and have deliveries performed in homely rooms which intensify the feeling of security, with due regard to the psychic and sensational sphere of intimacy for a woman. The psychological training of all co-workers appears to be of foremost importance. In this connection it is surprising what wonders a skilful and sympathetic female helping hand works, winning by a mere trifle the thanks of mothers. WITTGENSTEIN, intentionally considering local conditions, coined the term of "cultivated stationary domiciliary delivery".

The *visual experience*—by the way also considering female curiosity to some extent—induced us to use the *mirror* for selfobservation during the second stage of labour. The mirror, as a familiar "tool" of the fair sex, plays a psychologically interesting part anyhow. We use it as an auxiliary for the promotion of labour and devotion to parturition. Its application often strengthens the contact to the child and the confidence of the expectant mother in the obstetrician who comments upon the events during labour thus elucidating them to her. Not infrequently, the image of the child forcing its way through into daylight is highly welcomed, thus making richer the experience of childbirth. According to the hitherto valid concept of parturition, consideration was given to pains, distress and sorrows the way through the "vale of tears"—in the *maturity process* of a woman. This might be true for the individual case. But we believe that in general we have to value far higher the proud delight of a mother in her own achievements obtained by labour and the blissful experience "on her way to an individual being herself" (E. KRETSCHMER). By a qualified optimistic attitude towards parturition the desire for and the will to have a child are intensified and the regal way to motherhood is widened and paved.

He who aims at psychologization of obstetrics aspires after an intensification of psychic values, broadening and deepening of the emotional sphere during the experience of parturition. Co-operation in the materialization of this "guiding image of eutocia" will gradually effect a change and a new attitude towards the event of "natural childbirth" which I have tried to outline as a sort of "conversion". For the purpose of mutual co-operation of couples, obstetrics might obtain new fruitful contents in future, ranging between dampening of the exaggerated technical functional desire of male intellect and better consideration of female psychic though not at all extremistic interests.

Nemo obstetricus nisi physiologus – et psychologus!

Author's address: DR. R. HELLMANN, *Hamburg 20*, Heilwigstrasse 105 (Germany).

Neurosis and Psychosomatic Disorders in Out-Patients

P. Sainsbury, Chichester

The purpose of this investigation was to see whether the relative levels of two personality factors, neuroticism and extraversion, would distinguish patients with diseases commonly classed as psychosomatic from patients with other diseases; that is, those in which the psychological component is not usually considered important.

As physicians outside the psychiatric field are chary of the concept of psychosomatic disease, my intention was to design an experiment which might provide the kind of objective evidence for psychological determinants in physical disorders which the general physician might accept and find meaningful. With these aims in view I have taken two defined and measureable factors of personality, Eysenck's (1947) neuroticism and extraversion, and then stated simple hypotheses of the relation of each to psychosomatic disorder. Scores on the two factors were then obtained in unselected out-patients and related to diagnosis.

Neuroticism is defined as the general emotional lability of a person, his emotional over-responsiveness, and his liability to neurotic breakdown under stress. *Extraversion* refers to the outgoing, uninhibited, sociable proclivities of a person (Eysenck, 1959).

The extensive experimental work by which these two independent dimensions of personality were identified may be found in Eysenck's books (Eysenck, 1947, 1952). The correlations found between neuroticism and certain constitutional characteristics such as body build or lability of the autonomic nervous system are particularly relevant to this investigation.

Hypotheses

1. That the level of *neuroticism* will be higher in patients with psychosomatic diseases than in a control group without psychosomatic diseases.

2. If psychosomatic diseases arise from a prolongation of the physiological effects of emotion, patients with psychosomatic diseases will be more dysthymic, and therefore less *extraverted*, than a non-psychosomatic control group; for EYSENCK has shown that dysthymics (e.g. reactive depressions and anxiety states) are introverted. Were one to favour the alternative view that the somatic disorders in these patients are hysterical (i.e. conversion) symptoms then EYSENCK would predict that they would be as, or more, extraverted than the controls, because he also found hysterics are extraverted.

Methods and procedure

Through the kind co-operation of the Consultants working in the clinics at two General Hospitals in Chichester we were able for two months to ask all out-patients aged 20–59 to complete the Maudsley Personality Inventory while they were waiting to see the doctor. A small proportion of patients escaped us, but these omissions appeared to be of a random kind. We therefore examined a typical series of out-patients, unselected except for age.

The surgeon or physician, after seeing the patient, entered his diagnosis on the questionnaire. The diagnoses were then classified into four groups:

Psychosomatic diagnoses
Possibly psychosomatic diagnoses
Control diagnoses, and
Neurotic ones.

The composition of these groups was decided in advance, and it is important to emphasise that the patient's scores were not known when his diagnosis was classified.

We used an operational criterion of what was to be considered a Psychosomatic diagnosis. The diagnoses included in the Psychosomatic group were those given a chapter or paragraph heading by at least 2 of 6 writers of standard works on psychosomatic medicine (ALEXANDER, 1950; DUNBAR, 1948; HALLIDAY, 1943; HAMILTON, 1955; O'NEIL, 1955; WEISS AND ENGLISH, 1957).

Table 1 lists the *psychosomatic* and *possibly psychosomatic* diagnoses

Table 1

PSYCHOSOMATIC *Diagnosis occurred 8 or more times*		POSSIBLY PSYCHOSOMATIC *Diagnosis occured 8 or more times*
Asthma	Acne Vulgaris	Cervical Erosion
Coronary Disease	Alopecia	Chalazion
Diabetes	Eczema (End. and	"Herniated Disc"
Hypertension	Exogenous)	Lupus Erythematosus
Peptic Ulcer	Fungus Infections and	Low Back Pain
Rheumatoid Arth.	Sweating	Obesity
Pulmonary T. B.	Lichen Planus	Pain (No organic basis
Thyrotoxicosis	Pruritus	found)
Chronic Nasal Infection	Psoriasis	Sterility
Dysmenorrhoea	Seborrhoeic Derm.	
Leucorrhoea	Urticaria	
Irregular Menstruation		
Menorrhagia		

which occurred 8 or more times in our sample and which are there-fore the principal conditions included in these two groups.

The *possibly psychosomatic* group includes: 1. those diagnoses in which psychological factors are considered to play a part by some authorities, including the Consultants who co-operated with us; 2. a group of disorders which, though often clearly due to an extrinsic cause, also contain many cases where a typical history and physical signs are not obtained, or where the symptoms are inexplicably prolonged, as for example, with the diagnosis prolapsed intervertebral disc; and 3. patients in whom no organic cause for the symptom was found. The possibly psychosomatic disorders are a somewhat arbitrary

Table 2. Controls. Diagnosis which occurred 8 or more times

Appendicitis	Pregnancy
Cholecystitis	Prolapse
Deafness	Skin Infections
Ear Infections	Tumours, Benign
Fractures	Varicose Veins
Hemorrhoids	Warts
Hernia	———
Injuries	Carcinoma
Osteoarthritis	Poliomyelitis
	Rheumatic Heart Dis.

selection; their claim to consideration is that the diagnoses were placed in this group without prior knowledge of their scores.

Table 2 lists the principal *control* diagnoses, that is the remaining diagnoses which occurred 8 or more times. I have sub-divided the list; those below the line are conditions of a very chronic or serious nature which I will refer to presently.

The last group, the *Neurotic* one, was largely composed of Anxiety States and Reactive Depressions.

The questionnaire

The Maudsley Personality Inventory (M.P.I.) is a questionnaire of 48 items. It was devised by EYSENCK to provide a more valid and a briefer measure of the two personality factors neuroticism and extraversion than other scales used for this purpose. EYSENCK selected 261 items from the latter scales and by an item analysis found the 24 items which best discriminated on neuroticism and the 24 which best discriminated on extraversion. These items make up the M.P.I. Each may be answered *yes*, *no*, or ?. The appropriate *yes* or *no* scores 2 points, and the ? one point. The maximum score on neuroticism and on extraversion is therefore 48 points each.

The scales have a satisfactory reliability. They have been standardised by EYSENCK (1959) on a representative sample of the population of England (1800). The mean scores on *neuroticism* of various neurotic populations are consistently and significantly higher than the mean of the normal sample. *Extraversion* scores are found to be lower in the dysthymics than in the hysterics, as EYSENCK predicted they would. The scales have therefore been satisfactorily validated and this is their most important attribute from the point of view of this experiment.

A feature of the M.P.I. which particularly suits it to our purpose, apart from its brevity, is the form of the questions. None of them refer to somatic symptoms, so that the patients presenting symptoms at the clinics will not increase his scores on the personality factors, nor will the anxiety of visiting the doctor and the consequent physiological symptoms of palpitations, tremor, etc. contribute to the score.

Findings

1,352 patients between the ages 20–59 filled up the questionnaire while waiting in one of the 11 clinics. Table 3 gives the number of

Table 3. Totals for Clinics and Diagnostic Groups

Clinic	Control	Psycho-somatic	Neurotic	Poss: Psycho-somatic	Total
Medical	50	61	1	10	122
Chest	10	57	0	0	67
Diabetic	0	22	0	0	22
Skin	49	148	0	23	220
Physical Med.	55	45	0	71	171
Orthopaedic	112	4	0	54	170
Surgical	115	15	0	19	149
Eye	36	8	0	13	57
Ear, Nose and Throat	51	25	0	2	78
Gynaecol.	66	68	0	35	169
Psychiat.	2	6	115	4	127
Total	546	459	116	231	1352

patients in our four diagnostic groupings who successfully completed
the form in each clinic.

Neuroticism

Table 4 shows the number of patients in the four groups, and
the means and standard deviations of their Neuroticism scores. I have
added for comparison the mean and S.D. of EYSENCK's quota sample.

Table 4. Neuroticism

	Number	Mean neuroticism	S. D. N.
Controls	546	18.4	10.8
Psychosomatic	459	23.8	10.3
Possible psychosomatic	231	23.1	10.9
Neurotic	116	32.0	9.2
Control Gen. Pop. (EYSENCK 1959)	1800	19.9	11.0

The significance levels of the differences found between the
Neuroticism means of the groups are shown in Table 5.

Patients with psychosomatic and with possibly psychosomatic
diseases both have very significantly higher scores on Neuroticism
than do the controls; but lower scores than the neurotics from the

Table 5. Levels of significance of differences between groups: Neuroticism

	Controls	Psychosomatic	Possible Psychosomatic
Psychosomatic	.001	—	—
Possible Psychosomatic	.001	N. S.	—
Neurotic	.001	.001	.001

psychiatric clinic. There is *no* difference between the psychosomatic and possibly psychosomatic groups on Neuroticism.

These differences are not accounted for by the age and sex distributions of the different populations. Among the psychosomatic group, however, there were more patients who had made previous attendances at the clinics. It is therefore possible that the high level of neuroticism in the psychosomatic group may be a consequence of the duration of their illness with the result that they have reacted neurotically to the prolonged stress it has imposed.

This possibility was investigated by extracting from the control group all those patients with *chronic disabling and prognostically serious*

Table 6. Chronicity of disease and neuroticism

	Chronic or Serious Dis.	Controls	Psychosomatic
Number	67	546	459
Mean Neuroticism	19.0	18.4	23.8
S. D.	9.1	10.8	10.3

illnesses. The mean Neuroticism score of these seriously ill or disabled patients was 18.96, which is not significantly different from the controls (Table 6). Chronicity, therefore, does not account for the high N found in the two psychosomatic groups.

Extraversion

The findings on the Extraversion factor are shown in Table 7 which gives the means and S.D.'s of the four groups; again EYSENCK's control quota sample is included.

It may be seen in Table 8 that the psychosomatic group is significantly less extraverted than the control, as also is the neurotic group; but the possibly psychosomatic group has a level of Extraversion which does *not* differ from the controls.

The results so far support our original hypotheses. In an un-

Table 7. Extraversion

	Number	Mean Extraversion	S. D. E.
Control	546	25.7	8.5
Psychosomatic	459	23.2	9.7
Possible Psychosomatic	231	26.0	8.9
Neurotic	116	21.4	10.1
Control Gen. Pop. (EYSENCK 1959)	1800	24.9	9.7

Table 8. Levels of significance of differences between groups: Extraversion

	Control	Psychosomatic	Possible Psychosomatic
Psychosomatic	.001	—	—
Possible Psychosomatic	N. S.	.001	—
Neurotic	.001	.05	.001

selected sample of out-patients we find that those with psychosomatic diagnoses score higher on Neuroticism than do the control patients. The psychosomatic patients, like the neurotics, were also more introverted than the controls; a finding which would support our contention that they are dysthymic, that is to say, their symptoms are likely to be associated with anxiety or depression and the consequent disturbance of physiological function. The *doubtfully psychosomatic* group are also higher on neuroticism than the controls; and they are significantly more extraverted than the clearly psychosomatic group. This result would be consistent with a hysterical explanation for some of their symptoms, which is not unlikely, as the commonest diagnoses in the *possibly psychosomatic* population were such conditions as "herniated disc" and pains with no discernible organic basis.

Diagnoses, neuroticism and extraversion

The scores on Neuroticism and on Extraversion for each diagnosis listed in the psychosomatic, possibly psychosomatic, and control groups provides some support for this.

Table 9 lists the 22 psychosomatic diseases which occurred 8 or more times. It also shows their means on neuroticism and on extraversion, and the levels of significance of the differences from the control's. With the exception of Peptic Ulcer, Coronary disease, Pruritus and Acne, they are consistently and significantly more neu-

Table 9. Psychosomatic diseases which occurred 8 or more times

Diagnosis	No.	Neuroticism Mean	P	Extraversion Mean	P
Dysmenorrhoea	9	29.2	.001	24.9	NS
Urticaria	10	27.2	.01	20.8	.01
Leucorrhoea	13	27.1	.005	24.9	NS
Fungus infections	9	26.4	.005	24.1	NS
Alopecia	17	26.4	.001	23.1	NS
Asthma	14	26.1	.01	20.9	.05
Eczema	32	25.0	.005	23.0	NS
Menorrhagia	32	24.8	.001	23.4	.05
Seborrhoeic Derm.	23	24.8	.01	21.7	.025
Psoriasis	28	24.8	.005	23.5	NS
Hypertension	19	24.7	.005	21.2	.05
Diabetes	37	24.5	.005	21.0	.025
Pulmonary T. B.	54	24.3	.001	21.9	.01
Irregular Mens.	12	24.3	.005	23.1	NS
Dermatitis	17	23.9	.025	24.6	NS
Chronic Nasal Inf.	14	23.3	.05	22.4	NS
Thyrotoxicosis	14	22.2	.05	23.7	NS
Rheumatoid Arth.	42	22.0	.05	25.1	NS
Pruritus	13	21.5	NS	23.5	NS
Peptic Ulcer	22	21.4	NS	24.6	NS
Acne Vulgaris	9	19.4	NS	27.2	NS
Coronary Disease	12	15.9	NS	26.0	NS
Control Patients	546	18.4	—	25.7	—

rotic than are the controls; and in only one instance, Coronary disease, is the mean neuroticism score less than the control's.

The patients with psychosomatic diagnoses are also less extraverted than the control (with the exception again of Coronary disease and Acne). The diagnoses in which the mean level of extraversion is *significantly* lower are: Diabetes, Hypertension, T.B., Seborrhoeic Dermatitis, Menorrhagia and Urticaria.

I would particularly like to draw your attention to the following conditions: Diabetes, the various Menstrual disorders and Leucorrhoea, Pulmonary T.B., and Rheumatoid Arthritis; although they are frequently considered psychosomatic diseases, I do not know of any controlled experimental studies which establish the psychological component. Since this investigation was begun, however, KISSEN (1958) has also shown that patients with Pulmonary T.B. present more psychiatric problems than does a control group.

All the diagnoses in the *possibly psychosomatic* list (except Chalazion) also have a higher level on neuroticism than the controls, those with low back pain, cervical erosion, herniated disc and sterility significantly so; but they *differ* from the previous list of psychosomatic disorders in that all of them, except low back pain, have a level of Extraversion at, or above the control level (see Table 10). As the combina-

Table 10. Possibly psychosomatic diseases which occurred 8 or more times

Diagnosis	No.	Neuroticism Mean	P	Extraversion Mean	P
Sterility	8	28.4	.01	25.6	NS
Cervical erosion	15	24.4	.01	27.7	NS
Low Back Pain	43	23.3	.01	23.4	NS
Lupus Erythematosus	10	22.3	NS	25.8	NS
"Herniated Disc"	37	21.8	.05	25.8	NS
Obesity	9	21.8	NS	26.7	NS
Pain (No organic basis found)	30	20.7	NS	25.9	NS
Chalazion	12	16.2	NS	28.2	NS
Control Patients	546	18.4	—	25.7	—

tion of high Neuroticism and high Extraversion is found to be peculiar to hysterics, it is again worth considering whether the list of *possible* psychosomatic diseases differs from the psychosomatic list in that hysterical mechanisms are determining the symptoms in the one, and physiological dysfunction of emotional origin in the other.

Lastly, we come to the *control* group (see Table 11). The psychosomatic diseases were high on Neuroticism and low on Extraversion in nearly every diagnosis. The diagnoses in the control list, however, differ from the control group as a whole in only a few instances; in two diseases Neuroticism was significantly high, and in two or possibly three, Extraversion was significantly high; in one it was significantly low.

The exceptions are of interest, however. Patients with Warts are significantly more emotionally unstable; but also significantly more extraverted than the control patients. The repeatedly commented upon observation that Warts may be charmed away suggests that this hysterical pattern may not be spurious.

I was also interested in the fracture patients who, as a group, are significantly more extraverted than the remainder of the controls. This may throw a little rational light on the concept of accident-

Table 11. Control diseases which occurred 8 or more times

Diagnosis	No.	Neuroticism Mean	P	Extraversion Mean	P
Appendicitis	12	19.2	NS	23.8	NS
Cholecystitis	8	21.3	NS	24.8	NS
Deafness	8	17.4	NS	30.0	.01
Ear Infections	20	20.9	NS	26.5	NS
Fractures	51	18.3	NS	28.1	.05
Hemorrhoids	9	23.0	NS	26.0	NS
Hernia	19	18.7	NS	25.2	NS
Injuries	60	19.0	NS	25.8	NS
Osteoarthritis	25	19.4	NS	25.1	NS
Pregnancy	13	20.6	NS	25.0	NS
Prolapse	25	24.2	.05	20.4	.01
Skin Infections	14	13.6	NS	26.1	NS
Tumours, Benign	22	15.0	NS	23.3	NS
Varicose Veins	20	17.1	NS	27.9	NS
Warts	8	29.1	.01	32.9	.01
Carcinoma	16	22.31	NS	21.7	NS
Rheumatic Heart Disease	10	19.00	NS	21.9	NS
Poliomyelitis	9	15.8	NS	26.7	NS
Control	546	18.4	—	25.7	—

proneness. That the liability to fracture is associated with more than normally outgoing and uninhibited tendencies in the personality seems entirely reasonable.

Finally the E and N scores of the patients with uterine prolapse reflects the pattern of the psychosomatic patients: neuroticism is high and extraversion is low. KROGER AND FREED (1951) in Psychosomatic Gynaecology observe a relation between prolapse, hypotonus of the pelvic muscles, and emotion.

Conclusions

There are many psychosomatic studies in which relations are sought, and claimed, between specific types of personality and particular psychosomatic diseases (DUNBAR, 1943; HALLIDAY, 1943). The consensus is, however, that the similarities in personality are more evident than the differences. We find that patients with many different psychosomatic diseases are characterised by high scores on neuroticism. It may therefore be that the failure to find real differences in the personality profiles of the different diseases is because previous workers were describing a variety of traits common in neurotics: dependency, repressed hostility, and so on.

The extraversion factor may further distinguish dysthymic neurotic personalities and hysterical neurotic personalities among patients with psychosomatic diseases. Examples of the former might be hypertension, eczema, or menorrhegia; and of the latter, back. pains with atypical symptoms of a prolapsed disc, warts and sterility.

Acknowledgments

I wish to thank the Consultants, Staff and Management Committee of the Royal West Sussex and St. Richard's Hospitals, Chichester, for their generously given help; also PROF. H. J. EYSENCK for allowing us to use the Maudsley Personality Inventory and for unpublished data on it.

I am very indebted to Miss PAT RAY who assisted me in collecting, recording and computing the data.

Bibliography

ALEXANDER, F.: Psychosomatic Medicine (Allen und Unwin, London 1950).

DUNBAR, F.: Psychosomatic Diagnosis (New York 1943).

DUNBAR, F.: Synopsis of Psychosomatic Diagnosis and Treatment (C.V. Mosby, St. Louis 1948).

DUNBAR, F.: Emotions and Bodily Changes (Columbia University Press, New York 1954).

EYSENCK, H.J.: Dimensions of Personality (Kegan Paul, London 1947).

EYSENCK, H.J.: The Scientific Study of Personality (Routledge and Kegan Paul, London 1952).

EYSENCK, H.J.: The Manual of the Maudsley Personality Inventory (In the Press 1959).

HALLIDAY, J.L.: The Concept of Psychosomatic Affection. Lancet 2: 692 (1943).

HAMILTON, M.: Psychosomatics (Chapman and Hall, London 1955).

KISSEN, D.M.: Emotional Factors in Pulmonary Tuberculosis (Tavistock Publications Ltd., London 1958).

KROGER, W.S., and FREED, S.: Psychosomatic Gynaecology (Saunders, London 1951).

O'NEILL, D.: A Psychosomatic Approach to Medicine (Pitman, London 1955).

O'NEILL, D.: Modern Trends in Psychosomatic Medicine (Butterworth, London 1955).

WEISS, E., and ENGLISH, O.S.: Psychosomatic Medicine, 3rd Ed. (Saunders, London 1957).

Author's address: DR. P. SAINSBURY, Medical Research Council, Clinical Psychiatry Research Group, Graylingwell Hospital, *Chichester* (England).

The Place and Recognition of Emotional Factors in the Etiology and Treatment of Chronic Non-Specific Colitis

R. West, Dorrington Grove

In 1930, C.D. Murray first drew attention to the emotional sensitivities and immaturities of character which occur in ulcerative colitis. Subsequently Wittkower (1938) showed, in 40 cases, that, by his (Freudian) approach to character, these sensitive character-types were diverse. Wittkower classified the character-types of his patients into obsessional and hysteric, there being both men and women in the first of these groups and only women in the second (hysterical) group (of 12 cases).

Long before the time of this approach observant clinicians had been aware of a gradation between a severe and often intractable ulcerative colitis and a so-called "mucous" or "muco-membranous" colitis, which latter was, at least by 1920, generally considered to be either entirely of nervous origin or much associated with nervous factors (c.f. Price's "Textbook of Medicine", 1922). Thus there was early recognition of the importance of emotional factors in the colonic dysfunctions and disease which have come to be united under the title of "chronic non-specific colitis", whether it presents with colonic spasm or actual ulceration, whether with the passage of mucus, or blood, or both. But an adequate understanding of just what in the "psyche" predisposes to these conditions—which may have infective, allergic, chemical, biochemical and endocrine, or enzymatic components (Brooke, 1954)—remained elusive, as indeed has any precise understanding of the physical mechanisms of the disease. Ulcerative colitis presents us with a profound and intricate psychosomatic relationship. Students of its various components must make advances where they can, each along his own line, until a suitable combination of fact and theory can acceptably bring our findings together. This uncoordinated advance has gone on now for many years.

On the physical side the following early findings still appear to be relevant to the issue of causation. First, a causal relationship between colonic spasm and ulcer formation was found to occur experimentally in dogs (LIUM AND PORTER, 1939). The agent of the colonic spasm could be mechanical irritation, acetylcholine or other parasympathomimetic drug, or toxic irritants such as that of dysentery toxin. The ulcers could form quickly. Relaxation of colonic musculature allowed such ulcers to heal. An early experimental observation introducing the psyche was that fright can blanche the colonic mucous membrane of the dog and can do this without the mediation of adrenaline (DRURY ET AL., 1929). Eventually it was established by direct vision that the exposed human colon can become congested and hyperfunctioning as a result of mixed feelings ("conflict, a desire to please, and resentment"). Associated with such sustained hyperfunctioning is increased fragility of the mucous membrane—so that minor traumata result in haemorrhage and ulceration (GRACE, WOLF AND WOLFF, 1951). Ways in which toxaemias and chronic infection might operate upon tissues thus debilitated have often been considered but have remained unsatisfactorily proven since the pioneer attempts of BARGEN (1924) to establish his "diplostreptococcus" as a satisfactory and specific cause of the lesions of ulcerative colitis (BACON, 1958).

On the psychological side, the character-type most generally associated with the long-lasting and intense colonic hyperfunctioning found in chronic diarrhoea and ulcerative colitis gradually became more closely defined. According to PAULLEY (1950) colitis occurs in an excessively dependent, parentally (usually maternally) controlled individual who is never outwardly aggressive, though he (or she) is often querulous, nursing a dull, prolonged resentment rather than expressing overt anger. Excessively sensitive, the ulcerative colitic type broods for months over real or imagined wrongs or insults. If a man, he may be effeminate and is usually fastidious. Immature emotionally (as noted earlier by CULLINAN, 1938), they are often frankly childish. The drunkenness, separation or death of a parent was often a precipitating cause of an attack of colitis. GRACE, WOLF AND WOLFF's (1951) version of this is: "a character at first sight one of passivity and acquiescence. Superficially mild, bland and sweet, there is evidence of underlying feelings of great anger and hostility".

Meanwhile, cases were investigated psychoanalytically and some of these yielded to psychotherapy in varying degrees.

Where deep levels of the unconscious mind—those of obsessions and phobias—were involved, no analyst expected results to be quick or complete. Hysterics should theoretically have yielded more quickly to treatment; and it is interesting that no division such as WITTKOWER suggested appears to have been reported on the treatment front. Perhaps hysterical symptoms, where such symptoms presented, always covered deeper problems, more distorting to the Ego but not detectable at first interview? This explanation would fit the two-layered character described by GRACE, WOLF AND WOLFF and by PAULLEY. At any rate, in more recent work references to hysteria have fallen into the background. Deep analysis also eroded the other large category of the "obsessional neurotic". Thus DANIELS (1940, 1942, 1944) reported character-types "more deeply narcissistic in their failures" and therefore "more psychotic than neurotic in their outcome". Psycho-analysis here revealed the physical symptoms of colitis as being "equivalent to" (i.e. a seemingly necessary alternative to) psychotic depression and melancholia. Indeed, the physical symptoms of ulcerative colitis were sometimes found to yield temporarily to treatment, only to be converted suddenly into these their psychotic "equivalents". I reported one such event in a short series of three cases which were treated by analytical therapy (WEST, 1946). In 1945 LINDEMANN (confirmed later by SPERLING, 1946; GROEN, 1947; PAULLEY, 1950; MUSHATT, 1954 and KIRKETERP, 1957) pointed to the sudden aggravation of a colitis by the loss of a key figure of the patient's life through bereavement, the psychogenic mechanism being considered (LINDEMANN, 1945) to be an increase of unconscious guilt and rage. Such an event—the loss of a father—preceded the fatal psychotic depression in the case to which I have just referred.

Such findings naturally require that great caution should be exercised in any case of ulcerative colitis which worsens under psychotherapy. An intensification of symptoms under treatment is likely to indicate that deep emotional pressures are increasing under exploratory anamnesis. Many psychiatrists guard against such an event by avoiding any genuine *analysis* of the patient's mental state. Instead they are content to support the existing Ego of the patient, taking his side, trying to express his unvoiced resentments for him, trying to guarantee him reliable emotional support and protection, never allowing him to feel forsaken (GROEN AND BASTIAANS, 1951). GRACE, PINSKY AND

WOLFF (1954) concluded that relief of stress in this sort of way gave better therapeutic results than did the then (antibiotic) medical treatment. Probably *deep* analysis, if undertaken at all, should begin and proceed as far as possible during an intermission of the disease. Since analysis of the Ego is, in fact, an attempt to put right the faulty character of the patient, it is dangerous to make this attempt while a patient is acutely ill, physically and mentally, essentially because of the precarious adaptation of that distorted Ego. Furthermore, the very real danger of worsening matters by attempted psychotherapy is a warning against *incautious* psychological interference of any kind in all cases of ulcerative colitis. Physicians skilled in their art have instinctively felt this danger: it is an emotional response that has often gone too far and turned them against the making of any serious psychiatric approach to patients with ulcerative colitis under their care.

It is not difficult to see how complex and potent doctor-patient relationships build up in ulcerative colitis! On the part of the medical (and nursing) staff frustration and an almost overwhelming urge towards *activity* in the face of actual or potential calamity: on the part of the patient attitudes which at once appeal and antagonise, a mixture of acquiescence and resistance such as has precipitated many a ward decision to abandon uncertain medical for more radical surgical treatment. In the 1940's, the medical treatment of ulcerative colitis was "expectant", symptomatic, and rather helpless. Surgical treatment, on the other hand, often gave dramatic relief. To such treatments the doctor increasingly turned.

Since 1950 two factors have tended to confirm a trend away from attempting to investigate the emotional life of patients with ulcerative colitis. One of these was the maintained good results of surgery (in England we have an enthusiastic "Ileostomy Association" with an ever growing membership). The other was the favorable response to cortisone or other steroid therapy. Large-scale trials with steroids showed that cortisone by mouth exerted a very favorable effect upon first attacks, nearly half of the patients so treated being essentially symptom-free after only a few weeks' treatment (TRUELOVE AND WITTS, 1954, 1955; KIRSNER ET AL., 1954, 1957; SKLAR ET AL., 1957; MALTBY ET AL., 1956).

Cortisone has, however, proved generally unable to prevent cases of ulcerative colitis from relapsing (TRUELOVE AND WITTS, 1959). In their recent report, TRUELOVE AND WITTS describe corticotrophin as having a "much superior" action to oral cortisone on such relapsed cases, though that drug proves more prone than oral cortisone to be associated with the relapse of first treatments and with complications such as "hypercortisonism, mental disturbance, moniliosis and serious complications of peptic ulcer". Such observations suggest that corticotrophin is merely a remedy of "greater potency". Doomed as both seem to be first to aid and then to fail the patient, cortico-trophin is found to do both these things more thoroughly than does the direct use of adrenal steroids, natural or synthetic.

It is for psychiatrists—and particularly those with analytical experience—to ask themselves certain questions at this juncture. How sure are we of our own ground? First, do we *know* that ulcerative colitis consistently afflicts people of abnormal character-type and abnormal and peculiar sensitivity to their emotional environment? Is this mental abnormality an essential feature of non-specific colitis? The psychoanalyst is accused of reporting few cases! Alas! he sees few cases (at deep levels) to report; but those he does see may be very impressive. In the international literature the reports are numer-ous, as recently collected bibliographies shew (see e.g. MUSHATT, 1954). To the psychologically observant physician there can, I think, be no doubt at all about the abnormality of character build of most cases—I would be inclined to say of every case—of non-specific colitis *. Next, do the onset of symptoms coincide, with any great regularity, with peculiar emotional stresses in the life of the patient? Yes! Anyone who will learn to take psychological case-histories is sure of that: though, alas! many physicians eschew or have never been taught this art. But can we help to clarify the success of steroid therapy and its present limitations? Can we account for the just satis-faction of the surgeon in his frequent and maintained cures, by ileo-stomy, colostomy and colectomy? More important, can we learn to co-operate more fully with both physician and surgeon to the ad-vantage of the patient with ulcerative colitis? Only, I would submit, if we make our findings as plain and as assimible as possible. It will also greatly help if we can more regularly follow up psychogenic theory by psychotherapeutic practice.

Evidence of the existence of a typical susceptible character-type and of the emotional precipitation of symptoms ought to be obtainable

---

* MITSCHERLICH is to be endorsed when he says (in this Conference) that specificity of deep conflicts are to be found more consistently than their over-lying, and sometimes facilely drawn, character "profiles", which may or may not bear a constant relationship to such deep conflicts.

from every series of cases of ulcerative colitis. This evidence is usually not very difficult to elicit. Here follows a summary of a one to three interview investigation of 8 consecutive cases that passed through medical or surgical treatment according to the choice of the physicians and surgeons of a general hospital in an English Midland city last year (1958). The cases were seen at follow-up interviews and the total time spent with the 8 cases was not more than 12 hours. All the patients are from a female ward.

Criteria. In allocating categories to patients in respect of their mental and emotional responses some definitions are necessary: however arbitrary this may be it improves communication between medical colleagues. A frank and confidential case-history, obtained (in a quiet room and not behind ward screens!) by the physician, nurse or student most fitted by ability for this task—but best of all by the physician who is treating the patient—will enable a technically superficial account of attitudes, habits and events to be adequately recorded in terms of character-type and precipitating emotions. The deep analyst too can use the following scale, though he will weight responses somewhat differently and find it difficult not to question the meaning of superficial responses and to suppress his desire to pass on, in anticipation, to deeper categories whose emotional vigour only he can evaluate.

1. The term *"Obsessional"* includes the following subdivisions:— evident obsessiveness in thought or action; perfectionism; undue overt sense of guilt; clear evidence of unconscious guilt, whether defensive (as in veiled resentments against loved ones) or compensated by aggressiveness; sado-masochism. 2. *"Hysteria"* denotes *either* a physically demonstrative emotional hypersensitivity (if with overt apprehensiveness this may be called anxiety hysteria), *or* a somatic conversion of this (conversion hysteria). Frankly overt anxiety is simply called "anxiety". 3. *"Psychotic"* denotes a massive withdrawal of vital emotions combined with fixed perceptive failures.

Character types. Of these 8 cases, and using the above criteria, 5 were classed as "obsessional", the group being composed of one frank obsessional, one perfectionist, two with overt guilt and one sado-masochist. The 3 remaining cases gave a presenting diagnosis within the hysterical category (hysteria 1, anxiety hysteria 1, anxiety 1). I am confident that all of these so-called hysterics had deeper problems of aggressiveness than this surface diagnosis could take note of. In this series there was no sign of the ulcerative colitis being a psychotic equivalent. But all the patients were in a state of remission when they were interviewed by me.

Precipitating emotional factors

7 of the 8 cases showed these clearly. They may be epitomized seriatim as:—1. marriage forced by pregnancy, 2. *First time:* death of father, *second time:* a wooing but married business chief, 3. *First time:* worries of finance and early marriage problems, *second time:* death of a brother-in-law, 4. professional worries (care of children), 5. a culmination of marriage tensions, 6. *First time:* mother hospitalized, *second time:* husband's illness (peptic ulcer), 7. "any worry brings on the colitis". The remaining (8th) case was a perfectionist obsessional in whom the first onset of symptoms had followed immediately upon the birth of a "much wanted" baby. A second interview might perhaps have elicited if, and under what circumstances, this also was a precipitating situation.

Medical treatment

5 of the 8 patients had been given cortisone, prednisolone or A.C. T.H. All had responded temporarily. The 3 cases that had been given steroid treatment for the first time over a year ago had all relapsed within the year, one of them to respond to a second course of steroid (3 months ago), another, after relapsing twice on steroid, to be given a successful ileostomy 7 months ago, with complete absence of symptoms to date. In the third a colostomy was performed followed by an excision of the rectum, again with complete success. Of two cases whose first steroid treatment started less than one year ago, one—a case of spontaneously remitting colitis of 11 year's duration—remitted in 3 months and has remained well for 9 months since, the other—a first onset in an unmarried woman of 30 (the sado-masochist)—remitted 9 months ago but began to bleed again recently under the strain of difficult decisions in a personal relationship across the sexes.

Surgical treatment

This has been resorted to in 3 cases only: 1. In one, an ileostomy (September 1958) in a girl of 19 with severe colitis of 2 years duration (following two relapses on Prednisolone) has given complete relief. Since this operation the patient, previously a perfectionist, has "not worried at all about whether it will come back" (which she had done before), "but only about getting a new house to live in".

2. In the second case, after 30 years of recurrent severe ulcerative colitis, which was treated generally in 1928 and 1932 and by transfusions in 1948 and 1955, colostomy was performed four years ago followed by excision of the rectum. The results are excellent, the patient can "eat anything except some fruits", and, whereas previously "any worry caused colitis", there are now no worries at all to do this. 3. In the third surgical case colitis had lasted on and off for 23 years. An operation for fissure in ano "cured" her for 2 years, general medical treatment kept the disease at bay for 10 years, after which a colectomy was done (August 1957). Since then, the patient has done well, with increasing weight, and she is able to eat things she could not eat during the previous twenty years. A perfectionist in type, she adapted herself only slowly to the conditions of a permanent colostomy.

The psyche in treatment

Ulcerative colitis being a psychosomatic affection, we must ask what emotional changes accompany, a) its radical cure by surgery? and b) its temporary remission with steroid therapy? In the first place, all of these 8 patients agree that they are emotionally quite different when their physical disease remits. The mechanism of the emotional change is, however, open to discussion.

1. *In surgical treatment:*

Surgery can do at least three different things to the psyche of the patient with ulcerative colitis. 1. It can provide a solace for masochistic needs, particularly so if it includes a colostomy or an ileostomy. 2. It is an authoritative interference of high degree. 3. It physically alters the region of the symptoms, perhaps even removes that region from the body altogether. Here arises a question of great interest beyond our present knowledge: "How far can an unavoidable return to physical health in a psychosomatic illness carry a return to mental health along with it?"

Of the small series reported in this paper, the three patients who were given surgical treatment all held their operation and their surgeon in high regard. All have lost not only worries but much of their disposition to worry. Case 1. (Hysteric, after ileostomy) comments:

"Perhaps I kept bringing it back by worrying if it would come back? Since that operation I just don't worry at all". Case 2. (Anxiety, treated by colostomy, followed by excision of the rectum): This patient was able to date the onset of her colitis from a particular incident, a minor injury done to her, in spite, twenty-three years ago! Thereafter, "Whenever I began to worry about anything, the colitis came back. I have been less of a worrying type since I had my operation."

Case 3.: This patient continues to be anxious about various things but repudiated a suggestion that she was ever a worrying type of person.

2. *In steroid therapy:*

Whatever their total actions on the body may be, the outstanding characteristic in all diseases in which the steroids are employed is that they flood the diseased part with physical—and the mind of the patient with mental—betterment during their period of maximum impact. Usually this is at their first effective employment. Thereafter efficacy tends to wane and the initial euphoria may be replaced by depressive trends of feeling and thought, with an accompanying regression in the local physical condition. From the psychological point of view, the action of steroids seems very much that of a temporarily sustaining drug, of which we have known many earlier examples in medical history. Permanent change in ulcerative colitis, as in any other psychosomatic affection, requires, not mere sustenance, but a radical physical alteration of the soma at the seat of election of the illness and an associated and permanent alteration of the psyche itself.

The achievement of these two changes is a collaborative matter. The number of long-standing cases—30 to 50 per cent in some series (BROOKE, 1954)—which ultimately develop a carcinoma coli, often obscurely and often of high malignancy, provides an additional urge to return these ailing persons to full mental and physical health by quick and effective means. For severe cases it seems that at present these means are usually surgical. But a really good co-ordination of steroid treatment with a psychotherapy that aims at relieving deep anxiety has yet to be set over against the results of modern surgery. It is hardly reasonable to expect that continued steroids without psychotherapy could permanently alter both the bodies and the minds of patients who suffer from ulcerative colitis.

Bibliography

BACON, H.E.: Ulcerative colitis (Lippincott, Philadelphia/Montreal 1958).

BARGEN, J.A.: Experimental studies on the etiology of chronic ulcerative colitis (preliminary report). J. Amer. med. Ass. *83*: 332 (1924).

BROOKE, B.N.: Ulcerative colitis and its surgical treatment (E. & S. Livingstone, Edinburgh/London 1954).

DANIELS, G.E.: Treatment of a case of ulcerative colitis associated with hysterical depression. Psychosom. Med. *2*: 276 (1940).

— Psychiatric aspects of ulcerative colitis. New Engl. J. Med. *226*: 178 (1942).

— Nonspecific ulcerative colitis as a psychosomatic disease. Med. clin. N. Amer. *28*: 593 (1944).

DRURY, A.N.; FLORY, H., and FLOREY, M.E.: The vascular reactions of the colonic mucosa of the dog to fright. J. Physiol. *68*: 173 (1929).

GRACE, W.J.; WOLF, S.G., JR., and WOLFF, H.G.: The human colon (Heinemann, London 1951).

GRACE, W.J.; PINSKY, R.H., and WOLFF, H.G.: The treatment of ulcerative colitis. II. Gastroenterol. *26*: 462 (1954).

GROEN, J.: Psychogenesis and psychotherapy of ulcerative colitis. Psychosom. Med. *9*: 151 (1947).

GROEN, J., and BASTIAANS, J.: Psychotherapy of ulcerative colitis. Gastroenterol. *17*: 344 (1951).

KIRKETERP, P.: Colitis ulcerosa medicinsk og psykosomatisk belyst. Saertyk fra Nord. Med. *58*: 1066 (1957).

KIRSNER, J.B., and PALMER, W.L.: Ulcerative colitis: therapeutic effects of corticotrophin (ACTH) and cortisone in 120 patients. Ann. intern. Med. *41*: 232 (1954).

KIRSNER, J.B.; BICKS, R.O., and PLAMER, W.L.: The treatment of ulcerative colitis. Arch. intern. Med. *99*: 642 (1957).

KIRSNER, J.B.; SKLAR, M., and PLAMER, W.L.: The use of ACTH, cortisone, hydrocortisone and related compounds in the management of ulcerative colitis: experience in 180 patients. Amer. J. Med. *22*: 264 (1957).

LINDENMANN, E.: Psychiatric problems in conservative treatment of ulcerative colitis. Arch. Neurol. Psychiat. *53*: 322 (1945).

LIUM, R., and PORTER, J.: Etiology of ulcerative colitis. I. the preparation, care and secretions of colonic explants in dogs. Arch. intern. Med. *63*: 201 (1939).

MALTBY, E.J.; DICKSON, R.C., and O'SULLIVAN, P.M.: The use of ACTH and cortisone in idiopathic ulcerative colitis. Canad. Med. Ass. J. *74*: 4 (1956).

MURRAY, C.D.: Psychogenic factors in the etiology of ulcerative colitis and bloody diarrhea. Amer. J. med. Sci. *180*: 239 (1930).

MUSHATT, C.: In Wittkower and Cleghorn: Recent developments in psychosomatic medicine. p. 346 (Pitman, London 1954).

PAULLEY, J.W.: Ulcerative colitis. A study of 173 cases. Gastroenterol. *16*: 56 (1950).

— Psychotherapy in ulcerative colitis. Lancet *ii*: 215 (1956).

PRICE, F.W.: Textbook of the practice of medicine (O.U.P., London 1922).

SKLAR, M.; KIRSNER, J.B., and PALMER, W.L.: Problems in the management of ulcerative colitis, with particular reference to ACTH and the adrenal steroids. Ann. intern. Med. *46*: 1 (1957).

SPERLING, M.: Psychoanalytic study of ulcerative colitis in children. Psychoanal.
    Quart. *15*: 302 (1946).
TRUELOVE, S.C., and WITTS, L.J.: Cortisone in ulcerative colitis. Preliminary
    report on a therapeutic trial. Brit. Med. J. *2*: 375 (1954).
— Cortisone in ulcerative colitis. Final report on a therapeutic trial. Brit. Med.
    J. *2*: 1041 (1955).
— Cortisone and corticotrophin in ulcerative colitis. Brit. Med. J. *1*: 387 (1959).
WEST, R.: Psychotherapy of ulcerative colitis. Lancet *ii*: 899 (1946).
WITTKOWER, E.: Ulcerative colitis. Personality studies. Brit. Med. J. *2*: 1356 (1938).

Author's address: DR. R. WEST, Dorrington Grove, near Shrewsbury, Shropshire (England).

Psychoanalysis of Myxedema
A Case Report

H. G. MANTHEY, Hamburg

It is generally recognized that emotional factors play a decisive part in the genesis of hyperthyroidism and that the treatment of this disease is greatly assisted by psychotherapy.

Myxedema on the other hand seems to be in an exceptional position, and has hitherto been discussed from the somatic point of view only. BLEULER has already critically questioned whether we are confronted in this case with a scientific prejudice and taboo delaying the investigation of the problem.

Therefore, we have paid special attention to Myxedema in our psychosomatic studies of disturbances of the thyroid gland. In the course of 5 years we succeeded in investigating in full the cases of 8 patients and in treating 2 of them over a long period. In all these cases it seemed that the emotional factor played an important and decisive part in the development as well as in the progress of the disease. Because of the fundamental importance of our findings we feel we are justified in submitting a detailed report on a case history in order to point out the psychosomatic relations. Since the treatment is not yet completely finished our statements must for the present be considered as provisional.

The subject of the investigation is a nurse, now 39 years old, who, at the beginning of 1955, was treated at our hospital for a serious primary myxodema. The usual treatment with thyroidin resulted in a quick recovery of the normal physical functions.

The preliminary stages of the disease began in February 1952, following her first sexual intercourse with a married man (the patient was at that time 32 years old). She reacted with a strong feeling of guilt and the fear of becoming pregnant, although the menstruation continued in the regular manner. These ideas were supported by symptoms which at that time consisted of a swollen abdomen, nausea and chronic constipation. Those around her also drew similar conclusions. After 9 months of these complaints which were accompanied by extreme anxiety and restlessness, the changes typical for myxodema set in, namely shaggy hair, swollen face, general feebleness and apathy. The patient felt greatly deformed and regarded her disfiguration clearly as a punishment. She retired more and more from her surroundings, so that only in 1955 did it become possible to make a definite diagnosis and to treat her in the hospital.

As a result of the physical therapy the patient quickly recovered her normal appearance and regained some of her energy, yet in comparison with former times she felt a lack of energy and became more easily exhausted. Also in her moods she continued to be very unstable, (*subdepressive*) and liable to obsessive ideas and a strong feeling of guilt. She had not dared to entrust her inner conflicts to anybody and often felt the fear that the doctors would bring up the subject. In October 1957 she was sent to us from our clinical hospital, by a colleague who took part in our series of psychosomatic investigations.

Here the patient reacted at first with considerable resistance, but after her first discussions showed signs of relief which influenced her condition in a very positive way. She then decided to become an analytic psycho-therapy outpatient, the treatment to be at her own expense. Ever since then she has been coming regularly thrice a week and up to now, during a period of 18 months, she has been analysed for a total of 180 hours. The continuation of the treatment with thyroidin was left to the patient herself. It was arranged that regular physical examinations would take place every 6 weeks.

The following facts from her biography are important: The patient was born in 1920, as the 3rd child, and typical late arrival in a family. She was in fact unwanted and undesired because at her birth the two elder children were already 14 and 15 years old. Her father is said to have been an outsider with a weak character, having difficulties in his social relations. He worked as a commercial clerk, yet being

principally occupied with his private interests he took little interest
in his family. She was supposedly her father's pet, but she can hardly
remember him, since he died when she was 6 years old. The mother
had been extremely active, strict and pointedly moralistic; she always
worried in an exaggerated way about the patient, who as a child was
already rather wild, impulsive and even agressive. The patient felt
that her mother obviously did not want her. She suffered considerably
from the aggressions of the other two children, especially from those
of her elder sister, who showed herself to be extremely jealous of her.

After the death of her father she showed herself in strong need
of security with clearly defined fear for her mother. The mother
suffered at this time from heart-trouble and often talked about death
and dying. The patient had been distinctly boyish, wild and agressive
during her childhood, but became at that time considerably calmer,
more self-controlled and showed at school already an overemphasized
conscientiousness, but was unsure of herself in her work. Her relations
with boys led quite early to sexual games, which troubled her conscience
with a strong feeling of guilt. She had never been instructed in the facts
of life, but she always felt unduly reprimanded and morally controlled.

She never really felt herself to be a girl but rather a hybrid and
suffered accordingly from anxious imaginings. She was clearly opposed
to her menstruation as well as her physical development. She thus
remained physically infantile; it is rather characteristic that only a
year after the analysis her breasts developed. After having finished
school the patient became a trained children's nurse and remained
from her 17th year onward in the same home for Mothers and
Babies, where she has worked for more than 20 years. Here she saw
mothers with their illegitimate children, which intensified her fear of
and opposition towards sexual problems, pregnancy and birth.

A decisive inroad was brought about by the death of her mother,
who died unexpectedly at the beginning of the war. This left a deep
impression upon her; the patient was at that time 24 years old. From
then onward her fear and feeling of guilt intensified; yet on the other
hand, she felt relieved at having escaped from her mother's control.

Ever since she has been living with her sister, who wants to take
the part of the mother—which the patient, however, violently opposes.
Several times the patient sought the acquaintance of men. However
she never had intimacy with any of them. As late as 1952 and only after
4 years relationship with a married man—which was in the beginning
purely platonic—did she have sexual intercourse for the first time.

A profound ambivalent relation towards the mother combined with anxiety, notably fear of death, marks the main conflict. The patient's psycho-sexual development is grossly disturbed which led to male identifications. She felt to be a hybrid. The conflict with the married friend clearly carried an Oedipus character and set strong agressive impulses to work which had to be rebutted. Each attempt to disengage herself from her infantile condition led to regressive reactions. The ambivalent part of the mother was later transferred to the elder sister and to headnurses in the *children's home*. Contrary to the condition resulting from hyperthyroidism, where the maturity is being accellerated and where the thyroid gland reacts accordingly, in this case owing to excessive demands—a regression is taking place which extends also to the functions of the thyroid gland. We have observed the same reaction-patterns in the other patients suffering from myxodema. The psychoanalysis means in this case an aftermaturing whereby the typical psychosomatic reaction-patterns have to be disengaged. During the therapy the patient clearly continued to develop and at the same time her obsessive neurotic reactions could be more and more diminished. She is now entering a new relationship which will probably continue.

The physio-therapy applied at the same time continued as follows: the patient reduced the dose of thyroidin after 6 weeks, since her troubled conscience had been greatly relieved at the beginning of the treatment. After 3 months she discontinued the treatment. The result was a slow but continuous rise of the basic metabolism. From March 1958 she stopped taking any medicaments for 4 months. In this period her state of health showed marked fluctuations, influenced by the course of the analysis. In July 1958 a new friendship with a married man brought a definite relapse, showing the typical myxoede-matic symptoms. There was another relapse following her visiting the mother of an early friend, which again stirred up her emotional feelings towards her own mother. On each occasion the treatment with thyroidin lasted only a short time. Since the end of October the patient again ceased taking any medicaments. The basic metabolism still shows slight fluctuations in a hypothyreotic sense, but typical myxoedematic complaints no longer exist.

I hope to have demonstrated that also in hypothyroidism there may be a close relationship between the physical and emotional side and that psychotherapy may be of great importance in these cases. The rapid therapy success of a physical therapy cannot solve the emotional conflicts, but very often activates and intensifies them. In the cases where the psychoanalysis is successfull the question should be asked whether a further substitution-therapy must be applied at all. The answer of course will be different according to each individual case, but common to all will be general questions concerning the autonomy of physical processes and the limits of the ability to influence them.

However this may be, the case just reported was meant to illustrate that there is no need to be pessimistic about these possibilities.

Author's address: DR. H. G. MANTHEY, II. Medizinische Universitätsklinik, *Hamburg-Eppendorf* (Germany).

From the Psychosomatic Research Unit at the Wilhelmina Gasthuis, Amsterdam

Comparison of the Social Setting and Behaviour of Patients with Bronchial Asthma, Coronary Occlusions and Healthy Subjects

J. M. VAN DER VALK*

The hypothesis of psychosomatic specificity should be tested by different methods. When we state that there are certain specific traits in the personality of patients with a psychosomatic disease, we should be able to predict the behaviour of patients with the disease, in certain situations. That can be the psychological test-situation, as used by BARENDREGT (1957). In this "pilot study" we tried in how far the common life situation might be a suitable test.

Method

We used data, collected by social workers by means of an inquiry.

The social workers who made the report did not know the predictions nor did they at that time have enough knowledge about the psychosomatic concepts to know the contents of the hypotheses.

---

* We are grateful to the sociologist DRS. S. DE JONGE and the social workers: Miss M. SNOEK, Miss D. OOSTDIJK and Mr. L. J. BARENDSE for their cooperation.

The reliability of the answers could be controlled to some extent by comparing the results from the inquiry with information obtained on other occasions, such as:

a) the history taken during the stay in hospital,

b) notes from psychiatric interviews with some of the patients and

c) in a few patients the results from a similar inquiry made by an other investigator about a year earlier.

This showed only slight variations in the answers given on different occasions, at least on the subjects discussed in this paper.

Material

There were three different groups:

1. 101 patients (64 males and 37 females) who had been in hospital for bronchial asthma.
2. 15 patients (all males) who had been in hospital because of a coronary occlusion.
3. 38 healthy subjects (19 males and 19 females) who had not consulted their family-doctor during the last five years, never had any important disease or chronic ailment, never had consulted a psychiatrist, and came from the same population as the hospital patients.

All patients were visited one year or more after their discharge from the hospital. None of them had had psychotherapy for their disease. The mean ages for the groups asthmatic or healthy males or females were all between 43 and 47 years. The mean age of the patients with coronary thrombosis was much higher, 61 years. This difference can not be of great importance for the data pertaining to the earlier life-history of the patients.

Most coronary patients got their first complaints only at middle-age, whereas two-thirds of the asthmatics had their first attack only as adults (Fig. I). That means, that some of the findings were related to what happened *before* the present illness.

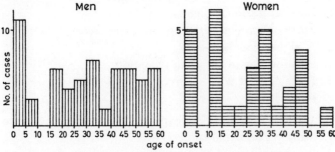

Fig. I. Age of onset of bronchial asthma in our patients.

Hypotheses

According to GROEN (1950) and BASTIAANS and GROEN (1955) patients with bronchial asthma have some specific personality traits:

1. Marked egocentricity.
2. A tendency towards impatient and impulsive behaviour.
3. A tendency towards domineering and tyranny which is usually most manifest in the limited environment of the family.
4. A diminished capacity to adapt to unfavourable life situations.
5. A marked narcissistic vulnerability and emotional hypersensitivity.
6. A great need for love and affection, which is often hidden behind pseudo-indifferent or even aggressive behaviour.
7. Stubborness, which may lead to conflicts with authoritative figures towards whom they behave ambivalently, showing a tendency to act by protests or against advice.
8. Strong reactions of jealousy and rivalry, which often make the patients difficult individuals in their social contacts.
9. A difficulty in solving interpersonal conflicts by "talking it over", by "giving and taking", or another form of regulated aggressive discharge.
10. A disturbed psychosexual development. Most asthmatics mature late.

KITS VAN HEYNINGEN (1959) describes some personality traits of patients with coronary occlusions. He has found among other things:

1. A marked tendency to work hard.
2. Conflict-situations with a severe and strict father or with father-figures.
3. A need for activity, also *out*side the professional sphere.

Compared with the healthy control-group and with patients with other diseases, we therefore expected the *asthmatic* group to show:

1. Less persistence in school-training.
2. Less professional success.
3. More difficulties with superiors and colleagues.
4. A higher marriage-age.
5. Less interest in community activities.
6. Little contact with relatives and
7. Few friends.

On the other hand we expected the *coronary* groups to show:

1. More professional success.
2. A tendency to work hard.

3. Many activities outside their work.
4. Some difficulties with authorities and (male) relatives, and
5. More social contacts.

Results

In the next tables some results of the inquiry are shown, mainly from the male groups.

The number of patients in each group is not the same in every table. In the beginning fewer questions were asked than in later interviews and therefore the information about nearly half of the asthma patients is not complete. Furthermore we had to omit patients from the tables occasionally when the information on a certain subject was inadequate.

Although in most cases the groups are too small for any definite conclusion, the figures nevertheless give an idea of the direction in which the differences may lie. Where possible P-values were computed with the likelihood ratio test of the indepence hypotheses.

Table 1 gives the number of persons that were normally working at the time of the inquiry.

Table 1

Work	Men		
	A	C	H
Normal	30	4	17
Part-time	1	1	—
Not working	25	7	—
Retired	6	3	2
	62	15	19

In all tables   A =   asthma patients
               C =   coronary patients
               H =   healthy subjects

Difference in distribution: "Normal working" versus "Part-time" and "Not working" statistically significant for A versus H and C versus H (P<0.001).

(In all tables: A = asthma patients, C = coronary patients, and H = healthy subjects).

40% of the asthmatics and 47% of the coronary patients were not working. In the coronary patients this was because they were medically declared unfit for work. Four of them told how they had asked the doctor not to reject them. Most notworking asthmatics however gave no reason why they had stopped work. Sometimes they simply said that they disliked their job. In many instances they were living on what the wife or other family members earned. There were cases where one got the impression that the patient made some money by irregular work, and did not want to tell it.

Table 2 shows how many asthmatics disliked their work. Most of them said so without hesitation. The coronary patients on the other hand stressed their eagerness to work even when they were not very fond of their job.

Table 2

Attitude towards work	Men		
	A	C	H
Positive	21	15	18
Negative	40	—	1
	61	15	19

Difference in distribution statistically significant for A versus C and A versus H (P<0.001).

Table 3 gives the number of severe difficulties in the sphere of work. Many healthy subjects and coronary patients had no serious problems whereas many asthmatics had conflicts with superiors and colleagues. Interhuman difficulties in the coronary group were mostly due to conflicts with superiors when a patient had fought for the rights of his colleagues or his group even with neglect of his own position.

Table 3

Occupational difficulties	Men		
	A	C	H
No difficulties	14	6	13
Interhuman difficulties	33	3	4
Too heavy	4	2	2
Illness	10	4	—
	61	15	19

Difference in distribution: No difficulties/interhuman difficulties statistically significant for A versus H (P<0.001).

That asthmatics often stopped work, as mentioned, could be a result of the illness. In *table 4* however a same tendency is shown in

Table 4

Schooling	Men		
	A	C	H
Only Primary School	12	10	6
Secondary schooling, finished	1	2	12
Secondary schooling, not finished	6	1	1
	19	13	19

Difference in distribution: Secondary schooling finished/not finished statistically significant for A versus H (P<0.001).

the attitude towards schools. This table includes only asthma patients who acquired the disease as adults so *these figures refer to a period when all subjects in the three groups were healthy*. Still 32% of those who later acquired asthma did not finish their secondary training, that means the largest majority of those who started this type of education. In the coronary group there were some individuals who had wanted further training but were forced by their parents to earn money at an early age.

For *table 5* the professional level of each subject was compared with that of the father. (The scoring of this professional level was done according to a classification list of the Institute of Social Research of the Netherlands Population (Isonevo). The investigator had no information as to which diagnostic group the subject belonged.) For comparison some other diagnoses are included in this table.

Table 5

Professional level	Men, compared with the father		
	+	=	—
Essential hypertension	5	4	1
Ulcerative colitis	4	7	—
H Healthy subjects	7	10	1
Rheumatoid arthritis	3	6	1
C Coronary thrombosis	4	7	4
Peptic ulcer	5	8	5
A Bronchial asthma	5	25	8
Pulmonary tuberculosis	1	11	5
Thyreotoxicosis	1	6	5

Difference in distribution statistically significant for A versus H (P<0.03).

Apparently the asthmatics had been less successful than the healthy controls in reaching a higher occupational level than their father. For the coronary group we had predicted a better result than was found.

After all these data it is interesting to see in *table 6* how few asthmatics complained of financial difficulties. Even when they were found to live in rather poor circumstances it sometimes did not seem to affect them.

Table 6

Financial difficulties	Men		
	A	C	H
No difficulties	13	2	9
Difficulties in the past	5	—	1
Moderate difficulties	3	9	8
Situation difficult or bad	5	4	1
	26	15	19

Fig. II gives the age of marriage of the married men and women in our groups. The mean age is lower for the asthmatics than for the other groups. This is opposite to what we predicted. There were some male asthmatics however who had hesitated a long time before marrying. In the coronary group there was a marked tendency not to marry without a sound financial basis.

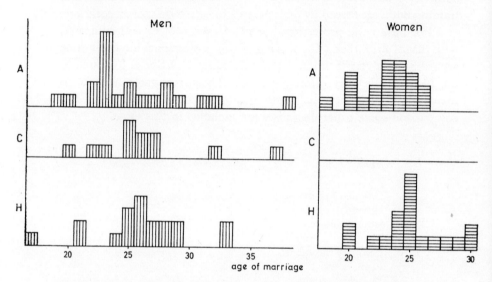

Fig. II. Age of marriage of married man and women in the different groups. A = asthma patients   C = coronary patients   H = healthy subjects

Table 7 shows that there was much more contact with relatives in the healthy group than in the groups of patients.

Table 7

Contact with relatives	Men			Women	
	A	C	H	A	H
Good	22	4	16	13	14
Moderate	15	4	2	11	3
Bad	2	3	1	1	—
None	23	3	—	11	—
	62	14	19	36	17

Difference in distribution statistically significant for A versus H for both men and women (P<0.001) and for C versus H (P<0.01).

In *table 8* the lack of social contacts of the asthmatics is still more pronounced. Of the asthma patients of both sexes 72% said to have

Table 8

Social contact	Men			Women	
	A	C	H	A	H
No difficulties	4	10	18	—	18
Disappointed	—	4	1	1	—
Bad	16	1	—	11	1
	20	15	19	12	19

Difference in distribution statistically significant for A versus C and A versus H (men) and for A versus H (women) (P<0.001).

no friend at all. *(Table 9)* Membership of societies was also rare among these patients *(Table 10)* and the majority never went out *(Table 11)*.

Table 9

Friends	Men			Women	
	A	C	H	A	H
None	44	1	1	27	4
Few	17	10	11	7	13
Many	1	3	7	2	2
	62	14	19	36	19

Difference in distribution statistically significant for A versus C and A versus H (men) and A versus H (women) (P<0.001).

Table 10

Member of societies	Men		
	A	C	H
No member of societies	57	6	8
Member of one society	6	8	5
Member of more societies	—	—	6
	63	14	19

Difference in distribution statistically significant for A versus H (P<0.001).

Table 11

Going out	Men			Women	
	A	C	H	A	H
Never	42	1	2	23	2
Sometimes	11	12	12	10	13
Often	5	1	5	1	4
	58	14	19	34	19

Difference in distribution statistically significant for A versus C and A versus H (men) and for A versus H (women) (P<0.001).

Table 12 gives the number of hobbies of our subjects. Over 50% of the asthmatics had no hobby at all, whereas each coronary patient had at least one hobby. (In the female groups 27 out of 37 asthmatic women had no hobby but only 6 out of 19 healthy females, again a statistically significant difference (P<0.01).

Table 12

Hobbies	Men		
Number of hobbies	A	C	H
0	33	—	2
1	17	5	5
2	8	7	10
3	4	—	1
4	1	2	1
5	1	—	—
	64	14	19

Difference in distribution statistically significant for A versus C and A versus H (P<0.01).

Table 13

Reading	Men			Women	
	A	C	H	A	H
Seldom or never	44	4	10	28	10
Only newspaper	5	1	4	—	—
Often	14	9	4	8	7
	63	14	18	36	17

Difference in distribution statistically not significant.

Table 14

Smoking	Men		
	A	C	H
Heavy	12	9	3
Moderate	11	6	11
Not at all	39	1	4
	62	15	18

Difference in distribution statistically significant for A versus C, A versus H and C versus H (P<0.01)

Table 15

Use of alcohol	Men		
	A	C	H
Heavy	—	3	—
Moderate	3	5	5
Occasionally	9	3	14
Never	49	4	—
	61	15	19

Difference in distribution statistically significant for A versus C and A versus H (P<0.001).

Although many asthmatics have few activities, even in reading they show no more or even less interest than the other groups. *(Table 13)*. In this respect the coronary group differs from the others.

Table 14 and *table 15* give information on the smoking and drinking habits. The asthmatics appear to use less alcohol and tobacco than the healthy group. Some coronary patients on the other hand declared rather proudly to have been "always a heavy drinker" or "a heavy smoker". Some others had decreased their consumption lately but boasted of the amounts they had been used to in former days.

In this paper we will not go into the statistically more complicated problems like changing of jobs, number of divorces and many others data.

Conclusions

With the exception of the age of marriage of the asthmatics and the professional level of the coronary patients, all differences found were in the predicted direction and often statistically highly significant. In this way they support the hypotheses mentioned in the beginning. Some of the differences originated through incidents preceding the onset of the disease, thus sustaining the hypothesis of the preexistence of some of the personality traits.

Many objections can be made against the methods and the results of this pilot study. It nevertheless seems worth while attempting a validation along these lines of the description of personality traits, in patients with psychosomatic illnesses, as deduced from the biography of individual patients.

Bibliography

BARENDREGT, J.T.: A cross-validation study of the hypothesis of psychosomatic specificity. J. Psychosom. Res. *2*: 109 (1957).

GROEN, J.: Asthma bronchiale seu nervosum. (Scheltema & Holkema, Amsterdam 1950).

BASTIAANS, J., and GROEN, J.: Psychogenesis and psychotherapy of bronchial asthma. In: Modern Trends in Psychosomatic Medicine (Ed. O'Neill) (Butterworth, London 1955).

KITS VAN HEIJNINGEN, H.: Some notes on the psychiatric aspects of patients with coronary occlusions. Fortschr. Psychosom. Med. *1* (1960).

Author's address: Dr. J.M. VAN DER VALK, Reijnier Vinkeleskade 70, *Amsterdam-Z* (Netherlands).

Some Notes on the Psychiatric Aspects of Patients with Coronary Occlusion *

H. KITS VAN HEIJNINGEN, Amsterdam

In this paper I would like to show some psychiatric aspects of patients with coronary occlusion. The data are derived from 13 biographical anamneses of married male patients, aged between 48 and 68 years, of the Wilhelmina Gasthuis Amsterdam.

It is my aim to advance psychodynamical understanding of personality traits we found and to arrive at characteristics which might be accessible for psychological tests.

The most prominent feature FLANDERS DUNBAR (1) found in her patients with this disorder, was their history of excessively strenuous work. Although our patients are all from a relatively low social level—and not so distinguished looking as DUNBAR's—we found that they showed very definitely the same attitude towards their work. When they were their own masters, they worked very hard indeed; when they were employed, they boasted of their performance and stressed the importance of their position and the trust put into them by their superiors.

This attitude assumes all the more significance when we found too, that occlusion occurred so often when there had been a set-back in their work, a loss in their income, a decrease of prestige in their profession.

We got the impression that working hard was not an activity

* From the Psychosomatic Research Unit at the Wilhelmina Gasthuis, Amsterdam.

carried on just because it was needed, or because it was enjoyed in itself, but was a form of activity with a different meaning, that is, to subserve other needs: it seemed to stand for creativeness on the one hand, but on the other hand to ward off uncertainty or insecurity. A dream may illustrate this point: in it the patient loaded a boat single-handed with 400 tons of coal in one hour—just to show off in front of his subordinates what it was really like to work hard.

Now supposing that working hard is a specific feature of such patients and has to do with their emotional make-up, we should look for corroboration. I think we can find such corroboration in the description those people gave of their fathers: 8 out of 11 patients who had known their fathers, described them as: working hard, working day and night, always busy. In 2 of the 3 remaining cases the mother was described in the same way. In preparing our psychological tests to distinguish coronary patients from patients suffering from other psychosomatic disorders the father-image will play an important part. There is more reason to do so, because the second feature frequently in the description of these fathers—7 out of 11 cases— is that they were: hot-tempered, stern, strict, severe, beating and thrashing their children.

Now it seems probable that working hard, being active, has to do with their father's identification and is closely connected with warded off feelings of aggression and fear towards him.

This leads us to consider the way these patients are dealing with aggression. This aggression is directed against persons of authority, e.g. the schoolmaster, the priest, the boss. They often say: I can stand anything but unfairness. But in their actual behaviour they suppress their aggression towards others. They will tell you how they manage to behave calmly while inwardly they feel like killing. In line with this way of dealing with aggression we often found fantasies of accidents, dreams of killing and being killed, of blood and fighting. One patient dreamt that he massacred the Russian Czar and his whole family. FLANDERS DUNBAR also refers frequently to fearfull dreams and nightmares of these patients.

Attention has to be drawn to the fact that these patients experience aggression as fighting *bodily*. This physical experiencing, this direct mental connection of aggression with motor activity, I think, determines in a specific way the link between their emotions and the patho-physiology of their heart. Their preoccupation with motor activity can also be demonstrated by the frequent use of terms like: busy, brisk, calm, fussy, quiet, etc. in descriptions of other people or themselves. In the dream of the man who loaded the coalboat single-handed, his work—although he was actually a clerk—was also experienced as an enormous *physical* achievement.

In addition another feature found in such patients should be mentioned: their pseudo-virile attitude, their tendency to appear unaffected both physically and mentally. Physically they sometimes boast of their previously excellent health, their sportive performances. More typical, however, is their denial of anything they regard as weak. They must seem to be strong and sturdy no matter how. To what extremes they might go, is shown in PROF. J. GROEN's story of a man complaining of pain in his chest. Physical examination revealed no pathological findings. He was told, however, to be careful. The patient answering: "I see, you think me a hysteric", raced his bike over Amsterdam bridges—and promptly contracted coronary occlusion.

Our patients denied frustrations and they especially denied feelings of dependence. One patient denied to mind that his beloved wife had to go to hospital because of dementia. He denied to mind her being transferred to an asylum without warning. He just shrugged his shoulders at her not recognising him during his last visit. "If I minded all that I could not live" he said. Returning from this visit he got coronary occlusion. We think that denial is one of the main mechanisms of defense of these patients and that BETTINA WARBURG in her discussion with ARLOW (2) was right saying "that their exaggerated pseudo-independence did not only conceal their continuous struggle against father-figures, but also their strong unsatisfied dependent wishes." Biographical anamneses describe mother's main quality most frequently as: tenderness. She was looked upon as a lovely sweetheart, a darling giving everything you wanted. Often there are associations about receiving food. Passive receptive feelings are prominent here and we expect to find them in psychological tests too. In this respect there seem to be factors common with ulcer patients, the more so as ulcers are not infrequently encountered in the life history of coronary patients.

Although such patients have these passive receptive feelings towards their wives, the description of them is quite unlike that of their mothers. They look upon their wives as: always busy, fussy (7 out of 13); aggressive, hot-tempered (7 out of 13); dominating, humilating (6 out of 13); frigide (5 out of 13). In fact 10 out of 13 descriptions of the wives showed at least 2 of these features. One only mentioned fits of hot-temper, another extreme jealousy, another again gave a short description of his wive and refrained from any criticism. I will not try to formulate psychodynamic hypotheses on these data, but will desdribe two other traits.

Firstly their inhibited sexual attitude towards their wives before and after marriage, as contrasted with the rather early sexual activities of these patients, the sexual relations with girlfriends before and often during marriage.

Secondly the way they deal with money. Out of 10 biographical anamneses which gave sufficient data on this subject, there were 7 in which the patient stated that he left money matters entirely to his wife, praising her as a good businesswoman. In the remaining 3 cases the patients complained bitterly that their wives could not handle money at all.

A final word about the situation in which coronary occlusion occurred in our patients. I record one case that shows most of the features we may consider as characteristic for that situation. This patient, aged 59, was recently put on a pension because the bank which employed him for many years, underwent reorganisation. With one of his older colleagues he had often severe quarrels. He was his real enemy and remained at the bank with considerably increased salary. The patient's wife was very hot-tempered and recently quarrelled with her husband's family. Although very upset the patient could not do anything about it and had to meet his family secretly. One day the patient, meeting a friend who also worked at his bank, discussed his enemy hotly and in great anger. They then came to a place where a women's boat race was in progress. They cycled along the waterside to keep up with the rowing boats. The patient soon lagged behind his friend and all the others, mostly boys. Although he felt a pain in his chest, he tried his utmost to keep up the pace. Finally, the pain becoming intolerable he had to give up. In hospital a recent coronary occlusion was diagnosed.

Finally, it can be stated that although in most of our patients coronary occlusion occurred during emotional and physical stress; severe attacks of angina pectoris and probably coronary occlusion can occur *also* during rest or sleep. This stresses the necessity for further research on the phenomenology of aggression, fear, and other feelings and on the interrelations of these emotions with motor activity in patients with coronary occlusion.

Bibliography

Arlow, J.A.: Identification mechanisms in coronary occlusions. Psychosom.
    Med. *VII*: 4 (1945).
Dunbar, F.: Psychosomatic diagnosis (Hoeber, New York 1943).

Author's address: Dr. H. Kits van Heijningen, Bachplein 9, *Amsterdam* (Netherlands)

Psychosomatic Investigations on Patients
with Heart Complaints, Respectively on a Physical
and Non-Physical Basis

M.R. van Alphen de Veer, G.A. van Andel, W. Holst,
C. v. Norren and P. J. Willems, Eindhoven

In the past years in the Netherlands psychosomatic research has
been concentrated on psychosomatic specificity and in this respect
the investigations of Barendregt should be mentioned. For that
purpose Barendregt has used well defined groups of psychosomatic
patients, e.g. asthmatics and patients suffering from ulcerative colitis
and duodenal ulcer. It must be said, however, that also persons with
the more vague diagnosis of psychoneurosis and psychosomatosis
and groups of healthy people have been the object of his statistical
research. In order to prove psychosomatical specificity he made use
of the Rorschach test and of tests on neuroticism and sociability
designed respectively by Eysenck and Heron.

The correlation of psychological and physiological data have
been lately studied by van der Valk in his investigations on the
electrical skinresistance. Recently there is a dispute going on about
the value of clinical prediction in psychology. The experimental

statistical method has been opposed to the method based on intuition and experience, a well known antithesis of long standing.

We would not meddle with these discussions, but prefer to present an investigation originated from daily clinical praxis as we medical men understand it.

In industry the physician is often confronted with patients complaining of the heart, which might be of physical or nervous origin. Complaints such as palpitations, heartache, oppression, tightness of the chest often point to a physical origin, a coronary disease, an infarctus or hypertension. On the other hand they may be due to nervous or functional troubles and then we find patients with anxiety, neurotics and those who are overconscious of their bodily functions.

Common believe is that patients with a coronary occlusion often have been exposed to physical and mental stress which may be caused by the worksituation. Hard-working well adjusted individuals who control themselves well, are not seldom in this group. They may also show agressive tendencies. On the other hand in the nervous group maladjustment and social difficulties would be often signalized. All these patients offer problems in the field of psychosomatic medicine. On the one hand there is agression, on the other hand anxiety, two fundamental qualities which have been described by Alexander.

Now we intended to perform a detailed physical and psychological examination of these patients in order to get an insight into the pathogenesis of their illness and into their personality structure. If we could get a clear clinical conception of the different aspects, this would provide us perhaps with a means of predictionary value in those cases which remained vague as to diagnosis and prognosis.

We must emphasize that we did not take well defined groups of psychosomatics and psychoneurotics as Barendregt did. We started from daily medical praxis.

We made a classification as follows:

Group A: 28 persons with heartcomplaints with coronary occlusion or infarctus. Average age of the group 47.8 years.

Group B: 28 persons with heartcomplaints without physical symptoms. Average age of the group 38.8 years.

Group C: 25 persons. Healthy, well-adjusted people without heart complaints. Average age of the group 36.5 years.

The subjects were male people, all working in different departments of the Philips Glowlampworks in Eindhoven.

We failed to make the average age of the three groups equal which is a disadvantage.

Our methods of investigation were:
a) Physical and cardiological examination. We used electro-cardiography and vectorcardiography.
b) Biographical anamnesis and study of the worksituation.
c) Cornell Index test, a questionnaire.
d) Estimation of the I.Q. and the Rorschach test.
e) Measurement of skin resistance.

ad b) and c) The data of the biographical anamnesis and of the Cornell Index Test were brought into a rating scale, in which we distinguished different fields of adaptation. The items were the physical condition, judged objectively and subjectively (by the patient); the emotional adaptation, i.e. the psychological balance; the adaptation to the family; the adaptation to the job, judged objectively and subjectively; the social adaptation; the evaluation of the Cornell Index Test in the number of negative responses; the description of youth and how the subject experienced it. Finally the course of his life was judged in the sense of a sthenic or an asthenic attitude, the aptitude of being with reality, the aptitude for integration and persistence in the face of difficulties, or the reverse.

With the exception of the objective physical condition and the Cornell Index Test data must be seen as an interpretation by two investigators who scored separately. The psychologist who gave the Rorschach test was not informed as to the classification of the testees into three groups, nor was he acquainted with the data of the biographical anamnesis.

The electrical skin resistance was measured during 15 minutes in a condition of rest. After that period a stimulus was given twice, by switching the electrical light off and on. We measured
a) the skin resistance every minute and
b) the integral of the fluctuations in the skin resistance, known as the psychogalvanic reflex.

By an integrating connection the size and duration of every psychogalvanic reflex may be added to the foregoing reflex and so we get the total amount of activity, i.e. the product of size, duration and number of all psychogalvanic reflexes. With another counter we could count the number of reflexes.

1. From the biographical anamnesis and the Cornell Index test

taken together in our adaptationscale, combined with some data of the Rorschach test we got the following results.

A. *Adaptation:* (points 3, 4, 5 of the scale)

	good	bad
Group A	15	13
Group B	14	13
Group C	23	2

There was no difference in adaptation between groups A and B.

B. *Emotional balance:*

	good	bad
Group A	17	11
Group B	9	18
Group C	25	0

Emotional balance was better in group A. $\chi^2 = 3.9$
$$P = .05$$

C.	agressivity	anxiety	Hyper sensibility of the autonomic nervous system
Group A	17	12	8
Group B	17	16	9
Group C	5	3	3

There was no difference between the groups A and B. With group C there was a significant difference.

D. A clear distinction of the occurence of introversion-extroversion in both groups was not to be made. Nor showed the data of youth and of course of life any marked differences between the groups A and B.

A next point which was investigated is the distribution of age and intelligence of the three groups under investigation.

The following results were obtained:

	A	B	C	
age	47.8	38.8	36.5	years

The differences between A and B, and between A and C are significant. The difference between B and C is not significant.

The intelligence score obtained on the WECHSLER-BELLEVUE SCALE (Verbal) showed the following results

	A	B	C
IQ (WAIS)	107,6	107,8	105,6

The differences between the groups are not significant.

2. The measurement of the skin resistance showed the following picture:

A. *The initial level of skin resistance*

The initial level of s.r. was divided in 3 categories: "high" is an initial skin resistance higher than 80 K Ω, "average" between 80 and 40 K Ω, and "low" below 40 K Ω.

The distribution was as follows:

	A	B	C
high	16	3	5
average	10	11	18
low	1	9	2
			75

Calculations were made to see whether this distribution differed from a random distribution

χ^2 (corrected) was 20,5 these differences are significant, P < 01.

Because the average age of group A is significantly higher than the average of the other group, difference in initial level of skin resistance might be due to this age-difference. When we take into consideration only people over 40 years of age in the three groups we get this division.

	A	B	C
high	14	2	3
average	9	9	6
low	1	2	1
			47

To see whether this result differs from a random distribution χ^2 was calculated. It is (corrected) 7.4, P = .10.

From this result it seems that the originally found very significant differences might be due to the age factor, although there is a trend which indicates that the organic group has a higher initial level of skin resistance than a group of neurotic and normal subjects.

B. Increasing and decreasing levels of skin resistance. During the 15-minute period the general resistance level shows fluctuation. If the difference between initial and final level of s.r. is 10 K Ω or more, this will be called increase or decrease (depending on the direction of the difference). Differences of less than 10 K Ω are considered as constant level of s.r.

The distribution was as follows:

$\chi^2 = 3,6$. The differences between the groups are not significant. Increase or decrease of level of s.r. gives no indication to which group the subject belongs.

	A	B	C
Increase	11	10	14
Constant	15	14	9
Decrease	1	1	2
			77

C. By means of an integrator switching device it was possible to count the total psychogalvanical activity of the subject. The integrator counted number, duration and amplitude of reflexes exhibited during the 15-minute period. The total activity was classified: "high" activity above 750 units, "average" 250–750 units, low below 250 units (the calibration of the apparatus was such that 250 units roughly equal one Kilo Ohm). We combined the measures initial level of skin resistance and total reflex activity. This gave the following results:

	A	B	C
High initial resistance + low activity	12	1	3
Low or average initial resistance + high activity	2	7	4
			29

χ^2 (corrected) 10,6 $P < .05$

The group of functional complaints differs significantly from the organic group in these combined measurements.

D. The P.G.R. on light stimulus.

The decrease of skin resistance after switching the roomlights off and on was determined. Average decrease was determined.

The following results emerged:

		A	B	C
subaverage	s.r. decrease	4	I	I
average	s.r. decrease	22	20	21
large	s.r. decrease	I	4	3
				77

$)(^2 = 1.3$. There are no significant differences in reaction to the light off and on-stimulus.

3. Rorschach results

The psychologist did not know the medical diagnosis when giving and scoring the Ro.

The Rorschach results were scored in two ways:
a) a structural interpretation
b) a quantitative scoring and comparison of different categories.

a) structural interpretation:

	Group		
	A	B	C
arterioscler. + depressive	I I	–	4
Ro.-classification			
Neurotic	4	13	3
Normal	10	12	17
			74

$)(^2 = 11.1$ significant 5% level.

b) scoring of separate categories.

Use was made of
1. the general organic syndrome, described in R. BOCHNER AND F. HALPERN.
2. the organic syndrome from BOHM.
3. Rorschach's neurotic factors and
4. ZULLIGER's anxiety syndrome.

The purpose of this comparison of separate scoring categories was to see whether the above-mentioned syndromes could be found in our groups. Most of the signs mentioned by these authors did not differentiate between the three groups.

The only differences which were found are:

	A	B	C
N	25	25	24
Average N of answer	17.6	19.5	21.—
A	59%	51%	54%
At	10%	9.5%	6%
Reject	5	5	2
Shocks (color shading)	6	13	—

None of these differences (except shocks) are significant. All other categories, including movement and color, showed no difference at all.

This raises the question whether the syndromes given by the above-mentioned authors constitute a basis for differentiating between organic, neurotic and normal groups. A clear-cut answer cannot be given because our groups are not large enough to obtain a statistically significant answer and because the classification of our subjects on the basis of a medical examination did not exclude the possibility of having neurotic personalities in the organic and in the normal groups.

In looking back on our investigations once again we think that our clinical division into a physical group, a functional group and a healthy group has been useful in the field of psychosomatics.

Our hypothesis regarding the differences in repressed agressivity, anxiety, introversion-extraversion and adjustment were not confirmed. The physical and the functional group were much more homogenous in various aspects as our supposition has been. Taken together, both groups differed considerably from group C., in that sense, that they contained more neurotic and nervous persons.

However, groups A and B show among themselves also differences. Emotional Stability is greater in group A and the structural Rorschach and the Shock for colour are different too. Apart from that the separate Rorschach categories seemed to be of little value for this psychosomatical investigation.

On the contrary the measurement of the skin resistance proved to be of great value. The combination of a high skin resistance and a low integral psychogalvanic activity was seen frequently in group A and this was highly significant.

The reverse a low or medium skin resistance combined with a

high integral psychogalvanic activity was seen more frequently in group B. This was also significant.

Two cases from group B and one case from group C which belonged psychologically to group A, afterwards showed indeed the skin resistance pattern of group A.

In the measurement of the skin resistance and of the psycho-galvanic integral activity as now described we see a valuable method for prediction as to the belonging of a special case to the physical or the functional group.

Bibliography

Bochner, R., and Halpern, F.: The clinical application of the Rorschachtest. p. 193–196 (New York 1942).

E. Bohm's Lehrbuch der Rorschachpsychodiagnostik. p. 289 (Hoeber, Bern 1957).

Rorschach's neurotic factors. p. 260–261 (Psychodiagnostik, 4e, 1941).

Zulliger's anxiety syndrome. p. 257–258. Der Tafeln-Z-Test (Bern 1954).

Barendregt, J. T. en Groen, J.: Een statistische bewerking van het Rorschach-materiaal van patienten met colitis ulcerosa. Ned. T. Psychol. 8: 469–489 (1953).

Barendregt, J. T.: Cross-validatie van een toetsing van de hypothese der psychosomatische specificiteit. Ned. T. Psychol. 11: 1–9 (1956).

Barendregt, J. T., Aris-Dijkstra, M., Diercks, L. M., en Wilde, G. J.: De Rorschachtest als middel tot toetsing van de hypothese der psychosomatische specificiteit; een cross-validatie. Ned. T. Psychol. 13: 173–195 (1958).

Barendregt, J. T.: Lijders aan psychosomatische kwalen als sociaal aangepaste neurotici. Ned. T. Geneesk. 102: 2044–2046 (1958).

Valk, J. M. van der: Onderzoekingen over de electrische huidweerstand; med. Diss. (Amsterdam 1958).

Authors' addresses: Dr. M. R. van Alphen de Veer, Dr. G. A. van Andel, Dr. W. Holst, Dr. C. van Norren and Dr. P. J. Willems, Willemstraat 22 A, *Eindhoven* (Netherlands).

Hypochondria in Duodenal Ulcer

A. Stenbäck, Helsinki

In 1948, Ryle described five varieties of nosophobia:

1. Fears about an existing illness or injury and its possible import; about the tolerability of anticipated pain; and about confinements, anaesthetics and operations which are, for the patient, an occasion of trauma and a common cause of dread and apprehension.

2. Fears of inheriting a disease, particularly epilepsy, insanity, cancer, and tuberculosis.

3. Fears of acquiring diseases, particularly those due to well-known types of infection.

4. Fears connected with a *non-existent disease* which a patient nevertheless imagines or suspects (usually *on the basis of some subjective symptom*) that he has already acquired.

5. Fears of death or dying considered as the final malignity of illness and, in the latter case, too widely suspected of involving painful or distressing experience.

When speaking of hypochondria I refer to the fourth type of nosophobia. According to the definition applied by me, hypochondria is a groundless fear of having a disease.

Robinson (1937) stated that hypochondria is very rare in duodenal ulcer patients, whereas Gainsborough and Slater (1946) took the opposite view. Obviously, such conflicting statements depend upon several factors. Different definitions of hypochondria and cultural differences between the patient series studied may be contributory causes of diverging results. The inability to detect hypochondria not infrequently depends upon theoretical bias and/or methodological approach. In his monograph "Pain and Pleasure", Szasz (1957) called attention to the surprising lack of psychoanalytical contributions to the problem of pain. Anxiety, aggressiveness, libido, etc. have been submitted to penetrating and comprehensive investigations, whereas pain and hypochondria were left untreated. It is not surprising that investigations with a sociological approach mostly overlook the problem of pain, although one can speak of a "sociology of pain". But in the investigation of the individual motivation, the disregard of the emotional significance of pain is more surprising.

This disregard is not due to the above-mentioned theoretical bias alone, but also depends upon the patient's unwillingness to disclose his hypochondriac fears. The patient reveals his hypochondriac fears only when he is completely sure that the doctor will not make him an object of derision by saying that he is suffering from a self-imagined illness. There is nothing so humiliating to the patient as to be regarded by the doctor as belonging to the group of "malades imaginaires" so masterfully described by MOLIÈRE. On these grounds there is need of a skilful as well as of a respectful interview technique for obtaining information concerning hypochondriac fears.

In this paper hypochondria is employed, as mentioned above, to designate an ungrounded fear of having a disease. Not always, but frequently, the hypochondriac fear arises in connection with an experience of pain. This paper deals only with this hypochondriac fear which has arisen in connection with the pain elicited by dyspeptic distress, duodenal ulcer, or other somatic illness. The hypochondriac psychotophobia induced by the experience of anxiety was not subjected to methodological investigation.

An unselected series of 50 patients with duodenal ulcer was studied. With two exceptions, all patients were an unselected series of inpatients admitted to departments of internal medicine (Table 1).

Table 1. Frequency of hypochondria in 50 patients with duodenal ulcer

Hypochondria: total	35
Starting point epigastric pain	29
epigastric pain or disease	18
both epigastric and other pain	12
only other pain	6
only epigastric pain	17
Generalized hypochondria	1
Health pedant	1
Not hypochondriac personality	48

Severe hypochondria was found in 35. In 29 patients the epigastric pain was the starting-point of the hypochondriac fear. In 18 patients there was hypochondria with other pain or somatic disease as starting-point. Amongst the 35 patients with hypochondria, there were 12 patients with hypochondria directed not only towards the epigastric pain but also towards other pain or disease. There were 6 patients who treated the epigastric pain in an adequate, non-hypochondriac way but experienced fear of other somatic diseases. It has to be especially emphasized that only in one patient was the hypochondria generalized so that the patient is to be designated a hypochondriac personality. One patient was a health pedant. The remaining 48 were not hypochondriac personalities. In those patients in whom hypochondria was found, it was limited to one or a few body-parts, and it began *after* the patient had felt the pain that was the focus of the hypochondriac concern.

Table 2. Types of hypochondria

Types of hypochondria	Starting-point both epigastric and other pain	only epigastric pain	only other pain
Cancerophobia total	24	10	2
cancer of stomach	15	10	
cancer of lung	4		
tumour of brain	2		
tumour of spine	3		
cancer of colon			1
cancer of urinary bladder			1
Visceral diseases	3	2	2
Pulmonary tuberculosis	2		1
Fatal heart attack	4		
Syphilodophobia	1		
Psychotophobia	3		

Table 2 shows the distribution of the different types of hypochondria. The most conspicuous finding is the high frequency of cancerophobia, especially cancerophobia of the stomach. Obviously, there are many reasons for this predominance of cancerophobia. First of all, severe pain is likely to give rise to a fear of severe disease. Cancer is a malignant disease, and is to be feared for that very reason. The propaganda carried out in order to promote the detection of cancer in the early stages, is apt to produce quite a lot of groundless cancerophobia. Nevertheless, this publicity about cancer, although not without risks, is hardly the most effective producer of cancerophobia. In a number of cases the background and localization to which the hypochondriac fear attached were traced to the death of a close relative: mother, father, sibling, or friend. One cancerophobic patient stated that his mother died of stomach cancer after being treated for peptic ulcer for five years. Another hypochondriac complaint, the fear of sudden death from heart disease, was observed in patients who had witnessed to the sudden death of a relative from heart disease.

In a series of patients with hypertensive cardiovascular disease, DUNBAR (1948) observed that more than 98 per cent had been closely exposed to serious cardiovascular disease in parent, sibling, or friends, and half of them to sudden deaths of parents, siblings or friends, at an early age. "This fact is stressed here, says DUNBAR, because of the marked effect of such exposure on the psychic component in the patient's preparation for illness". I suggest that this preparedness for illness, produced by close contact with an ill person, be named *disease introjection*.

In another paper (STENBÄCK, 1959) I have reported observations on severe conflict situations in the period prior to the diagnosing of duodenal ulcer (Table 3). Here attention will be drawn only to the

Table 3. Pre-ulcer conflict groups

Content of pre-ulcer conflict	Number
Sexuality and marriage	5
Illness and death	19
Material existence (loss of job, or home, economic misery, difficulty in gaining livelihood, disablement)	17
Self-assertion in occupation and in relationship to other persons (The go-getter conflict)	8

hypochondriac group "illness and death". In 19 patients i.e. in about half the patients with hypochondria, the hypochondriac fear of having a severe illness started, for one reason or another, before their habitual dyspeptic distress had changed into a pain with the clinical characteristics of ulcer pain later confirmed roentgenologically to be due to ulcer.

HÖJER-PEDERSEN, in his monograph (1958), emphasized the preponderance of anxiety and obsessive personality traits in an ulcer patient group. As far as hypochondriac patients are concerned, my findings are on the same lines as his, although I have concentrated not on the form but on the content of the obsessive rumination of the patients. Obviously the importance and frequency of hypochondria are due to cultural factors varying from one culture to another. Another feature in the hypochondriac pre-ulcer conflict as well as in the other pre-ulcer conflicts was the *existential* character of the conflict. The term "existential" is not used here in a philosophical sense; it is only used to stress *a specific meaning* of the conflict to the patient, the meaning that the patient experiences his difficulties as so severe that his existence, his life, is threatened by the factors and circumstances in which he is living. It was observed that as long as the conflict was weak only dyspeptic distress was produced but when, for one reason or another, the conflict changed and became strong, life-threatening, "existential", then a duodenal ulcer developed.

GARMA (1950) put forward the hypothesis that the pathogenic factor is the internalized bad mother who, from within, devours the patient. When this highly symbolized terminology is translated into ordinary psychiatric language, his hypothesis proves in some respects similar to ours; in the organism, a life-treatening process is taking place.

When summing up the results of psychosomatic research on duodenal ulcer, MIRSKY (1958) emphasized that there is *nothing specific* about the social situation prior to the precipitation of the disorder. The only inference that can be made, according to MIRSKY, is that it is the *specific meaning* of the environmental event to the particular individual that determines whether or not the event is responded to as if it were a noxious one.

Our study emphasizes that the hypochondriac significance of pain is one of several factors involved in the etiology of duodenal ulcer.

Bibliography

DUNBAR, F.: Psychosomatic diagnosis (New York 1948).

GAINSBOROUGH, H., and SLATER, E.: A study of peptic ulcer. Brit. M. J. *2*: 253 (1946).

GARMA, A.: On the pathogenesis of peptic ulcer. Internat. J. Psychoanalysis *31*: 53 (1950).

HOJER-PEDERSEN, W.: On the significance of psychic factors in the development of peptic ulcer (Copenhagen 1958).

MIRSKY, I.A.: Physiologic, psychologic, and social determinants in the etiology of duodenal ulcer Amer. J. Digest. Dis. *3*: 285 (1958).
ROBINSON, S.C.: Role of emotions in gastro-duodenal ulcers. Illinois J. *71*: 338 (1937).
RYLE, J.A.: Nosophobia. J. ment. Sci. *94*: 1 (1948).
STENBÄCK, A.: Gastric neurosis, pre-ulcer conflict, and personality in duodenal ulcer. To be published.
SZASZ, TH. S.: Pain and pleasure (New York 1957).

Author's address: DR. A. STENBÄCK, Frederiksgatan 68 A, *Helsinki* (Finland).

Psychosomatic Medicine and Phaenomenological Anthropology

L. VAN DER HORST, Amsterdam

Speaking about psychosomatic medicine and phaenomenological anthropology brings us to two distinct fields of thinking and research.

It is not my intention to discuss these doctrines; I will only indicate the organic relation between both.

On a certain level psychosomatic medicine holds that there is reciprocal interaction between body and mind. But under a more principal aspect in psychosomatics we are faced with an endeavour to regard disease not as a purely local phenomenon, but as a disturbance in the complete co-ordination of the human being. This is a vital factor in psychosomatics. But in our daily clinical work we take account of two essentially different matters. We speak of psychic and physiologic attributes. We use somatic and psychogenetic factors.

It may be that in our days the conditioning of a disease is shifting from the anatomical basis to a more psychological approach as for instance in the problem of Parkinsonism. Fifty years ago JELGERSMA demonstrated the atrophy of the basal ganglia and separated the

Parkinsonian pictures from the neurotic states. Now DR. LIT argues that we have to deal with psychasthenic individuals, who capitulate under certain social or psychogenetic factors.

In psychosomatics we are willing to accept it, but this does by no means alter the principles of medical methodology, for we treat psychic in the same way as somatic processes. They are objective data, things which we handle on the same level, and we suppose that they may influence each other.

We cannot flatly deny the existence of a relation between psychic and physiologic, although the contact mind-body remains a problem. It is too deeply ingrained in our stubborn folklore to be exorcised by an act of will or negation. In psychosomatics we take account of these reciprocal relations between body and mind, but it is not all. It means that illness under the psychosomatic aspect needs a specific anthropological concept. We all can distinguish the objects, with which we have to deal, in psychic and somatic.

But whether it may be psychic or somatic things, it belongs to the same objectivated sphere. To this sphere, these objects, which I *have*, I take my position as a possessor. They all belong to me: my head, my hand, my inner organs as well as my feelings and notions, my ideas and memories. You may collect these things under the notion "it", I should prefer to call it "myself". This "self" is in a curious way correlated with the "ego". So I can distinguish in my inner experience an "ego" and a "self", although they are never separated absolutely; they appear together always.

In this way we intend to bring psychic and somatic under one factor; however, this does not mean that we leave the dualistic way of thinking. In contemplations everyone had to deal with two instances: there are all the available objects, concrete, achieved, finished, irrevocable, and beside it there is in my inner experience a creating factor, regulating, temporalising, achieving—without getting achieved—, an organising instance, working, revolting, completing without being at any time completed, it is the spirit, the I ingraspable, not objectable.

In this way, the idea of human being, the concept is also dualistic but in quite another way as the Cartesian concept. I may mark these both, one from the other, but I cannot separate them. I never see them isolated one from the other, on the contrary, there is between I and self an identification-tendency. In normal circumstances a healthy person is what he has, nevertheless: he knows that he has his body, his feelings and emotions, his purposes; but he does not realise it. He is his body, his feelings, his purpose, and so on.

The sick man appears as a being who has something, something wrong that he carries about with him as an object. He has something. Such an existence as duality is very evident in the experiences of pain. The patient is a unity and yet in pain he becomes aware of his body and loses his natural unity with himself. Pain drives to reflection. In pain the body reverts to the outer world, forces us to give up our natural I-self unity, sets us in opposition to our body, accentuates our eccentric position. The same is true of every hindrance, whether it be disturbed sleep, hampered speech, fatigue or sickness. This is the tragedy of sickness and pain. It shatters the original bond with the body, confronts the doctor with a mutilated man and the patient with himself. In sickness man is set face to face with himself, with the eccentric structure; he realises the dualty of his existence and anticipates what the future holds, i.e. the loss of his body in death.

Unfortunately the medical practioner often adapts his treatment exclusively to the objective condition. Thus it can happen that the doctor does indeed treat pneumonia, but does not see the threat to the patients broken existence, nor does he examine the life-history resulting in the pneumonia. He knows about the difference between healthy and sick, but does not deepen it.

Every doctor knows from experience that sickness as such only appears in its full form when something has lasted for a certain time. If a man, who in the midst of life is admitted to hospital for operation, lies broken in bed only two days later, it is not that a certain organ is simply operated, but the person is confronted with his body. So we distinguish two important moments in illness: a body or psychic life that we try to cure, and a personality, who knows about his having a disturbed body or mind. But at the same time: he is this body. The grade of personalising the sickness may be very different. But at any rate: there is an instrumental and a personal aspect; but these two aspects are interwoven in such a way that we cannot separate them completely.

Under this anthropological conception we can presume something of the psychogenesis of somatic disease. Disease is no longer considered the language of an organ psychically expressing something, it is a specific way-of-being, inherent in the sick man. Viewed from this angle, a sick man is an entirely different person from a healthy one. Man as he exists, stands in the world in all kinds of relationships, but these relationships, this world he creates himself. In his being ill he also finds a mode of existence, which he himself designs and which is, to him, an attempt to exist in the situation in which he finds himself.

When formulated in this way psychosomatic medicine is undoubtedly under the influence of the modern trends in anthropology, notably HEIDEGGER's Daseinsanalyse and SARTRE's existentialism. They correspond with each other in that both of them imply a rupture with the Cartesian dualism. Existence means: man as he exists, body-mind, with its rational and irrational relationships, with his affectivity, volition, disposition, corporality, sexuality, age, what he has done and his intentions, with his being linked to everything that is inherent in being human. Disease is not an accident, but a response to an encounter, a response to a "vocation", to an appeal which reaches man as he is standing in the world. We have to respect this response, although when viewed from another angle this response would be called disease. Therefore we cannot take the syndromes and symptoms away from our patients with impunity. We have met with very remarkable evidences of this in our psychosomatic investigations. I may refer to the case of a man with ulcerative colitis, who almost recovered owing to our psychosomatic treatment. This patient, however, did not find an attitude to life in this situation that should render an existence easier than it had been prior to our taking away his colitis. This man, no longer accepting life in the form we had forced upon him, committed suicide.

The mode of existence in disease is often a restorative endeavour, or at least the realisation of the possibility of retreating from one's relationships, one's consolidations. Man is as it were the producer of his own suffering.

This cannot be approached by the ordinary scientific methods. In psychosomatics the suffering befalls man according to his personal life. The anthropological trend bases itself on the conception that every somatic suffering is a fixation of the "self", e.g. the psychosomatic totality. Traumatism and conflict, infection and degeneration furnish the opportunity for man to retreat from his relationships, to regress, to be fixated to other conditions that are not congruous with, and are not a response to the relationships of life in which the average man of his age is living. Effective utilisation of such opportunities causes a fixation. The physician wishes to free the individual from these fixations by taking away the regression. To achieve this objective datum the physician and the surgeon employ prescription and knife.

A number of people remains, however, who cannot be treated by physicians and they are called psychoneurotics or organic neurotics in whom it is not possible to take away the fixation without anthropological approach.

When using the term fixation we presuppose an arrest in development, an anchoring to the past or to the present, or at least the introduction of the concept of time. The fixated human is taken out of time. The anthropological view intends to loose fixations, or to remove possibilities of fixations, also with the aid of drugs or by means of the knife.

In this, psychosomatic medicine encounters the mystery of illness. In psychosomatics we have to deal with two divergent schools of thought, the Cartesian and the anthropological. The former tries to arrive at a genetical consideration of the phenomena as well as in the psychic field, and to a certain extent, it has a causal way of thinking. Medical science, which is based upon the "Daseinsanalyse" or upon existentialism, or, when expressing it in our words, upon phaenomenological anthropology, holds the view that the symptom is a revelation of being human. It is a fixation which psychosomatic medicine tries to understand in all its manifestations, but not without the co-operation of the patient, who is likewise responsible for his suffering, not as a datum acquired by means of thinking and founded on rational insight, but as a revelation of his mode of being. Illness is a retreat or a flight, or a captivity—at any rate a withdrawal.

The many problems concerning the conception of mankind facing us here, will not be solved for the time being; they constitute the object of anthropological reflection. The way in which the anthropological trend in medicine treats the problems often requires a specific way of formulation. The question is whether this way of thinking is still amenable to scientific practice inasmuch as in science one always tries to reach communicable and discussable data. Our congress may contribute to this purpose.

Author's address: PROF. DR. L. VAN DER HORST, Psychiatrische en Neurologische kliniek, Wilhelmina-Gasthuis, *Amsterdam* (Netherlands).

The Psychic State of Patients Suffering from Parkinsonism

M. MITSCHERLICH, Düsseldorf

Within the framework of an investigation by the German Research-Association 70 patients with extrapyramidal disturbances of movement were examined and treated, 40 of whom had Parkinson's disease. They all had something in common, that is, a more or less compulsory-neurotic character. However, despite their common characteristics, one can distinguish, for example, between the psyche of a tic-patient and that of a patient suffering from Parkinson's disease. The extrapyramidal diseases are disturbances of movement. Of special importance for the development of the human motoric is the second year of a child's life. It is then that the child learns how to approach things and people and how to act; how to defend and how to assert itself.

Experience is governed predominantly by motorial impulses. Closely connected with these are actually the aggressive impulses. It is mainly the motoric aggressive tendencies which are inhibited through punishment or deprivation of love. Thus we find anxiety reflexes and feelings of guilt instead of dynamic processes. No healthy self-assurance develops, in its place step inferiority complexes and compensating pushing and ambitious behaviour. The affective life of the two year old influences the motoric system to a much higher degree than in later years. For example, one has only to think of a child's fits of rage.

Together with the motoric process the process of thinking, develops which in itself is motorial. FREUD used to call thinking "rehearsed action". Recent research (ALLERS AND SCHEMINSKY) showed the connection between thinking and somatic innervation.

Motoric and thinking processes are now at the disposal of the awakening Ego and can be utilised as well in the sense of the Ego as that of the Id. At the time of the motorial development the child faces the demands of the environment, and in toilet-training is confronted with the performance obligation. It is decisive whether these demands and the obligation can be coordinated with the own emotional needs or whether the child has to submit prematurely to a hard reality.

The extrapyramidal system regulates the muscle-tonus which primarily enables deliberate purposeful movement. It is adapted to the biological situations: the fight, the flight, the seizing of prey, love-making. Associated movement and miming are decisively influenced by these. It is particularly the extrapyramidal system which can translate affections, emotions and moods into deportment, and which can be stimulated by each affection.

The connection between psychic factors and illnesses of the central-nervous system was pointed out in 1925 by MOHR, and in 1927 by RABINER AND KESCHNER. In 1953 JELIFFE stated the warding off of animosity to be the decisive factor of the Parkinson posture. BOOTH discerned in 1950 that the patients in the premorbid stage show a strong urge for motoric activity and a great striving for professional independence. They hide sadistic impulses behind a social mask. He spoke of a religious attitude towards success. The animosity described by the aforementioned authors, which far exceeds the norm, is relatively easy to discover in every analysis. It is due to the undeveloped aggressivity.

The patients are lacking the belligerent attitude suited to their individuality in their thinking, their experiences, their utterances and in their actions. They do not possess the natural self-assertion necessary in life. Just as an unused muscle atrophies, so does the aggressive impulse if not put to use in life; and then, when urgently needed, it is not at the person's command. Repressed prematurely, it has kept the form of as at the stage of development. The motoric aggressive impulse of the 2-year old is indifferent and aims when opposed at total destruction or elimination. Well known utterances at this age are: "I'll eat you up", or: "I'll chop his head off".

Mostly the patients lack the ability to fight back which is generally acquired during life by others. This basic disturbance could be ascertained in the realm of motoric aggressiveness as well as in the oral one. For example, it was impossible to get patients, who wanted something, to address their wish to the relevant quarters and to fight until it was accomplished. I do not wish here to investigate the trans- ference- and identification-processes motivating such behaviour, but only the actual incapacity of the patients.

Take for example a man of sixty three, leading in his profession, who was unable to ask for permission to eat an hour later than the other patients. Within the framework of the clinic some remarkable situations occurred. The same patient experienced the mistake made by an assistant during a visit of the medical superintendent, when the former mentioned in error that the patient was leaving the clinic the next day, whereas it had been arranged that he was to go home only the next following day. Although the man noticed the mistake, he was unable to put it right. He endured the leave-taking-ceremony without saying a word.—These incidents had their good side too. My other colleagues and the superintendent noticed the extraordinary behaviour recurring frequently in Parkinson patients and realised that there existed a certain faulty control besides the organic distur- bances.

When the patients were questioned about their conduct, the frequently recurring answers were: "One must not disturb the existing order", or: "What would happen, if everybody would do as he pleases!"—The institutional order, be it that of the family, work or the hospital is taken more into consideration than their own needs or their own wishes. Through this they become too dependent on their environment and take too little notice of themselves.

JAKOB observed in this connection that the patients only register even their illness after having had their attention drawn to it. They speak of themselves as "one" whereas the psychically sound would say "I". It is remarkable that the depressive ones speak of "we" and the compulsory-neurotics of "one"; this is significant and reveals their attitude. Slightly exaggerating one could say, that the patients have not only identified themselves with very strict persons of their childhood world, but even with the standards of society itself. They have no opinion of their own. There exists only the opinion of society, and the highest values are: cleanliness, order, decency and punctuality, to name only a few. All the aforementioned are, however, of such a nature as to guarantee a smooth functioning. Yet, just those who are so anxious to adapt themselves to the Collective reveal in the choice of their words already the vehemently mounting aggressivity. Whilst they are too peaceable and too ready to compromise in their dealings with others, they say things like: "One cannot just take an axe and strike", or: "Well, in such and such a case, one could hit the other at once on the head with a hammer".—In contrast to the conduct just described and their inability to defend themselves and to prevail, stands their excellent functioning in their profession and their work. They are usually industrious, very exact, extraordinarily ambitious and anxious to get on. As part of an institution they can even give orders to a certain extent and assert themselves. Their achievement in their profession is decisive for their wellbeing; they are inclined to work also in their spare time, and they do not find pleasure in hobbies. Their recognition is based on their social achievement, and they lay great stress upon it. "All my life I could work like a horse, I knew no tiredness and I was inured to hardship"; they like to say things like this and repeat it often. The motto of their life is: To be active and efficient to devote oneself to one's family or to one's place of work. They achieve extraordinary performances, at the same time neglecting their own needs. A man aged 30 was employed in a factory and at the same time built up his own business. When this young man was not all too successful in his striving for his own business, his illness began.—A woman of 52 looked after a big family and carried on a business singlehanded.—The man of 63, already mentioned before, became ill when one of his colleagues was made his superior and restricted his travelling abroad, of which he was so fond.—Defeats or serious disputes in business-life not seldom precede the illness. BOOTH has pointed this out too.

Parkinson's disease usually begins with the tremor. Upon examination of this symptom, analysis did not show any difference between the various forms of the tremor. The situations of conflict in which it occurred predominantly were always the same.

A married woman of 54, who had been ill with a Hemiparkinson for 4 years, reported the following: She was the eldest child of a very industrious and successful butcher-couple. The parents had not known anything but their work, and she herself had to help them at an early age and was not allowed to play much. Through her strict upbringing she always had the feeling that her brother was treated better than she. She laid particular stress on the fact that she was not permitted to go to high school despite her talents and the requests of her school-teacher. At the age of 20 she fell ill with encephalitis, when 22 she married a quiet, good natured man. After her father's death she took over a tobacconist' shop and worked day and night. She always looked well after her family with 3 children, but never spared herself. Her one aim had been to give her children a better life than that she herself had led. In this she succeeded, and the children all had positions which were socially far above her level. One daughter took over the business because her illness made it impossible for her to carry on. It should be emphasized that the patient as a child had to obey absolutely, and that no opposition was allowed.

Obeying implicitly, however, means that children must suddenly put a stop to some activity they have begun. HARTMANN besides others has pointed out the damaging effect of such conduct, whereby motoric actions are suddenly interrupted, which in turn prevents affective manifestations, thus destroying the child's whole planning in an instant.

After the war the aforementioned patient had pity on a war-disabled man and took him into her shop to run a lottery-depot. One day she saw him help himself to fifty Marks from the till. At this moment she had a nervous breakdown, could not utter a single word, trembled all over and was completely beside herself. She had the feeling that she had lost the ground from under her feet. "I could have strangled him" she said, and in doing so she took hold of her own throat. The next day her right arm began to tremble. One can always detect the surging for—of very anarchical—aggressive impulses and at the same time the vehement resistance against these. Sometimes one finds disputes which even lead to physical violence, in which the patient receives blows, but cannot hit back. Sometimes it is a professional defeat, through which wild impulses against the culprit are set in motion, causing simultaneously strong feelings of guilt.

If one suggests hypothetical aggressive situations to the patients, the symptom becomes frequently aggravated. I would only mention in passing that each provocation of the patient's free will has the same effect.

It is important to define the quality of the impulses, which are always motoric and in contrast to those passive ones, aiming at quietude and security. Besides this definition of quality the condition of the motoric system is decisive. The muscle is ready to act, the innervation has taken place, the right tonus-position for aggression exists: Just then the inhibition and repression takes place. Perhaps now we understand better, that the disturbance of the Parkinson disease presupposes the potentiality of a certain readiness to act which is not realized. The conclusions reached are in line with the findings of F. ALEXANDER, which he discovered when the vegetative nervous system was sympathetically disposed. He correlated them to certain organic-neuroses. And here we see a similar happening in the neuro-muscular system: A permanent readiness to motoric action without the possibility to realize it. Processes of movement are in a position to loosen affective tensions. If the motoric is inhibited, an affective stoppage occurs as well. It is therefore not surprising that we found in our investigations into Parkinson's disease a permanent emotional tension.

As already mentioned, the affective life in the first two years is so closely connected with motoric processes that an inhibition of the latter causes a grave injury of the emotional life.

BOOTH speaks of a "certain coolness" of the patients.

It could be said of the Parkinson patients that they can put in a good deal of activity in connection with their work, but that they lack what BÜHLER called "die Funktionslust" that is pleasure for its own sake.

The disease was discovered and named in 1813, around the time of the Industrial Revolution. It might be interesting to note in this connection that it only occurs in the Western world and Japan, in other words in a world which increasingly restricts the joy of movement and play and focuses its attention more and more towards maximum achievements not only in work but also in sport.

Concerning the therapy I should like to point out briefly that in the case of a youth aged 21 who had suffered from encephalitis at 14, a social adaptation could be reached after only 45 hours of analytic treatment. Before he was unable to keep a job; he would leave his working place after receiving payment and would squander his earnings. What is astonishing is, that after treatment he now does not break a single bottle in his work as laboratory-assistant despite a severe Hemi-Parkinson, whereas before he used to cause a great number of breakages.

This should encourage us to try psycho-therapeutic treatment of post-encephalitic youth, naturally in selected cases.

Bibliography

1. ALEXANDER, F.: Psychosomatische Medizin, Verlag Walter de Gruyter & Co., Berlin 1951.

2. BERINGER, K.: Selbstschilderung eines Paralysis agitans-Kranken. Nerven-arzt *19*: 70 (1948).

3. BING, R.: Über einige bemerkenswerte Begleiterscheinungen der extra-pyramidalen Rigidität. Schweiz. med. Wschr. *7*: (1923).

4. BOSTROEM, A.: Der amyostatische Symptomenkomplex (Berlin 1922). Zum Verständnis gewisser psychischer Veränderungen bei Kranken mit Parkinsonsymptomen. Z. Neur. *76*: 444 (1922).

5. BÜRGER-PRINZ, H.: Motiv und Motivation (C. Holler, Hamburg 1950).

6. MAYER-GROSS, W.: Über Zwangssymptome bei Encephalitis lethargica und über die Struktur der Zwangserscheinungen überhaupt. Z. Neurol. *116*: 645 (1928).

7. BUYTENDIJK, F. J. J.: Über den Schmerz (H. Huber, Bern 1948).

8. BOOTH, G.: Psychodynamics in Parkinsonism. Psychosomatic Medicine *1*: (1948).

9. CHLOPICKI, W.: Über anfallweise auftretende Zwangserscheinungen im Ver-laufe von Parkinsonismus nach der epidemischen Encephalitis. Arch. Psychiat. *93*: 1 (1931).

10. CHRISTIAN, P.: Über «Leistungsanalyse» dargestellt an Beispielen aus der Willkürmotorik. Nervenarzt *24*: 1, 10 (1933).

— Wirklichkeit und Erscheinung in der Wahrnehmung von Bewegung. Z. Sin-nenphysiol. *68*: 151 (1904).

— Studien zur Willkürmotorik. Dtsch. Z. Nervenheilk. *167*: 237 (1952).

11. DERWORT, A.: Zur Psychophysik der handwerklichen Bewegungen bei Ge-sunden und Hirngeschädigten. Beitrag z. allg. Medizin (v. WEIZSÄCKER). (F. Enke, Stuttgart 1948).

— Bemerkungen zu den Ausführungen von HOLST und CHRISTIAN. Nervenarzt *24*: 1, 16 (1933).

— Über die Formen unserer Bewegungen gegen verschiedenartige Widerstände und ihre Bedeutung für die Wahrnehmung von Kräften. Z. Sinnenphysiol. *70*: 50 (1943).

12. DORER, M.: Veränderungen der physischen Struktur durch Encephalitis epidemica. Arch. Psychol. *98*: 1 (1937).

13. FISCHER, H.: Zwangsmässige Bewegungen bei Encephalitis epidemica. Med. Klin. 1924: *42* (1459).

14. FOERSTER, O.: Die Mitbewegung bei Gesunden, Nerven- und Geisteskrank-heiten (G. Fischer, Jena 1903).

— Zur Analyse und Pathophysiologie der striären Bewegungsstörungen. Z. Neur. *73*: 1 (1921).

15. FERENCZI: Thinking and Muscle Innervation. Int. Z. ärztl. Psychoanl. *5*: 102–103 (1919).

16. GROSS, K.: Reversibilität und Beeinflussbarkeit parkinsonistischer Syndrome. Schweiz. Arch. Psychiatr. *72*: 27 (1953).

17. JELIFFE, S. E.: Die Parkinsonsche Körperhaltung, einige Betrachtungen über unbewusste Feindseligkeit. Internat. Z. Psychoanal. *19*: 485–498 (1933).

18. LEONHARD, K.: Eigenartige Tagenschwankungen der Zustandsbilder bei Parkinsonismus. Z. Neur. *134*: 76 (1931).

19. LOTMAR, F.: Die Stammganglien und die extrapyramidalmotorischen Syn-drome. Monogr. ges. Neurol. Psychiat. (Julius Springer, Berlin 1926).

20. SCHALTENBRAND, G.: Die Beziehungen der extrapyramidalen Symptomen-
       komplexe zu den Lage- und Bewegungsreaktionen zum motorischen Haus-
       halt und zu den Stammganglien. Dtsch. Z. Nervenheilk. *108*: 209 (1929).
— Symptomatologie der extrapyramidalen Erkrankungen (mit Hassler) in Natur-
       forschung und Medizin in Deutschland (Dietrich Verlagbuchhandlung,
       Wiesbaden 1948).
— Psychologische Untersuchungen an Kranken mit Parkinsonismus nach
       Encephalitis epidemica. Psychol. Arb. (Kraeplin) *8*: 563 (1925).
21. SCHULTZ-HENCKE: Lehrbuch der analytischen Psychotherapie.
22. ZUTT, Z.: Die innere Haltung. Z. Psychiat. *73*: 52, 243–330 (1929).

Author's address: DR. M. MITSCHERLICH, Lindemannstrasse 40, *Düsseldorf* (Germany).

The Significance of "Valuing" for Psychology and Psychopathology

E. THIEMANN, Hamburg

As far as the time at my disposal allows, I should like to attempt
to indicate to you the significance of the human being's capacity to
take up a "valuing" attitude. Ever since Man has existed as a civilized
being he has known of the connection between "valuing", willing
and acting. This has resulted in the setting up of doctrines of ethical
values and religious systems. These systems were principally concerned with the setting up of absolute values intended to remain valid
for all time and in every situation. The new value theory which I
have taken as my basis has been laid down by M. EBERHARDT in
"Erkennen, Werten, Handeln" (Cognizing, Valuing, Acting),
Richard Meiner Verlag, Hamburg. This has now shown that absolute
values do not exist. The "true" can be cruelty; the "good" in one
case can be evil in another. That the "beautiful" is highly dependent
on the culture, the time and the perceiving individual is being experienced particularly vividly at the present day. But even if there is no
realm of absolute values we human beings can yet determine the value

or the worthlessness of an object fairly accurately, this "object" also possibly being friendship, honour, courage etc.

We human beings ascribe either a positive or a negative accent of value to every object to which the components of our consciousness take up a relation. The processes that lead to the formation of values are based on psychical functions of the human being. Every formation of a value is derived from direct and indirect valuing.

What do we mean by direct and indirect valuing? The older psychology described "valuing" as feeling with regard to objects All objects, such as things, processes, creations of a purely mental nature, feelings arising from conditions of the moment such as anger, worry, distaste, guilt, fear etc. possess a positive or a negative accent of value.

The human being values directly the fulfilment of all functions, that is the thought, sensory, motory and feeling functions. As a result of the great diversity of their natural tendencies human beings vary considerably as regards what kinds of functions they value positively or negatively and with what intensity they do this. It is, however, generally accepted that that behaviour proves directly *positive* which is suited to the capability of the functions at the moment.

I value as directly positive the scent of a newly bred but otherwise not very beautiful rose—in everyday language I say: "I am very fond of it". Following this experience, "the smelling of a newly bred rose", I value the rose differently to previously—a disposition to value this rose has been newly formed. We are speaking of indirect valuing. Alone the name of the newly bred rose has now a positive accent of value under these circumstances, although it may, on the other hand, be cheaply sentimental and therefore to be repudiated, that is, to be valued negatively.

If there were no such thing as indirect valuing we human beings could not act, could not strive for or will anything at all. We humans have been so created that we can only strive for and will the positively valued.

The child playing alone continues its play as long as it values playing positively. But what it chooses to do next will be decided by indirect valuing.–For example, it runs to its mother in order to ask her advice. And if she then suggests going shopping together the child immediately agrees to this, since "shopping" already possesses a very strong positive accent of value. There is a lot to be seen on the way, one is given extra sweets etc.

Every ability ready for application at the moment at a person's disposal arouses the necessity of its application. All the individual drives, including all functions available for application at the moment, can be collected together in the one drive to form the most highly "valued" overall function; in other words the human being is prompted by his internal drives to strive for the amount of activity and experiences suited to his condition at the moment. If this drive is not satisfied there arises a negative valuing of the overall function— that is in our opinion a pre-condition for the arising of psychogenic diseases.

A critical objection would be quite justified at this point: what evidence is there that the drive of the human being is directed towards an increase in the individual's wealth of functions? This would after all give one direction for all striving, willing and acting. My answer to this is as follows: "This is taught by self-observation". What overall function is "valued" most highly naturally varies considerably according to the conditions of the moment. It can be the most intensive mental or physical work; it can also be dozing or pleasant physical idleness. On one occasion we value the experience of a great work of art particularly positively, on another gay, sociable chatting.

The wealth of the human being's functions is greatly increased if he is able to value not only for his future ego but also for other people, that is to share in the experience of their fate. Alone the fact that a human being can value for his future ego increases his possibilities of action to an extraordinary degree; he can, at the moment, exercise functions valued strongly negatively for the sake of his future ego. The positive value of the goal then passes on to the means for its achievement, in themselves valued as negative. Sometimes the knowledge that an object was only valued positively or negatively as a means is lost, and the object retains the value in question as a value of its own. Thus, for instance, one of my patients values the company of his wife's brother very negatively. This value was then attached not only to his wife's brother himself but also to the latter's photograph. Every time he entered his wife's room, in which a photograph of the brother hung, he was put into an ill-humour.

Since the human being is also able to value not only for his future ego but also for other people, an entirely new dimension of valuing and thus also of willing and acting is opened up for him as it were.

We mentioned just now that there are no absolute values. But if, for instance, we so interpret the "good" that we can define it thus: good is all activity and experience that raises the positive value attached to the overall function of one or many persons without at the same time reducing the positive value attached to the overall function of other people, the "good" thus defined could also be called an absolute value. Speaking quite generally, everything can be called good which altogether increases the positively valued wealth of functions of the human being.

Similarly, the "expedient", the "health-promoting" is, within a limited field, always a value. That in certain situations that which is detrimental to health can, as a means to the attainment of an end with a strongly positive value, in itself be valued positively as self-evident.

In the course of life the human being can acquire an abundance of wrong values which altogether decrease the wealth of positively valued functions. We designate these values as deceptive values and the structure of valuations built upon them as deceptive attitudes. Every deceptive value or deceptive attitude can prevent the application of positively valued functions, and an excess of negatively valued functions leads to the overall function being negatively valued and thus to psychical disturbances which impair the mental and physical health of the human being.

For example, we find in many of our patients a course of action prompted by duty; "duty" is given a strong positive value and leads to an application of the individual's energies without regard for his own future well-being. The patients in question have not experienced the fact that a so much richer and more satisfying life is possibly the more "valuing" and acting are directed towards increasing the functional wealth of life as a whole. How many patients do we encounter who have, as the result of excellent abilities, attained a leading position in their work. If they are characterized not only by their ability but also by a strong sense of duty, they do more work than is good for them. They overtax themselves continually and yet will not be able to alter their mode of living, even if they have already gained the knowledge that they demand too much of themselves— their behaviour has become "a cherished habit" for them. Such people have often not recognized that they do not value themselves sufficiently as a means to be applied for the accomplishment of tasks going far beyond themselves.

Two years ago, in Copenhagen, I reported to you with reference to anorexia nervosa that we see in certain deceptive valuations the causative factors for the development of diseases. In the meantime I have been able to re-examine the validity of these views in the case of asthma bronchiale and the affective psychoses.

It is seen again and again that the positively valued functional forces (for example the romping of a child) are obstructed in their fulfilment by the deceptive valuations (for example being a well-behaved child)—their application is inhibited. The inhibiting factor is always derived from the first valuations to be acquired, and what is inhibited can be an external or internal behaviour and activity which is either the result of natural tendencies, and thus directly valued, or is based on first acquired valuations, and is consequently indirectly valued in the first place. It is in the strongly inhibited person that the process first arises which FREUD has designated as repression. If the overall function is valued positively only to a slight degree, the abilities ready for application, felt to be of strongly negative value on account of their not being used, can no longer be remembered since, "quite unnoticed", counter-valuations have come into being to prevent these ready abilities becoming conscious.

What disease arises depends on the specificity of the combination of the value attitudes and specific somatic dispositions causing it. In the case of asthma bronchiale we consistently established a negative valuation of the overall function, either strong or of long duration, resulting from the affirmation of a high "ideality" and a neglect of the directly valued functions, together with the simultaneous presence of the appropriate somatic dispositions. In the case of the psychoses —by the way all psychogenic diseases can turn into psychoses—the specificity consists alone, in our opinion, in the overall function being given a particularly strong negative value, this partly resulting from absolute hopelessness. This hopelessness is, in our opinion, based in some cases of heavy blows of Fate, in others on an extremely weak feeling of one's own personal value.

I have reached the end of my remarks. Perhaps I have been too theoretical; if so, I would ask you to refer to the works I quoted.

Author's address: Dr. E. THIEMANN, Dürerstrasse 6, *Hamburg* (Germany).

Index